ORAL HEALTH CARE FOR SOCIALLY DISADVANTAGED COMMUNITIES

DENTAL SCIENCE, MATERIALS AND TECHNOLOGY

Additional books in this series can be found on Nova's website
under the Series tab.

Additional e-books in this series can be found on Nova's website
under the e-book tab.

HEALTH CARE ISSUES, COSTS AND ACCESS

Additional books in this series can be found on Nova's website
under the Series tab.

Additional e-books in this series can be found on Nova's website
under the e-book tab.

DENTAL SCIENCE, MATERIALS AND TECHNOLOGY

ORAL HEALTH CARE FOR SOCIALLY DISADVANTAGED COMMUNITIES

FEBRONIA KOKULENGYA KAHABUKA
EDITOR IN CHIEF

EMIL NAMAKUKA KIKWILU
ASSOCIATE EDITOR

IRENE ANDERSON KIDA
ASSOCIATE EDITOR

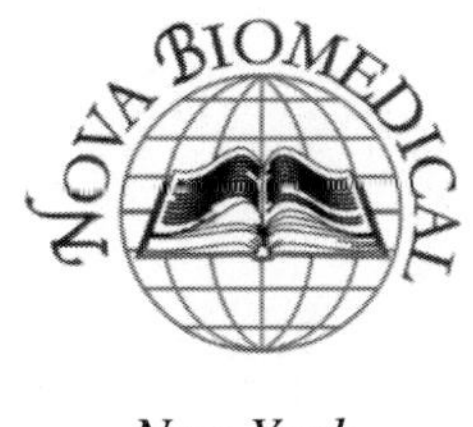

New York

NOTICE TO THE READER

Library of Congress Cataloging-in-Publication Data

Oral heatlh care for socially disadvantaged communities / editor, Febronia Kokulengya Kahabuka.
    p. ; cm.
 Includes bibliographical references and index.
 ISBN 978-1-62948-287-3 (softcover)
 1. Dental public health. 2. Community dental services. 3. People with social disabilities--Dental care. I. Kahabuka, Febronia Kokulengya.
 [DNLM: 1. Dental Care. 2. Health Services Accessibility. 3. Poverty. WU 29]
 RK52.O68 2011
 617.6--dc23
                2011027361

Published by Nova Science Publishers, Inc. † New York

Contents

Preface

The aim of this book is to provide readers in a single cover, the current information on common oral diseases and conditions and their management in socially disadvantaged communities.

The book summarizes the available evidence signifying that social disadvantage is a strong risk factor in oral health, and therefore the need of addressing the social inequalities in the efforts to improve oral health among populations. The book further unveils the influence of major socio-behavioral risk factors in oral health and oral health care and the importance of oral health intervention as well as common risk factors approach at population level.

From chapter three onwards authors have outlined features and treatment modalities of oral ailments, and proposed feasible options for socially disadvantaged communities. This part of the book talks about approaches in the management of dental caries at all levels of its development and progression, a summary of the classification, epidemiology and management of periodontal diseases and a discussion on surgical conditions of the oral and maxillofacial region and associated challenges.

The last half of the book present oral health care to special groups: children, the elderly and people living with HIV/AIDS and winds up with a chapter on prevention of oral diseases and conditions. In this part, the dental development and oral diseases and conditions that affect children are discussed. In addition, myths and practices detrimental to child oral health is explained to enable readers understand and appreciate the need to discourage them. Different types of malocclusions are presented, and limitation of their management discussed. The burden of oral diseases in the elderly is highlighted, and the need for home-based care and outreach programmes indicated. A detailed outline of the classification, diagnosis and management of oral lesions associated with HIV/AIDS is presented. The last chapter summarizes preventive interventions for oral diseases and conditions applicable in socially disadvantaged communities.

We believe that the book will serve as a useful reference material for undergraduate and postgraduate students. It may also be a good source of information for academicians, as well as practicing dentists willing to serve socially disadvantaged communities.

The Editors express their sincere appreciation to Dr Moshi K. Ntabaye for valuably guiding and providing critical comments to authors.

The Editors

In: Oral Health Care for Socially Disadvantaged Communities   ISBN: 978-1-62948-287-3
Editors: F.K. Kahabuka, E.N. Kikwilu and I. Anderson © 2013 Nova Science Publishers, Inc.

Chapter I

Social Disadvantage and Oral Health

Emil N. Kikwilu
School of Dentistry, Muhimbili University of
Health and Allied Sciences

1.1. Introduction

Social disadvantage is a complex term that refers to a social group of individuals, families and societies occupying the lower end of the socioeconomic status scale in relation to others. The differences in the social strata within the socioeconomic status scale are mainly attributable to the differences in the material possession of necessities of life, and the abilities to manage the environment in which one lives. Those occupying the high end of the socioeconomic status possess material necessities and abilities to manage their environment. On the other hand, those occupying the lower end of the scale are deficient of material necessities of life and have low abilities to manage their environment. The lack of necessities of life and abilities to manage ones environment predispose individuals, families and societies occupying the lower end of the socioeconomic status scale to diseases and ill health.

There are complex social processes that place individuals, families or societies at any point of the socioeconomic status scale. Although each one struggles to reach at the top of the socioeconomic scale, many find themselves at the bottom of the scale. The struggle in the relationship between the haves and have not makes those individuals, families and societies that fall to the lowest end of the socioeconomic status scale be classified as socially disadvantaged.

Of recent, social disadvantage has gained much of the international attention because of its relationship with poor health and oral health in particular. In this chapter, different forms of social disadvantage are defined and their relationships with oral health discussed using the current literature. The chapter enables a reader to gain a deeper understanding of the different forms of social disadvantage and their interrelationships. In addition, a reader will be able to understand the influence of social disadvantage on oral health. Since social disadvantage negatively affects oral health as well as utilization of dental services, it is the sincere hope of the writers that a reader will appreciate the need for reducing social disadvantage among societies as prerequisite for improving oral health and reducing inequalities in oral health.

1.2. Definitions of Terms
Related to Social Disadvantage

Social disadvantage encompasses poverty, deprivation and social exclusion. In the following sections of the definitions of terms, we elaborate on the meaning of poverty, deprivation and social exclusion, to aide in clarifying what social disadvantage means. Poverty is a situation in which someone's income is so inadequate as to preclude them from having an acceptable standard of living. It exists when people's actual income is below a poverty line (Saunders et al 2007, p. viii). As Townsend argued, "Individuals, families and groups in the population can be said to be in poverty when they lack the resources to obtain the types of diet, participate in the activities and have the living conditions and amenities which are customary, or at least widely encouraged or approved, in the societies to which they belong. Their resources are seriously below those commanded by the average individuals or family that they are, in effect, excluded from ordinary living patterns and activities" (http://en.wikipedia.org/wiki/Peter_Townsend_(Sociologist).

In 1995, UN defined overall poverty as including lack of income and productive resources to ensure sustainable livelihoods; hunger and malnutrition; ill health; limited or lack of access to education and other basic services; increased morbidity and mortality from illness; homelessness and inadequate housing; unsafe environments and social discrimination and exclusion. It is also characterized by lack of participation in decision-making and in civil, social and cultural life. It occurs in all countries: as mass poverty in many developing countries, pockets of poverty amid wealth in developed countries, loss of livelihoods as a result of economic recession, sudden poverty as a result of disaster conflict, the poverty of low-wage workers, and the utter destitution of people who fall outside family support systems, social institutions and safety nets (UN 1995). Looked in the perspective of human right, the UN further described poverty as "a denial of choices and opportunities, a violation of human dignity". It means lack of basic capacity to participate effectively in society. It means not having enough to feed and clothe a family, not having a school or clinic to go to, not having the land on which to grow one's food or a job to earn one's living, not having access to credit. It means insecurity, powerlessness, and exclusion of individuals, households and communities. It means susceptibility to violence, and it often implies living on marginal or fragile environments, without access to clean water or sanitation (UN statement, 1998).

Deprivation exists when a lack of resources prevents people from accessing the goods and activities that are essential. In short, deprivation can be defined as an enforced lack of socially perceived necessities (or essentials). It involves going without because of lack of resources, and this explains the close link between deprivation and poverty as conventionally defined in terms of low income. In order to identify who are deprived, therefore, one needs to first identify in a society items that are regarded by a majority of the population as being necessity. Secondly, identify who does not have each of these items. Thirdly, distinguish between those that do not have each of the items because they do not want it, and those who do not have it because they cannot afford it. Those who fall in the later category are deprived, because they are unable to afford those items regarded as essential by a majority of the community. This means that deprivation should be viewed both by considering individual incomes in relation to the community in which people are located (Saunders et al 2007).

Social exclusion exists when people do not participate in key activities in society. Whereas deprivation focuses on what people cannot afford, what matters for exclusion is what people do not do. If we assume that there is a set of core activities which constitute participation in society, then an individual is socially excluded if two conditions are met: 1) an individual is not participating for reasons beyond his/her control, and 2) he or she would like to participate (www.aunt-sue.info/assets/files/Public...).

Social disadvantage encompasses poverty, deprivation and social exclusion which are distinct but overlapping concepts. Social disadvantage involves restricted access to resources, lack of participation and blocked opportunities (Saunders et al 2007, p. viii). The Townsend's explanation of who is in poverty, as summarized under definitions for poverty above (http://en.wikipedia.org/wiki/Peter_Townsend_(Sociologist), reveal components of deprivation (lack of resources to obtain the type of diet and living conditions and amenities) and social exclusion (failure or lack to participation in the activities) thus emphasizing that poverty, deprivation and social exclusion are overlapping concepts which describe the term social disadvantage.

In their national study to identify indicators of social disadvantage in Australia, Saunders et al 2007 revealed that there were distinct overlaps between poverty, deprivation and exclusion. The overlap differed among total Australian sample to that of low income people. The overlap was 5% in Australian sample, while it was as high as 37.4% among low income sample (Saunders et al 2007).

The differences and relationship between poverty, deprivation and disadvantage can also be explained in terms of process/cause and outcome. Poverty is used to define the outcome: an inability to share in the everyday lifestyles of the majority because of a lack of resources (often assumed to be disposable income). Disadvantage is similar, but used to describe a broader outcome of deficit, in all aspects of a person's life, not just material (Shucksmith, et al 2000). Social exclusion, however, is much more about the processes in operation causing the resultant circumstances and outcomes. It recognizes that these processes are complex and interrelated, constantly changing over time. It is a term coined more recently reflecting the shift in academic thought and government policy away from static accounts of people's (often material) circumstances towards a recognition of the complexities and cause and effect relationships involved (Room 1994, Peace et al 2001).

Since social disadvantage encompasses poverty, deprivation and social exclusion, socially disadvantaged groups or communities are communities or groups of people where several factors reduce the life chances and opportunities for people to thrive. In such communities or groups of people, there will be some similarities in lack or insufficiency of "essential amenities": housing, location, health and health care, education, employment, care and support, social and civic engagement and financial resources. The results of the focus groups discussion of the study which was designed to develop new indicators of social disadvantage among Australians clearly indicated that in socially disadvantaged groups there were outcries which indicated that the groups had difficulties in obtaining essential amenities. Statements such as "..it's very hard to go out and meet friends", "it's close to impossible because you can't afford to do things", "we barely survive week to week at the moment let alone having anything left over", "My issue with the government housing is that my partner and I have applied to get housing and she's been on the list for 10 years and still nothing, and we're not recognised as partners" point to obvious deficiencies in essential amenities (Saunders et al 2006).

1.3. Forms of Social Disadvantage and Their Relation to Oral Health

Poverty and General- and Oral-Health

Many studies have shown that poverty has direct association with general and oral health (Morris et al 1996, Stronks et al 1998, Sabbah et al 2009, http://www.sochealth.co.uk. Incomehealth/ch1.hmtl, Ecob and Smith 1999, Mackenbach et al 2004, Celeste et al 2009, Perera and Ekanayake 2008). In 1996, Morris and colleagues did show that the degree of deprivation was negatively associated with pass rate in secondary education, and positively associated with mortality and incidence of coronary heart diseases in England (Morris et al 1996). In the study by Stronks et al 1998, the association between equivalent income and health problems, as assessed by means of logistic regression, the relative risk of the highest income group was set at 1. The odds ratios indicated how much more likely it was for a person with a certain income to have a health problem compared with those in the highest income group. Both health complaints and perceived general health were statistically significantly related to equivalent income after controlling for confounders such as educational and occupational level. The odds ratios steadily increased with decreasing income, and the odds of the lowest income group was approximately three times as high as that of the highest income group. The odds ratios for chronic conditions also increased in lower income groups, although not statistically significantly and to a lesser extent than for the subjective indicators.

Similar findings were noted among American populations in relation to oral health (Sabbah et al 2009). Sabbah et al 2009 studied the effects of income and education on ethnic differences in perceived oral health, gingival bleeding, periodontitis and tooth loss among American adults. The probabilities of poorer oral health were higher among African-American, Mexican-Americans and other ethnic groups than in White Americans. Adjusting for income and education resulted in a reduction in the ORs for having poorer perceived oral health (44%), tooth loss (29%), gingival bleeding (61%) and periodontitis (30%) among African-Americans than White Americans. Similar reductions in risk were observed among Mexican-Americans and other ethnic groups. These findings indicated that education and income play an important role in ethnic differences in oral health.

The association between income and health has also been shown by comparing the life expectancy and GNP of different countries (http://www.sochealth.co.uk. Incomehealth/ch1.hmtl). In this analysis of poverty and health, two distinct pictures emerge. Among the less developed countries there is still a clear relationship between their average per capita income and measures of health such as average life expectancy. The higher the standard of living in these countries, the healthier they are. Although the relationship is not perfect, it is statistically strong and highly significant. However, among the much richer industrial - or post-industrial - countries, improvements in health are no longer strongly related to rates of economic development and increasing per capita incomes. This indicates that there is a threshold of the income above which the relationship fades away. Similar findings were recorded by Ecob R and Smith GD (1999) in UK, Mackenbach and colleagues (2004) in seven European countries and Dowd et al 2011 in USA. In the study by Ecob and Smith (1999), the indices of morbidity, both self-reported and measured, were approximately linearly related to the logarithm of income, in all except very high and low incomes. Doubling of income was associated with a similar effect on health, regardless of the point at which this occurs, provided this was within the central portion (10-90%) of the income distribution (Ecob and Smith 1999). In the inter-country study of seven European countries, Mackenbach et al (2004) revealed a similar relationship between income and health. A higher household equivalent income was associated with better self-assessed health among men and women in all countries, particularly in the middle-income range. In the higher income ranges, the relationship was generally curvilinear and characterized by less improvement in self-assessed health per unit of rising income. In the lowest income ranges, the relationship was found to be curvilinear in four countries (Belgium, Finland, The Netherlands, and Norway), where the usual deterioration of health associated with lower incomes levels off or even reverses into an improvement. In USA, Dowd and colleagues analysed three decades mortality data for adult Americans. The association was detected at lower income quartiles, with no linear association at higher income quartiles (Dowd et al 2011).

The fading away of the relationship between income and health improvement as the income reaches a certain limit was also shown in oral health of Brazilians by Celeste et al 2009. In their study, Celeste and Nadanovsky (2009) explored the shape of the relationship between income and two oral health outcomes (dental caries experience and periodontal health) in Brazil. The findings did indicate a linear relationship at lower levels of income. The relationship levelled off at higher levels of family income. These findings point to the need of identifying a minimum income for healthy living for each country as Morris et al 2000, 2007 did for England.

In oral health many researches have yielded results which show strong associations between income and oral health. In many countries where dental caries have been related with socioeconomic status of populations, dental caries prevalence and severity has been consistently shown to be lower among affluent individuals and families than their counterparts with lower economic status (Boyce et al 2010, Piovesan et al 2010, Lawrence et al 2009, Amaral et al 2005). Boyce and colleagues (2010) studied the stress-related psychobiological processes that might account for the high, disproportionate rates of dental caries, the most common chronic disease of childhood, among children growing up in low socioeconomic status (SES) families in the San Francisco Bay Area of California, USA. The researchers performed detailed dental examinations to count decayed, missing or filled dental surfaces and microtomography to assess the thickness and density of microanatomic dental compartments in exfoliated, deciduous teeth (i.e., the shed primary dentition). Cross-sectional, multivariate associations were examined between these measures and SES-related risk factors, including household education, financial stressors, basal and reactive salivary cortisol secretion, and the number of oral cariogenic bacteria. The results indicated that nearly half of the five-year-old children studied had dental caries. Low SES, higher basal salivary cortisol secretion, and larger numbers of cariogenic bacteria were each significantly and independently associated with caries, and higher salivary cortisol reactivity was associated with thinner, softer enamel surfaces in exfoliated teeth. The highest rates of dental pathology were found among children with the combination of elevated salivary cortisol expression and high counts of cariogenic bacteria. They concluded that socioeconomic partitioning of childhood dental caries may thus involve social and psychobiological pathways through which lower SES is associated with higher numbers of cariogenic bacteria and higher levels of stress-associated salivary cortisol.

Piovasan et al (2010) assessed the inequality in caries distribution and the association between socioeconomic indicators and caries experience of preschool children in a city in Brazil. A high inequality in the caries distribution with Gini coefficient of 0.8 and Significant Caries Index of 2.8 was observed. The children from low household income had the highest prevalence of dental caries, indicating that income was a strong predictor for the inequality in caries distribution in Brazilian preschool children (Piovasan et al 2010).

Likewise, Lawrence et al 2009 did show a similar pattern of dental caries experience among the low income and rich groups of kindergarten children of Aborigine and non-Aborigine origin. The Aboriginal children (low income) had 1.9 to 2.3 times the risk of having early childhood caries (ECC) (dmft>0), 2.9 to 3.5 times the risk of a dmft>3 and 1.8 to 2.5 times the risk of untreated decayed teeth after adjusting the prevalence ratios for child's age and sex, school's risk level and clustered-correlated data (Lawrence et al 2009). Amaral et al (2005) studied dental caries among 18-year-old males from Maringa, Brazil in 2005. Caries prevalence was 82.6% and the caries experience as determined by mean DMFT was 4.6. The worst results were observed in the groups of lower income and purchasing power (Amaral et al 2005). The adverse effects of low family income on oral health were also reported in Sri Lanka (Perera et al 2008, Skudutyte-Rysstad 2009). In their study, Perera and Ekanayake compared the level of perceived oral health to different socioeconomic indicators using hierarchical logistic regression models. The final model indicated that poor perceived oral health was significantly associated with low household income, not using dental services, presence of gingivitis, being aware about the presence of oral disease, presence of toothache and other oral symptoms and perceived need for dental care (Perera et al 2008). Skudutyte studied the associations between family income and occurrence of dental caries among adolescents in Sri Lanka. The findings did indicate that low family income was significantly associated with presence of dentinal caries among adolescents (Skudutyte-Rysstad R, 2009).

The ethnic differences in oral health status reported in many studies may also be attributed to the differences in levels of family income and not ethnicity per se. Sabbah et al 2009 did show reduced differences in ORs for oral health indicators after controlling the effects of income and education. The reductions were substantial for having poorer perceived oral health (44%), tooth loss (29%), gingival bleeding (61%) and periodontitis (30%) among African-Americans than White Americans (Sabbah et al 2009).

The adverse effects of low income on oral health have also been revealed in oral cancer studies (Conway et al 2008). In a systematic review and meta-analysis study that utilized forty-one studies which met inclusion criteria did show that compared with individuals who were in high SES strata, the pooled ORs for the risk of developing oral cancer were 1.85 (95%CI 1.60, 2.15; n = 37 studies) for those with low educational attainment; 1.84 (1.47, 2.31; n = 14) for those with low occupational social class; and 2.41 (1.59, 3.65; n = 5) for those with low income. Subgroup analyses showed that low SES was significantly associated with increased oral cancer risk in high and lower income-countries, across the world, and remained when adjusting for potential behavioural confounders (Conway et al 2008).

Michael Marmot (Marmot 2002) discussed the two ways in which income affects health: through a direct effect on the material conditions necessary for biological survival, and through an effect on the social participation and opportunity to control life circumstances. Poverty has been shown to lead to thin enamel as well as poor enamel maturation, which in turn predispose the tooth to high susceptibility to dental caries (Boyce et al 2010). Poverty was also associated with elevated basal salivary cortisol secretion which favours multiplication of cariogenic strains of bacteria (Boyce et al 2010). A person/family with low income finds it difficult to purchase essential materials necessary for living such as food, water, safe house, clothing, soap to wash ones clothing and body. Lack or deficiency of the above mentioned material things leads to poor nutrition and hygiene, which have been shown to predispose a person or family to ill health. That is why Marmot concluded that the fewer goods and services are provided publicly by the government/community, the more important individual income is for health (Marmot 2002). Reduced social participation and opportunity to control life circumstances rises among people or families with low income because of psychological and behavioral factors. Worries on how to feed a family, how to get money to pay rent, may predispose a person to cardiovascular ill health. Lack of opportunities for recreation facilities may lead to unhealthy behaviors such as playing on unsafe grounds leading to raised accidents and traumatic injuries. As Clarke et al (2009) noted: driving at excessive speed, driver intoxication, driver/passenger failure to wear seat-belts, and unlicensed driving were most prevalent in fatal collisions in the low socio-economic disadvantaged population (Clarke et al 2009). Psychological effects of low income predispose the disadvantaged people to indulge in risk behaviours such as smoking which have been shown to be a risk factor for developing oral cancer (Petti S 2009, Boing et al 2010, Goldstein et al 2010) and periodontitis (Laxman et al 2008,Bergström 2006, Calsina et al 2002). In France people residing in cramped housing with noisy and stressful environment or deprived neighbourhood, were found to be significantly more likely to be smokers than their counterparts living in less deprived neighbourhood (Peretti-Watel et al 2009), therefore they are at increased risk of developing oral cancers and periodontitis.

The association between poor oral health and poverty can also be explained by looking at the factors leading to oral diseases. In case of dental caries, one needs alternative snacks to those containing sugars. A poor person, family or community will have limited purchasing power to buy alternative snacks because in most occasions, sugared snacks are available in every communities at cheaper price compared to alternative non-sugared snacks. In addition, primary prevention requires regular use of fluoridated tooth paste. People living in poverty may find it difficult to purchase tooth paste on regular basis or consider tooth paste as luxury goods worth not considering for purchase because of budgetary constraints in relation to other essentials of life such as food, clothing and shelter. This fact is well illustrated in the findings from the global affordability study by Goldman et al 2008. In their analysis of the expenditure in tooth paste from 48: high-, middle- and low-income countries, Goldman et at 2008 compared and related the cost of fluoride toothpaste to annual household expenditure as well as to days of work needed to purchase the average annual usage of toothpaste per head. The findings did indicate that the proportion of household expenditure that was required to purchase the annual dosage of toothpaste increased as the country's per capita household expenditure decreased. Therefore it is difficult to have optimum utilization of toothpaste in low income countries unless deliberate efforts are made to ensure that toothpaste is affordable to all people. Summaries of the main findings of studies that show relationships between oral health versus poverty and/or deprivation are presented in table 1.

**Table 1.1 A sample of studies whose findings indicate that
social disadvantage adversely affects oral health**

No	Authors, subjects and country of study	Findings
1.	Mashoto et al 2010; school children in one region, Tanzania	Adjusted logistic regression odd ratios for rural adolescents (disadvantaged) versus their counterparts in urban for DMFT>0 were 1.2 (1.0-1.4) indicating more caries experience among rural compared to urban adolescents
2.	Da Rosa et al 2010; school children in the province of Quebec, Canada.	Dental caries experience was 6.9% higher when comparing schools in unfavourable socioeconomic environments to the most favourable ones [95% confidence interval (CI): 2.1, 11.7%].
3.	Boyce et al 2010; kindergarten children from varying socioeconomic backgrounds in the San Francisco Bay Area of California, USA.	Low SES, higher basal salivary cortisol secretion, and larger numbers of cariogenic bacteria were each significantly and independently associated with caries, and higher salivary cortisol reactivity was associated with thinner, softer enamel surfaces in exfoliated teeth.
4.	Piovesan et al 2010; preschool children in a city in Brazil.	The children with mothers having low level of education and from low household income had the highest prevalence of dental caries.
5.	Lawrence et al 2009; Aboriginal and non-Aboriginal kindergarten children in Ontario, Canada	Adjusted prevalence ratios for severe childhood caries S-ECC: (dmft>3) was 3.5 [2.6-4.9] indicating much higher caries experience among Aborigines (socially disadvantaged) compared to non-aborigine (p< 0.001)
6.	Delgado-Angulo et al 2009; children aged 12 years from 11 underserved communities in Lima, Peru	Children living in poor households were 2.25 times more likely to have dental caries (95% confidence interval: 1.24; 4.09), compared to those living in non-poor households.
8.	Tagliaferro et al 2008; 6-8 year old school children in Piracicaba, Brazil	In their 7-years follow-up of children aged 6-8 yrs, the risk of developing dental caries lesions was higher in children whose mothers' education was low (socially disadvantaged) {OR=2.87 (1.40-5.88)}
9.	Amaral et al 2005; 18-year old from Maringá province, Brazil.	Proportionately more Brazilian adolescents from low income families had 1 or more tooth decay than their counterparts from high income families {89.2 % vs 73.5%; (χ^2 =8.88; p=0.003)}.
10.	Sabbah et al 2009; adults in the USA.	The probabilities of poorer oral health were higher among African-American, Mexican-Americans and other ethnic groups than in White Americans. Adjusting for income and education resulted in a reduction in the ORs for having poorer perceived oral health (44%), tooth loss (29%), gingival bleeding (61%) and periodontitis (30%) among African-Americans than White Americans. Similar reductions in risk were observed among Mexican-Americans and other ethnic groups
11.	Celeste et al 2009; 15-19 year olds in Brazil	Mean decayed teeth= 3.70 (3.75) for lowest quartile, and = 1.30 (2.29) for highest quartile of social economic ranking respectively. Pearson correlation: decayed teeth vs income= -0.15, p< 0.001; decayed teeth vs social ranking= -0.25, p< 0.001.

Deprivation and Oral Health Status

Socially deprived persons find it difficult to utilize preventive services, and therefore suffer natural course of diseases. In developed countries, for example, populations residing in deprived areas have been shown to exhibit a greater burden of oral diseases than populations from affluent communities. The studies conducted in Australia (Jamieson et al 2006, Armfield 2007, Parker et al 2007, Jamieson et al 2007), Scotland (Levin et al 2009aandb), and Belgium (Vanobberge et al 2001, De Reu et al 2008) reveal this assertion.

In Australia, Armfield JM (2007) examined the relationship between prevalence of dental caries and six discrete area-based measures of socioeconomic status. The findings indicated a consistent linear relationship between caries prevalence and socioeconomic status with children having poorer oral health residing in areas of greater socioeconomic disadvantage. Children from more socioeconomically disadvantaged areas had higher odds of having either one or more decayed, missing, or filled teeth or four or more decayed, missing or filled teeth than children residing in areas of greater socioeconomic status. The odds of having DMFT>1 in 12-year-old children was 1.0 for 1st quartile of family income and 1.56 for 4th quartile of family income (Armfield 2007). In their study Parker and Jamieson did show that children who attended for dental care at Pika Wiya (from socially disadvantaged communities) aged 10 years or less had 1.8 times the mean dmft, 1.4 times the SiC and 1.4 times the SiC[10] of their counterparts attending for care at Port Augusta SDS (socially advantaged communities). Over half the children aged ≥6 years who attended Pika Wiya for dental care had caries experience in the permanent dentition compared with 38% of their Port Augusta SDS-attending counterparts. Children aged ≥6 years who attended Pika Wiya for dental care had 1.9 times the mean DMFT, 1.8 times the SiC and 1.6 times the SiC 10 of their similarly-aged Port Augusta SDS-attending counterparts. The findings from the study conducted by Jamieson and colleagues clearly show a distinct social gradient among indigenous and non-indigenous children respectively, whereby those with the highest dmft/DMFT levels were in the most disadvantaged SES category and those least disadvantaged had the lowest dmft/DMFT levels. Indigenous children aged 5 years had almost four times the dmft of their counterparts in the same disadvantaged category (p<0.05), while indigenous children aged 10 years had almost five times the DMFT of similar disadvantaged non-indigenous children (p<0.05) (Jamieson et al 2006). In 2007, Jamieson reported similar findings in Australian children whereby indigenous children aged <10 years had 1.6, 1.9, 1.6, and 1.4 times the percent dmft>0, mean dmft, SiC primary and SiC[10] primary respectively, of their non-indigenous counterparts. Also children aged 6+ years had 1.3, 1.7, 1.7 and 1.6 times the percent DMFT>0, mean DMFT, SiC permanent and SiC[10] permanent respectively, of their non-indigenous counterparts.

Living in deprived areas have been shown to be a predisposing factor for poor oral health among children in Belgium (Vanobberge et al 2001, De Reu et al 2008), increased risk for traumatic dental injuries (Glendeor 2009), and difficulties of recruiting children from deprived communities into school based fluoride rinsing programmes have been experienced in Edinburgh (Levin et al 2009a). Vanobberge et al (2001) did show that the mean dmft and dmfs values were the lowest for the most advantaged children (1.3/2.7) and were threefold higher in the least advantaged children (3.9/9.1). The prevalence of caries-free children was 2.5 higher among the highest SES families compared with the lowest SES families. In a logistic regression model adjusted for the stratification factors, the excess risk for caries in children increased with decreasing occupational level of parents.

Review article by Glendor U (Glendor 2009), did indicate that material deprivation was among the many factors which increased the risk of sustaining the traumatic dental injuries.

The reasons for this association may be explained based on the aetiology and prevention of oral diseases. Prevention requires sound knowledge of aetiology and informed decisions to avoid these aetiological factors. For example judicial use of sugar and sugar containing snacks/food stuff would highly reduce the occurrence of dental caries in populations. On the other hand effective regular tooth brushing with fluoridated tooth paste would eliminate the initiation and progression of periodontal diseases, in addition of preventing tooth decay. Deprived person has a reduced ability to routinely and effectively brush teeth, and access alternative diets conducive to oral health. Deprived communities and families cannot afford to purchase tooth paste on regular basis let alone purchasing a new tooth brush to replace an old one.

These deficiencies compromise the deprived person to self-control of oral diseases. Since social deprivation is characterised by limited participation in community activities, deprived people, communities and families will also be less knowledgeable on preventive measures, thus become powerless to take control over their oral health. Living in deprived areas is also associated with lack of recreation facilities such as safe play grounds, good roads, and well lit streets. Such environment predisposes residents to accidents and violence leading to traumatic injuries including dental injuries.

In less developed countries, however, the association is such that the higher the economic power, the more decayed teeth.

This is because the diet for poor people consist mainly unprocessed foodstuffs which are less cariogenic in nature. However, as purchasing power increases, diets change to more processed foodstuffs which are more cariogenic. This fact is illustrated by different epidemiological studies conducted in Tanzania since mid 1980s. Frencken et al 1986 reported clear differences in DMFT and deft between rural and urban children in one region in Tanzania. The average baseline D3MFT scores of the 7-, 8- and -9-yr-old urban and rural children were 0.27, 0.33, 0.35 and 0.04, 0.23 and 0.23, respectively; the average deft values were 2.9, 2.4, 2.6 and 1.4, 1.9 and 1.4. The permanent dentition was caries free (D3MFT = 0) in 80 and 89% of the urban and rural children, respectively. The researchers concluded that their findings reflected the national Tanzanian situation with higher caries prevalence in urban than in rural children.

Similar findings were reported in the national survey data that was collected in early 1990s. In the 1990 national survey clear differences were noted between rural and urban population, in which urban communities exhibited a higher DMF-T than their rural counterparts (Mosha et al 1992).

Similar picture was shown in the study conducted by Awadia and colleagues. In their study they investigated the role of predictors of caries experience among children in urban and rural areas of northern Tanzania. Logistic regression analyses indicated that subjects in the high-F and urban Arusha municipality were at a significantly higher risk of dental caries than children in the low-F areas (odds ratio [OR] 2.6). Controlling for ethnicity, children in urban areas were at higher risk for caries (OR 5.4) than children living in low-F rural Kibosho (Awadia et al 2002).

However, recent reports show mixed findings. In an extensive survey involving 5,532 adult Tanzanians from rural and urban cluster samples, no differences in mean DMFT were noted between rural and urban residents (both had mean DMFT= 3.3±4.4) (Sarita et al 2004). More recent studies among adolescents indicate a reversal of the picture. Mashoto and colleagues (2010) studied 1745 rural and urban adolescents aged 10-19 years who were attending government primary schools in one of the regions in Tanzania. Adjusted logistic regression odd ratios for rural adolescents versus their counterparts in urban for DMFT>0 were 1.2 (1.0-1.4) indicating more caries experience among rural compared to urban adolescents (Mashoto et al 2010).

Effects of Poverty and Deprivation on Utilization of Oral Health Services

Poverty and deprivation has been shown to impart negatively on the utilization of oral health services. Gilthorpe et al 1997 did show a significant difference in the utilization of oral surgical services in West Midlands, UK. Most deprived communities used emergency services more than less deprived communities, while less deprived communities used more of elective surgical procedures than more deprived counterparts. In the same study the utilization of inpatient services was more among people of higher economic status than those of low economic status (Gilthorpe et al 1997).

Lopez and colleagues reported similar findings in Chile where students who consulted a dentist because of symptoms were more likely to have a father without income (Lopez et al 2007). Lang et al 2008 revealed that people living in most deprived areas of England were more likely to use dental services when symptomatic than least deprived people (Lang et al 2008).

In Tanzania, adults residing in deprived areas (rural areas) were less likely to use oral health care facilities due to lack of money to pay for transport, and more likely to use self-medication and traditional healers as alternative to established oral health care facilities than their counterparts living in less deprived areas (urban) (Kikwilu et al 2008). In this study, it was concluded that living in rural areas, poverty and old age were important barriers to seeking oral urgent care.

Difficulties were noted in recruiting children for fluoride rinsing programmes in UK from deprived areas then in less deprived areas (Levi et al 2009a). Lang and colleagues (2008) used area deprivation index to study the effect of deprivation on utilization of oral health services. Those living in the most deprived 20% of neighbourhood, compared with those in the least deprived, had a relative risk ratio of 2.25 (95% conf interval 1.59-3.17) of using dental services only when symptomatic, rather than going for regular or occasion check-ups (Lang et al 2008). Data published by De Reu et al 2008 indicated that living condition had a significant influence on the health behaviour and care indices of the studied population of socially deprived adolescents. Table 2 summarises the studies and main findings that show the influence of social disadvantage on utilization of oral health services.

**Table 1.2. A sample of studies whose findings indicate that
social disadvantage adversely affects utilization of oral health services**

No	Authors, subjects and country of study	Findings
1.	Pavi et al 2010, adults in Greece	Results from Poisson regression analysis indicated that lower income level correlates to lower number of dental visits, while having visited for treatment (rather than for prevention) correlated to higher number of dental visits.
2.	Tramini et al 2010; patients in French public hospital	An evaluation of the results indicated that younger patients and people from lower socioeconomic groups used the emergency dental service more frequently. Unemployed people (OR = 1.60) and manual workers (OR = 1.86) were also more likely to use this service.
3.	Villalobos-Rodelo et al 2010; 6- to 12-year-old Mexican schoolchildren.	Higher unmet dental needs and lack of health insurance were associated with the experience of dental visits because of dental pain in the preceding 12 months. Boys who attended public schools had a 70% (95% CI = 1.29 to 2.23) higher probability of having had a dental visit in which dental pain was one of the main reasons for attendance, compared to boys attending private schools.
4.	Patel et al 2010; uninsured population in the United States	Compared to the uninsured, the insured had greater odds of having a dental check-up within the past year.
5.	Kaylor et al 2010 utilization of dental services by women of childbearing age in Ohio State, USA	Results of bivariate analysis showed that having a dental visit in the past year varied significantly by SES, low SES being associated with low utilization of dental services.
6.	Muirhead et al 2009; utilization of dental services among working poor Canadians	Independent predictors associated with visiting the dentist >1 year ago: paying for dental care with cash or credit (OR = 2.31; P < 0.001), and past welfare recipients (OR = 1.65; P = 0.03). Sacrificing goods or services to pay for dental treatment was associated with visiting the dentist within the past year. The predictors of visiting the dentist only when in pain/trouble were paying for dental care with cash or credit (OR = 2.71; P < 0.001), a history of an inability to afford dental care (OR = 1.62; P = 0.01).
7.	Maharani DA 2009, dental care utilization among Indonesian adults	The concentration index showed a significant concentration of dental care utilization among groups with higher socioeconomic status (SES). The horizontal inequity index illustrated higher unmet dental care needs among lower SES groups. Decomposition revealed that higher SES was positively associated with the likelihood of dental care utilization.
8.	Larson et al 2009; family income gradients in US children's health, access to care and use of services	Income gradient was noted for no dental visit: 30.3% for category below 100% FPL to 15.3% for category of 400% FPL or greater.
9.	Kikwilu et al 2008; barriers to use of emergency oral care facilities among adult Tanzanians	Rural residents (geographically disadvantaged) were more likely not to report for dental care due to lack f money for transport {OR=2.12 (1.34-3.36)}; dental clinic too far {OR= 5.31 (2.09-13.54)} than their counterparts in urban areas
10.	Lang et al 2008; dental service use among older people in England	Elders living in the most deprived 20% of neighbourhoods, compared with those in the least deprived, had a relative risk ratio of 2.25 (95% confidence interval 1.59-3.17) of using dental services only when symptomatic, rather than going for regular or occasional check-ups.

No	Authors, subjects and country of study	Findings
11.	Sohn et al 2007; dental care visits among low-income children, USA	Children with private dental insurance had four times higher odds of having visited compared with those who had no insurance (deprived).
12.	Lopez et al 2007; dental attendance among adolescents in santiago, Chile.	Students who had not visited a dentist during the past year were more likely to have a father without income (OD=1.8). Students who consulted a dentist because of symptoms were more likely to have a father without income (OD=1.4).
13.	Gilthorpe et al 1997; socioeconomic status of patients who underwent inpatient oral operations from 1989 to 1994 in West Midlands, UK.	There was a highly significant correlation between the use of oral surgery specialty and social deprivation (R2 = 0.69, P < 0.001), indicating that patients who avail themselves of inpatient oral surgery are from a higher socioeconomic group.

Concluding Remarks

The literature cited in this chapter strongly and consistently indicates that social disadvantage adversely affects oral health status as well as the utilization of oral health services leading to poor oral health of disadvantaged people. In turn, poor oral health adversely affects quality of life of individuals (Sheiham 2006, Floyd 2009, van Gemert-Schriks 2009, Jamieson 2010) and families (Barbosa et al 2009, Ratnayake et al 2005, Locker et al 2002). In order to improve quality of life, and therefore realize the millennium development goals (MDGs), governments need to eradicate social disadvantage among their people.

References

Amaral M.A., Nakama L, Conrado C.A., Matsuo T. (2005) Dental caries in male young adults: prevalence, severity and associated factors. *Braz. Oral. Res.*, 19:249-255.

Armfield JM. (2007) Socioeconomic inequalities in child oral health: a comparison of discrete and composite area-based measures. *J. Public Health Dent.* Spring; 67:119-125.

Awadia A.K., Birkeland J.M., Haugejorden O, Bjorvatn K. (2002) Caries experience and caries predictors--a study of Tanzanian children consuming drinking water with different fluoride concentrations. *Clin. Oral. Investig.*, 6:98-103.

Barbosa TdeS, Gaviao M.B.D. (2009) Evaluation of the family impact scale for use in Brazil. *J. Appl. Oral. Sci.*, 17:397-403.

Bergström J. (2006) Periodontitis and smoking: an evidence-based appraisal. *J. Evid. Based Dent. Pract.*; 6:33-41.

Boing AF, Ferreira Antunes JL, de Carvalho MB, de Góis Filho JF, Kowalski LP, Michaluart P Jr, Eluf-Neto J, Boffetta P, Wünsch-Filho V. (2010) How much do smoking and alcohol consumption explain socioeconomic inequalities in head and neck cancer risk? *J. Epidemiol. Community Health.* doi:10.1136/jech.2009.097691.

Boyce W.T., Den Besten P.K., Stamperdahl J, Zhan L, Jiang Y, Adler N.E., Featherstone J.D. (2010) Social inequalities in childhood dental caries: the convergent roles of stress, bacteria and disadvantage. *Soc. Sci. Med.*, 71:1644-1652.

Calsina G, Ramón J.M., Echeverría J.J. (2002) Effects of smoking on periodontal tissues. *J. Clin. Periodontol.*, 29:771-776.

Celeste R.K., Nadanovsky P. (2009) Income and oral health relationship in Brazil: is there a threshold? *Community Dent. Oral. Epidemiol.* 37:285-293.

Clarke D.D., ward P, Truman W, Bartle C. (2009) A poor way to die: social deprivation and traffic fatalities. Behavioural research in road safety. Queen's printer and controller of Her Majesty's Stationery Office, London, UK.

Conway D.I., Petticrew M, Marlborough H, Berthiller J, Hashibe M, Macpherson LM. (2008) Socioeconomic inequalities and oral cancer risk: a systematic review and meta-analysis of case-control studies. *Int. J. Cancer*, 122:2811-2819.

Da Rosa P, Nicolau B, BrodEur. J..M., Benigeri M, Bedos C, Rousseau M.C. (2010)Associations between school deprivation indices and oral health status. *Community Dent. Oral. Epidemiol.* Nov 20. doi: 10.1111/j.1600-0528.2010.00592.x.

De Reu G, Vanobbergen J, Martens L.C. (2008) The influence of social indices on oral health and oral health behaviour in a group of Flemish socially deprived adolescents. *Community Dent Health*, 25:33-37.

Delgado-Angulo E.K., Hobdell MH., Bernabé E. (2009) Poverty, social exclusion and dental caries of 12-year-old children: a cross-sectional study in Lima, Peru. *BMC Oral. Health*, Jul 7;9:16.

Dowd J.B., Albright J, Raghunathan T.E., Schoeni R.F., LeClere F, Kaplan G.A. (2011) Deeper and wider: income and mortality in the USA over three decades. *Int. J. Epidemiol.*, 40:183-88. doi:10.1093/ije/dyq189.

Ecob R, Smith G.D. (1999) Income and health: what is the nature of the relationship? *Soc. Sci. Med.*, 48:693-705.

Floyd B. (2009) Associations between height, body mass, and frequency of decayed, extracted, and filled deciduous teeth among two cohorts of Taiwanese first graders. *Am. J. Phys. Anthropol.*, 140:113-119.

Frencken J.E., Truin G.J., König K.G., Ruiken R.M., Elvers H.J. (1986) Prevalence of caries, plaque and gingivitis in an urban and rural Tanzanian child population. *Community Dent. Oral. Epidemiol.*, 14:161-164.

Gilthorpe M.S., Wilson R.C. and Bedi R. (1997) A sociodemographic analysis of inpatient oral surgery: 1989-1994. *Br. J. Oral. Maxillofac. Surg.*, 35:323-327.

Glendor U. (2009) Aetiology and risk factors related to traumatic dental injuries--a review of the literature. *Dent Traumatol.*, 25:19-31.

Goldman AS, Yee R, Holmgren CJ, Benzian H. Global affordability of fluoride toothpaste. *Globalization and Oral Health* 2008, 4:7 doi:10.1186/1744-8603-4-7. (http://www.globalizationandhealth.com/content/4/1/7) (Accessed on 1st March 2011)

Goldstein BY, Chang SC, Hashibe M, La Vecchia C, Zhang ZF. (2010) Alcohol consumption and cancers of the oral cavity and pharynx from 1988 to 2009: an update. *Eur. J. Cancer Prev.*, 19:431-465.

http://en.wikipedia.org/wiki/Peter_Townsend_(sociologist). *Definition of relative poverty.* (accessed on 1st March 2011).

Jamieson L.M., Armfield J.M., Roberts-Thomson K.F. (2006) Oral health inequalities among indigenous and nonindigenous children in the Northern Territory of Australia. *Community Dent. Oral. Epidemiol,* 34:267-276.

Jamieson L.M., Parker E.J., Armfield J.M. (2007) Indigenous child oral health at a regional and state level. *J. Paediatr Child Health.,* 43:117-121.

Jamieson L.M., Robert-Thomson K.F., Sayers F.M. (2010) Risk indicators for severe impaired oral health among indigenous Australian young adults. *BMC Oral Health,* 10:1. http://www.biomedcentral.com/1472-6831/10/1

Kaylor M.B., Polivka B.J., Chaudry R, Salsberry P, Wee AG. (2010) Dental services utilization by women of childbearing age by socioeconomic status. *J. Community Health.,* 35:190-197.

Kikwilu E.N., Masalu J.R., Kahabuka F.K., Senkoro A.R. (2008) Prevalence of oral pain and barriers to use of emergency oral care facilities among adult Tanzanians. *BMC Oral Health.,* 8.28 doi:10.1186/14/2-6831-8-28. (http://www.biomedcentral.com/1472-6831/8/28)

Lang I.A., Gibbs S.J., Steel N, Melzer D. (2008) Neighbourhood deprivation and dental service use: a cross-sectional analysis of older people in England. *J. Public Health* (Oxf). 30:472-478.

Larson K, Halfon N. (2010) Family income gradients in the health and health care access of US children. *Marten Child Health* J, 14:332-342. doi:10.1007/s10995-009-0477-y.

Lawrence H.P., Binguis D, Douglas J, Mckeown L, Switzer B, Fiueiredo R, Reade M. (2009) Oral health inequalities between young Aboriginal and non-Aboriginal children living in Ontario, Canada. *Community Dent. Oral. Epidemiol,* 37:495-508.

Laxman V.K., Annaji S. (2008) Tobacco use and its effects on the periodontium and periodontal therapy. *J. Contemp. Dent. Pract.,* 9:97-107. (review).

Levin K.A., Davies C.A., Topping G.V., Assaf A.V., Pitts N.B. (2009[b]) Inequalities in dental caries of 5-year-old children in Scotland, 1993-2003. *Eur. J. Public Health.,* Mar 23.

Levin K.A., Jones C.M., Wight C, Valentine C, Topping G.V., Naysmith R. (2009[a]) Fluoride rinsing and dental health inequalities in 11-year-old children: an evaluation of a supervised school-based fluoride rinsing programme in Edinburgh. *Community Dent. Oral. Epidemiol.,* 37:19-26.

Locker D, Jokovic A, Stephens M, Kenny D, Tompson B, Guyatt G. (2002) Family impact of child oral and oro-facial conditions. *Community Dent. Oral. Epidemiol.* 30:438-48.

Lopez R, Baelum V. (2007) Factors associated with dental attendance among adolescents in Santiago, Chile. *BMC Oral Health,* 7:4 doi:10.1186/1472-6831-7-4.

Macintyre S, Macdonald L, Ellaway A. (2008) Do poorer people have poorer access to local resources and facilities? The distribution of local resources by area deprivation in Glasgow, Scotland. *Soc. Sci. Med.,* 67:900-914.

Mackenbach J.P., Martikainen P, Looman C.W., Dalstra J.A., Kunst A.E., Lahelma E. (2005) The shape of the relationship between income and self-assessed health: an international study. *Int. J. Epidemiol.,* 34:286-293.

Maharani D.A. (2009) Inequity in dental care utilization in the Indonesian population with a self-assessed need for dental treatment. *Tohoku J. Exp. Med.,* 218:229-239.

Marmot M. (2002) The influence of income on health: views of an epidemiologist, does money really matter? Or is it a marker for something else? *Health Affairs,* 21:31-46.

Mashoto K.O., Åstrøm A.N., Skeie M.S., Masalu J.R. (2010) Socio-demographic disparity in oral health among the poor: a cross sectional study of early adolescents in Kilwa district, Tanzania. *BMC Oral Health*,10:7 (http://www.biomedcentral.com/1472-6831/10/7) (Accessed on 30th October 2010).

Morris J.N., Blane D.B., White I.R. (1996) Levels of mortality, education and social conditions in the 107 local education authority areas of England. *J. Epidemiol. Community Health,* 50:15-17.

Morris J.N., Donkin A.J., Wonderling D, Wilkinson P, Dowler EA. (2000) A minimum income for healthy living. *J. Epidemiol. Community Health.*, 54:885-889.

Morris J.N., Wilkinson P, Dangour A.D., Deeming C, Fletcher A. (2007) Defining a minimum income for healthy living (MIHL): older age, England. *Int. J. Epidemiol.*, 36:1300-1307.

Mosha H.J., Ngilisho L.A., Nkwera H, Scheutz F, Poulsen S. (1994) Oral health status and treatment needs in different age groups in two regions of Tanzania. *Community Dent. Oral. Epidemiol.*, 22:307-310.

Mtaya M, Brudvik P, Astrøm A.N. (2009) Prevalence of malocclusion and its relationship with socio-demographic factors, dental caries, and oral hygiene in 12- to 14-year-old Tanzanian schoolchildren. *Eur. J. Orthod.* 31:467-476.

Muirhead V.E., Quiñonez C, Figueiredo R, Locker D. (2009) Predictors of dental care utilization among working poor Canadians. *Community Dent. Oral. Epidemiol.*, 37:199-208.

Parker E.J., Jamieson L.M. (2007) Oral health comparisons between children attending an Aboriginal health service and a Government school dental service in a regional location. *Rural Remote Health.*, 7:625.

Patel N, Bae S, Singh K.P. (2010) Association between utilization of preventive services and health insurance status: findings from the 2008 Behavioral Risk Factor Surveillance System. *Ethn. Dis.* 20:142-147.

Pavi E, Karampli E, Zavras D, Dardavesis T, Kyriopoulos J. (2010) Social determinants of dental health services utilisation of Greek adults. *Community Dent Health.* 27:145-150.

Peace, R. (2001) Social Exclusion: A concept in need of definition? In *Social Policy Journal of New Zealand*, 16, 17-36,

Perera I, Ekanayake L. (2008) Factors influencing perception of oral health among adolescents in Sri Lanka. *Int. Dent. J.,* 58:349-355.

Peres K.G., Peres M.A., Araujo C.L.P., Menezes A.M.B., Hallal P.C. (2009) Social and dental status along the life course and oral health impact in adolescents: a population based birth cohort. *Health and Quality of Life Outcomes*, 7:95 doi:101186/1477-7525-7-95.

Peretti-Watel P, Seror V, Constance J, Beck F. (2009) Poverty as a smoking trap. *Int. J. Drug Policy.*, 20:230-236.

Petti S. Lifestyle risk factors for oral cancer. *Oral. Oncol.* 2009; 45:340-50.

Piovesan C, Mendes F.M., Ferreira F.V., Guedes R.S., Ardenghi T.M. (2010) Socioeconomic inequalities in the distribution of dental caries in Brazilian preschool children. *J. Public Health Dent.*, Aug 23.

Ratnayake N, Ekanayake L. (2005) Prevalence and impact of oral pain in 8-year-old children in Sri Lanka. *Int. J. Paediatr Dent.*, 15:105-112.

Room (1994) in Shucksmith, M. and Philip, L. Social Exclusion in Rural Areas: a literature review and conceptual framework, *Scottish Executive Central Research Unit*, 2000

Sabbah W, Tsakos G, Sheiham A, Watt R.G. (2009) The effects of income and education on ethnic differences in oral health: a study in US adults. *J. Epidemiol. Community Health.*, 63:516-20.

Sarita P.T, Witter DJ, Kreulen CM, Matee MI, van't Hof MA, Creugers NH. Decayed/missing/filled teeth and shortened dental arches in Tanzanian adults. *Int. J. Prosthodont.* 2004; 17:224-30.

Saunder P, Sutherland K, Davidson P, Hampshire A, King S, Taylor J. (2006). Experiencing poverty: the voice of low-income Australian. Towards new indicators of disadvantage project. Stage I: Focus group outcomes. *Social Policy Research Centre.* Sydney.

Saunders P, Naidoo Y, Griffiths M. (2007). Towards new indicators of disadvantage: deprivation and social exclusion in Australia. Social Policy Research Centre. Sydney.

Sheiham A. Dental caries affects body weight, growth and quality of life in pre-school children. *Br. Dent. J.* 2006; 201:625-626.

Shucksmith, M. and Philip, L. (2000) Social Exclusion in Rural Areas: a literature review and conceptual framework, Scottish Executive Central Research Unit.

Skudutyte-Rysstad R, Sandvik L, Aleksejuniene J, Eriksen H.M. (2009) Dental health and disease determinants among 35-year-olds in Oslo, Norway. *Acta Odontol. Scand.*, Feb;67(1):50-56.

Sohn W, Ismail A, Amaya A, Lepkowski J. 92007) Determinants of dental care visits among low-income Africa-American children. *JADA*, 138(3):309-318.

Stronks K, van de Mheen D.H., Mackenbach J.P. (1998) A higher prevalence of health problems in low income groups: does it reflect relative deprivation? *J. Epidemiol. Community Health*, 52:548-557.

Tagliaferro EP daS, Ambrosano GMB, Meneghim MdC, Pereira AC. (2008) Risk indicators and risk predictors of dental caries in school children. *J. Appl. Oral. Sci.*, 16:408-413.

Tramini P, Al Qadi Nassar B, Valcarcel J, Gibert P. (2010) Factors associated with the use of emergency dental care facilities in a French public hospital. *Spec Care Dentist.* 30:66-71.

UN (1998). Press ReleaseDEV/2188 OBV/66 Poverty as violation of human rights. Panel on poverty, human rights, development held in joint second and third committee meeting marks international day for eradication of poverty,16 October 1998.

United Nations (1995). Declaration on poverty. Report of the World Summit for Social Development. A/CONF.166/9 World Summit for Social Development 19 April 1995 Copenhagen, Denmark 6-12 March 1995.

van Gemert-Schriks M.C., van Amerongen E.W., Aartman I.H., Wennink J.M., Ten Cate J.M., de Soet J.J. (2010) The influence of dental caries on body growth in prepubertal children. *Clin. Oral. Investig.* Jan 29.

Vanobberge J.N., Martens L.C., Lesaffre E, Decleck D. (2001) Parental occupation status related to dental caries experience in 7-year-old-children in Flanders (belgium). *Community Dent Health*, 18:256-262.

Villalobos-Rodelo J.J., Medina-Solís C.E., Maupomé G, Lamadrid-Figueroa H, Casanova-Rosado A.J., Casanova-Rosado J.F., Márquez-Corona Mde L. (2010) Dental needs and socioeconomic status associated with utilization of dental services in the presence of dental pain: a case-control study in children. *J. Orofac. Pain.*, 24:279-286.

www.aunt-sue.info/assets/files/Public Definition of social exclusion. Accessed on 1st March 2011.

www.sochealth.co.uk/Incomehealth /chl.html. Socialist Health Association. Income and health. Accessed on 02/09/09.

In: Oral Health Care for Socially Disadvantaged Communities   ISBN: 978-1-62948-287-3
Editors: F.K. Kahabuka, E.N. Kikwilu and I. Anderson © 2013 Nova Science Publishers, Inc.

Chapter II

Oral Health and Care in Low-Income Countries

Poul Erik Petersen[1] and Nanna Jürgensen[2]
[1] World Health Organization, Global Oral Health Programme,
Geneva, Switzerland
[2] World Health Organization Collaborating Centre for
Community Oral Health Programmes and Research,
University of Copenhagen, Denmark

2.1. Introduction

The objectives of this chapter are to outline the burden of oral diseases worldwide with emphasis on the situation in low income countries, and to highlight the influence of major socio-behavioural risk factors in oral health and oral health care. Despite great improvements in the oral health of populations in several countries, global problems still persist. The burden of oral disease is particularly high on the disadvantaged and poor population groups in all countries and poor oral health has a profound effect on general health and quality of life. Oral diseases such as dental caries, periodontal disease, tooth loss, oral cavity cancer, HIV/AIDS related oral disease and oro-dental trauma are major public health problems worldwide. The diversity in oral disease patterns and development trends across countries and regions reflect distinct risk profiles and establishment of preventive oral health care programmes. The important role of socio-behavioural and environmental factors in oral health and disease are shown in a large number of socio-epidemiological surveys. In addition to poor living conditions, the major risk factors relate to unhealthy lifestyles (i.e. diet, nutrition, tobacco, alcohol, poor oral hygiene), and low availability and accessibility of oral health services. Several oral diseases are linked to chronic diseases primarily because of common risk factors. Moreover, general diseases often have oral manifestations (e.g. diabetes or HIV/AIDS). Worldwide, strengthening of public health programmes through implementation of cost-effective oral disease prevention measures and health promotion is urgently needed. The World Health Organization Global Oral Health Programme and the World Health Assembly

2007 have formulated strategies and policies for countries to adopt in order to improve the oral health for all people.

2.2. The Burden of Oral Disease

The two major dental diseases- dental caries and periodontal disease- have historically been considered the most important components of the global oral health burden and they contribute considerably to the economic burden related to health care. Despite great improvements in the oral health of populations in several high income countries, major problems still persist. Poor oral health is a serious problem in all countries among the disadvantaged and underprivileged population groups. Poor oral health may be a profound effect on general health. The experience of pain, problems with eating, chewing, smiling and communication due to missing, discoloured or damaged teeth have a major impact on people's daily lives and wellbeing. In addition, oral diseases restrict activities in school, at work, and at home causing millions of school and work hours to be lost each year the world over.

In low- and middle income countries of Asia and Africa, significant proportions of school-aged children suffer from oral health problems [1, 2]. In a report from Thailand, about half of 12-year old children suffered from pain or discomfort from teeth within the past year, one fifth of the children informed that they avoid smiling or laughing because of poor teeth, and one tenth of children missed school class due to dental pain [3]. In a study of Chinese adolescents [4], one tenth of students informed that they had poor teeth or gums; another one tenth reported that other children made fun of their teeth, and four out of ten students claimed that they had experienced toothache or symptoms during the past year. Recently, a study of 12-year-olds was carried out in Lao PDR, one of the low income countries of South East Asia [5]. This survey revealed that substantial proportions of the children had poor quality of life due to oral disease; most importantly, the study demonstrated considerable associations between high dental caries experience and tooth ache, several impairments of daily life activities, and absenteeism from school. In addition, having filled teeth was highly associated to urban location, having a literate mother, and having an advantaged socio-economic position while untreated decay was likely for children living in semi-urban location.

Similar studies of 12-year-olds were conducted in Africa. For example, in Tanzania, a survey indicated that one tenth of children had poor teeth and a high need for dental treatment [6]. Among their parents, the burden of illness seemed to be somewhat higher as four out of ten adults suffered from dental pain during the past year, and poor teeth had a negative impact on social relations and communication. In Burkina Faso, only one tenth of 12 year old children had experience of pain within the past year but six out of ten adults aged 35-44 years claimed that they had pain or discomfort from teeth [7]. Another study of people aged 15 years or more found that nearly two thirds of the Burkinabé suffered from dental pain and problems during 12 months [8]; the figure was somewhat higher for people with no education compared with people of high education.

2.2.1. Dental Caries

Dental caries continues to be a major health problem in most high income countries as the disease affects 60-90% of school-aged children and the vast majority of adults [1]. At present, the distribution and severity of dental caries vary in different parts of the world and within the same region or country [9-11]. Currently, for children at the age of 12 years, the level of dental caries is very low or low in most low income countries (Figure 2.1); dental caries experience (severity) in permanent teeth is measured by the Decayed, Missing due to caries and Filled Teeth index (DMFT) at the age of 12 years. Children of this age are one of the principal age groups recommended by the World Health Organization (WHO) for international comparisons [12]. Figure 2.2 illustrates the trends over-time in dental caries experience of 12-year-old children in countries. During recent years dental caries experience of children has grown significantly in several low- and middle income countries. In contrast to the situation in low and middle income countries, declines in caries prevalence and severity have been observed in many high income countries over the past 20 years or so [13].

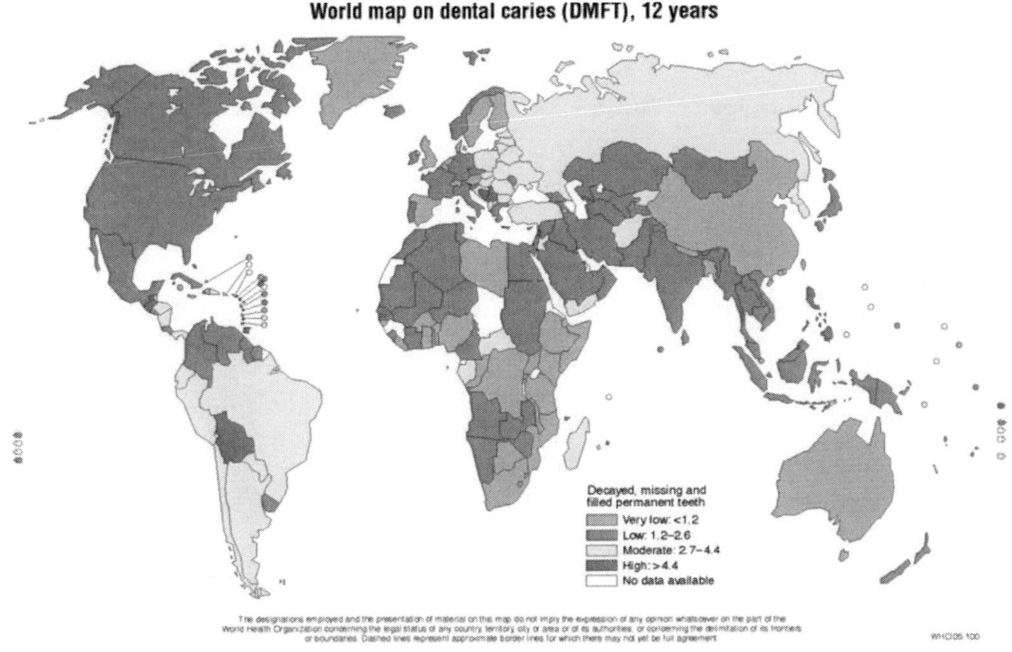

Figure 2.1. Dental caries levels (DMFT) of 12-year-olds worldwide [1].

Worldwide, the prevalence of dental caries is generally high among adults as the disease affects nearly 100% of the population in the majority of countries [13]. Traditionally, the burden of dental caries and tooth loss has been high among adults of industrialized countries and the poor dentate status remains a severe public problem to older people. Figure 2.3 outlines the global dental caries profile among 35-44-year-olds, as measured by the mean DMFT index [1]; unfortunately, a number of African and Asian countries have not update information on oral health status on adults. For the data available, dental caries experience figures are however rather low in poor countries of Africa and Asia. As for children, in most low- and middle income countries dental caries levels among adults have been low until recently but now dental caries prevalence rates and dental caries experience tend to increase in several of these countries [13].

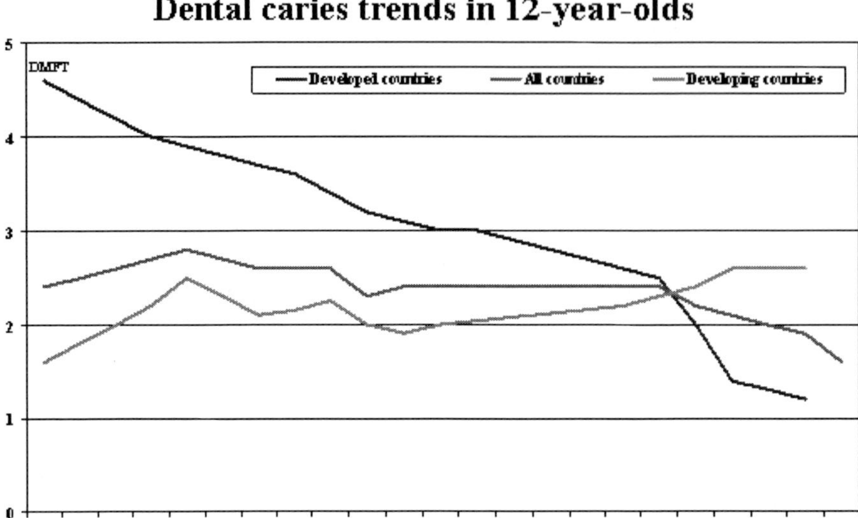

Figure 2.2. Changing levels of dental caries experience (DMFT) among 12-year-olds in developed and developing countries [1].

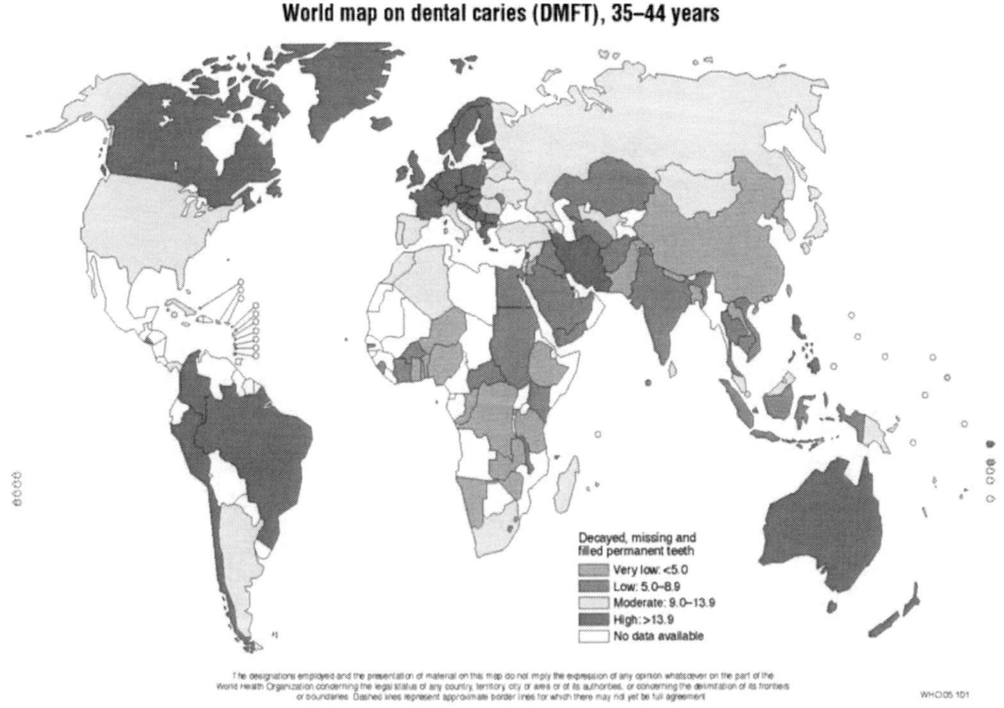

Figure 2.3. Dental caries levels (DMFT) of 35-44-year-olds worldwide [1].

Factors in Changing Patterns of Dental Caries

The current global and regional patterns of oral disease largely reflect distinct risk profiles across countries, which are related to living conditions, lifestyles and the implementation of preventive oral health systems. The significant role of socio-behavioural and environmental factors in oral disease and health is shown in a large number of epidemiological surveys [10, 11]. The importance of such risk factors in dental caries is shown worldwide for both children and adults. For high income countries and increasingly for low- and middle income countries studies carried out over the past 10-15 years have observed that the burden of disease, poor quality of life and the need for care are highest amongst the poor or disadvantaged population groups. The social inequalities particularly relate to poor education, low personal income or poverty, which have negative behavioural consequences. The poor life chances most likely lead to unhealthy life styles and low use of oral health services. In low- and middle income countries, the access to oral health care and prevention of oral disease is particularly critical for people living in remote rural areas.

The decline of dental caries observed in high income countries has been the result of a number of public health measures, including effective use of fluorides, adoption of healthy lifestyles and improved self-care practices, and changing living conditions. In low- and middle income countries, the increase in dental caries prevalence and severity is particularly due to the growing consumption of sugars and inadequate exposures to fluorides, coupled with a lack of tradition in oral self-care [14]. Population-directed fluoride programmes are still rare in low- and middle income countries but programmes such as salt or milk fluoridation are currently being established in some countries. In low income countries, the use of effective fluoridated toothpaste is expensive and not affordable to the vast majority of people. Several studies have documented the limited use of fluoridated toothpaste in these countries [15]. In Burkina Faso, surveys have shown that only some 5% of children aged 12 years make use of fluoridated toothpaste while this habit is observed for about one fifth of 35-44-year-olds [7]. In a number of middle income countries affordable fluoridated toothpaste is now available and the use of such toothpaste is on the increase [16].

2.2.2. Periodontal Disease

Tooth loss in adult life may be attributable to severe dental caries but also to poor periodontal health. Severe periodontal disease, which may result in tooth loss, is found in 5-20% of most adult populations worldwide [17]. According to the WHO Global Oral Health Data Bank, the principal symptoms of periodontal disease show only minor variation by WHO region or across national income [13]. In the majority of countries- poor or rich- adult people are significantly affected by signs of gingivitis or teeth with moderate periodontal pockets.

2.2.3. Oral Cancer

Cancer incidence and survival rates are clearly linked to socioeconomic factors [18]. Low-income and disadvantaged groups are generally more exposed to avoidable risk factors such as environmental carcinogens, alcohol, infectious agents, and tobacco use. These groups also have less access to the health services and health education that would empower them to make decisions to protect and improve their own health.

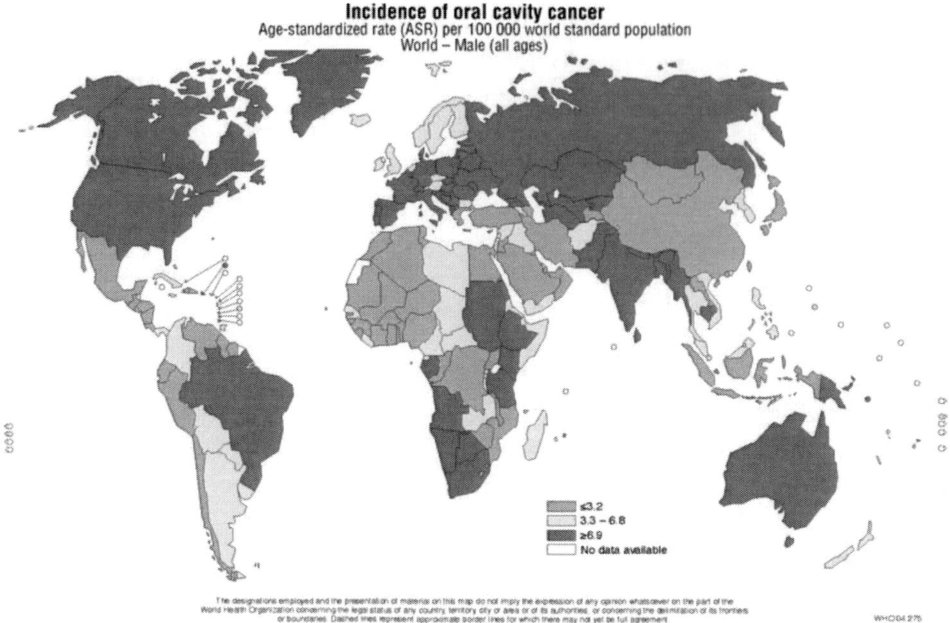

Figure 2.4. Incidence of oral cavity cancer among males (Age-Standardized Rate (ASR) per 100 000 world population) [19].

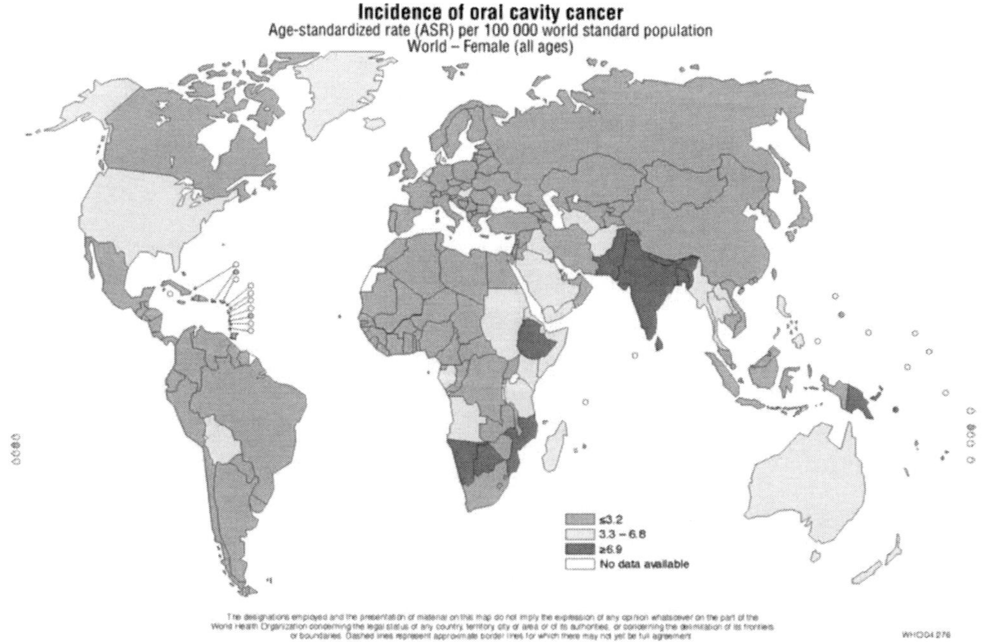

Figure 2.5. Incidence of oral cavity cancer among females (Age-Standardized Rate (ASR) per 100 000 world population)[19].

Figure 2.4-2.5 presents the incidence of oral cavity cancer in countries around the globe [19].The data are expressed in Age Standardized Rates ASR (per 100 000 world standard population). The incidence rate of oral cavity cancer firstly demonstrates high figures for men and populations of the industrialized world, partly reflecting a long tradition of smoking and excessive alcohol consumption. South-East Asia and certain African countries score high on incidence rates for both sexes; in these countries the high rates relate directly to risk behaviours such as chewing tobacco (e.g. betel nut or miang chewing, or the use of qat), in addition to smoking and use of alcohol. The risk of oral cavity cancer is particular high in cases where excessive alcohol and tobacco use interact. The Age Standardized Mortality Rate due to oral cavity cancer is generally higher for males than females. Moreover, the mortality rate is relatively low for many Western industrialized countries where health services are available to populations; however, relatively high rates are observed for low-and middle income countries and countries with economies in transition as access to health facilities here is limited.

2.2.4. Oral Health in HIV/AIDS

The HIV/AIDS pandemic affects millions of people worldwide and the highest burden of the disease is on the poor countries of Africa and Asia. Recently, UNAIDS and WHO has estimated that about 34 million people now are living with HIV/AIDS and about 23 million people with HIV are in sub-Saharan Africa [20]. A number of studies have demonstrated the negative impact on oral health of HIV infection [21]. Approximately 40-50% of HIV positive persons have oral fungal, bacterial or viral infections often occurring early in the course of the disease. Oral lesions strongly associated with HIV infection are pseudo-membranous oral candidiasis, oral hairy leukoplakia, HIV gingivitis and periodontitis, Kaposi sarcoma, and non-Hodgkin lymphoma. Dry mouth as a result of decreased salivary flow rate may not only increase the risk of dental caries but negatively impacts quality of life because of difficulty in chewing, swallowing and tasting food. The need for oral health care among HIV-infected people as regards immediate care and referral, treatment of manifest oral disease, prevention and health promotion is particularly high among the under-served, disadvantaged population groups of developing countries [21]. The poor oral health condition was confirmed in a recent Tanzania community survey of people living with HIV infection and the manifestation of the major oral lesions were established [22]. Moreover, it was shown in another report from Tanzania that the awareness of oral manifestations of HIV AIDS was lower than for the general symptoms of infection [23].

2.2.5. Noma-Cancrum Oris

Noma, debilitating oro-facial gangrene, is an important disease burden on certain developing countries, particularly in Africa and Asia (Figure 2.6) [24]. Noma primarily starts as a localized gingival ulceration and spreads rapidly through the oro-facial tissues, establishing itself with a blackened necrotic centre. About 70-90% of cases are fatal in the absence of care. Fresh noma is seen predominantly in the age group 1-4 years, although late stages of the disease occur in adolescents and adults. Poverty is the key risk condition for development of noma; the environment inducing noma is characterized by severe malnutrition and growth retardation, unsafe drinking water, deplorable sanitary practices, residential proximity to unkempt animals, and a high prevalence of infectious diseases such as measles, malaria, diarrhoea, pneumonia, tuberculosis and HIV/AIDS. Most infants and young children are left without any care of poor oral health and poor general health.

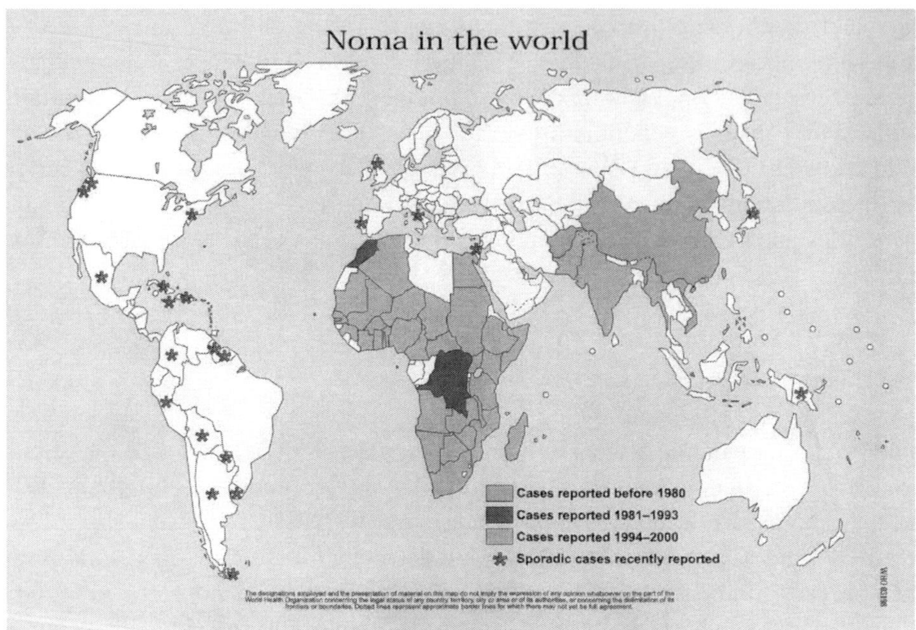

Figure 2.6. Cases of noma (cancrum oris) reported around the world [1].

2.2.6. Oro-Dental Trauma

In contrast to dental caries and periodontal disease, reliable data on the frequency and severity of oro-dental trauma are still lacking in most countries, particularly in low- and middle income countries [25]. Some countries in Latin America report dental trauma in about 15% of schoolchildren, while prevalence rates of 5-12% are found in children aged 6-12 years in the Middle East. In a recent study of 12-year-olds carried out in Laos showed that 7% had experienced dental trauma [5]. Furthermore, studies from certain industrialized countries have revealed that the prevalence of dental traumatic injuries is on the increase; current prevalence rates are ranging from 16% to 40% among 6-year-old children and in 4-33% among 12-14-year-old children [25]. An important proportion of dental trauma originates from unsafe playgrounds or schools, road accidents or violence. This is particularly the case in low- and middle income countries.

2.2.7. The World Health Survey

In 2003, WHO undertook the so-called World Health Survey (WHS) [26, 27].The WHS was a global survey covering the adult population aged 18 years or more and it was designed to collect national representative data on the state of health and on the performance of health systems; 72 countries with a total of 278,872 persons took part in the survey and data were collected by standardized personal interviews. The participating countries were categorized into low-, middle- and high income countries based on the Gross National Income according to the World Bank criteria. The WHS also included information on oral health status and intended to assess the capacity of the national health system, including the responsiveness of the oral health system within a country [27]. The oral health questions focused on key indicators, i.e. loss of all natural teeth; experience of problems with mouth or teeth within the past year, and accessibility of oral health care.

Figure 2.7 provides an overview of the global burden of oral disease according to national income level; the situation is illustrated for 65-74-year-olds as old-age people have accumulated experience of oral disease. Edentulism is found at high prevalence rate (35%) in upper-middle income countries whereas the figure at present time is low (10%) for low income countries.

In several industrialized countries older people often have had their teeth extracted early in life because of pain or discomfort, leading to reduced quality of life. Meanwhile, in many of these countries there has been a positive trend of significant reduction in tooth loss among older adults during recent years [28, 29]. At global level, a social gradient is observed as regards experience of problems with mouth/teeth. In low income countries about 40 % of older people report oral problems while this is the case for about 30% of people in high income countries.

Table 2.1 gives the country information from low income countries participating in the World Health Survey. Pakistan has the highest prevalence of edentulism and Ethiopia the lowest. Bangladesh has high proportion of older people with self-reported oral health problems while Myanmar has a low figure.

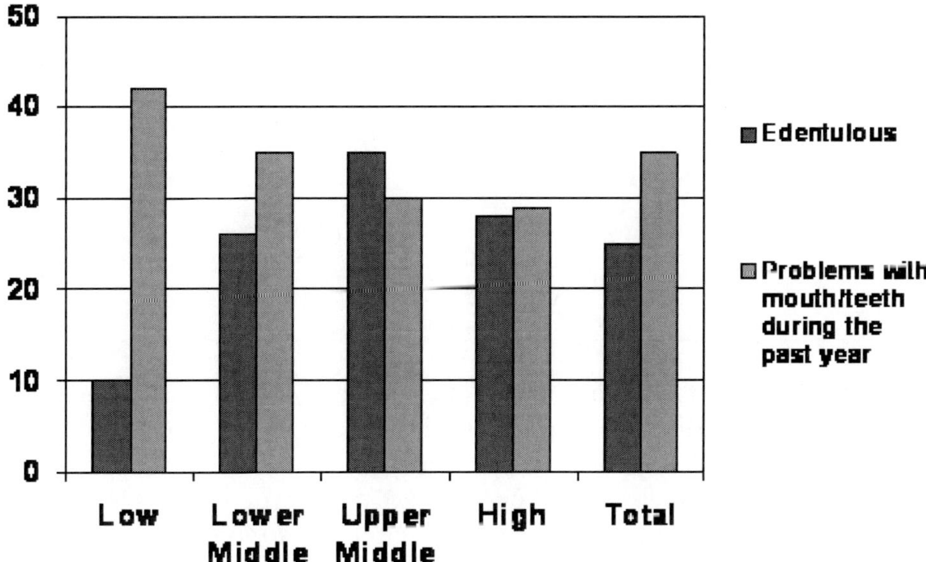

Figure 2.7. Percentage of 65-74-year-olds in low-, middle- and high income countries with no natural teeth and percentage of people having experienced problems with mouth/teeth during the past year [26,27] - The World Health Survey.

Table 2.1. Percentages of 65-74-year-olds in selected low income countries who have no natural teeth, having experienced problems from teeth or mouth during the past year, and persons who received oral health care [26, 27]

Persons with no natural teeth		Persons had problems with mouth/teeth		Persons who received oral care	
Country	Pct	Country	Pct	Country	Pct
Bangladesh	7,4	Bangladesh	56,8	Bangladesh	28,8
Burkina	5,4	Burkina	38,0	Burkina	15,6
Chad	24,3	Chad	52,3	Chad	15,2
Comoro	4,7	Comoro	26,9	Comoro	20,0
Congo	7,7	Congo	38,3	Congo	38,7
CotedIvorie	7,6	CotedIvorie	31,7	CotedIvorie	20,0
Ethiopia	3,4	Ethiopia	36,8	Ethiopia	9,3
Ghana	5,9	Ghana	32,1	Ghana	23,8
Kenya	5,0	Kenya	47,3	Kenya	21,7
Lao	9,4	Lao	30,0	Lao	20,3
Malawi	5,2	Malawi	59,7	Malawi	47,4
Mali	6,3	Mali	34,8	Mali	29,5
Mauritania	20,8	Mauritania	36,9	Mauritania	35,3
Myanmar	5,0	Myanmar	26,3	Myanmar	33,9
Nepal	9,6	Nepal	48,5	Nepal	12,7
Pakistan	28,1	Pakistan	45,7	Pakistan	54,6
Senegal	13,6	Senegal	35,5	Senegal	34,0
Vietnam	13,0	Vietnam	47,8	Vietnam	26,6
Zambia	5,2	Zambia	56,3	Zambia	28,3
Zimbabwe	8,0	Zimbabwe	48,3	Zimbabwe	35,1
Total	9,8	Total	42,2	Total	27,5

In order to highlight the responsiveness of the health system the participants were asked whether they received health care related to their oral problems. As shown in Figure 2.8, the global social gradient in health care is profound; in urban settings more than double the number of older people in high income countries receives care of their oral health problems as compared with people in low income countries. In addition, for low- and middle income countries, the survey demonstrates that people living in rural areas are less likely to have oral health care. This is in contrast to high income countries where equal proportions of older people living in urban and rural areas receive care in case of problems with mouth or teeth. The World Health Survey documents huge differences in oral health across countries and regions; in addition, considerable intra-country disparities are shown by education, gender, and age.

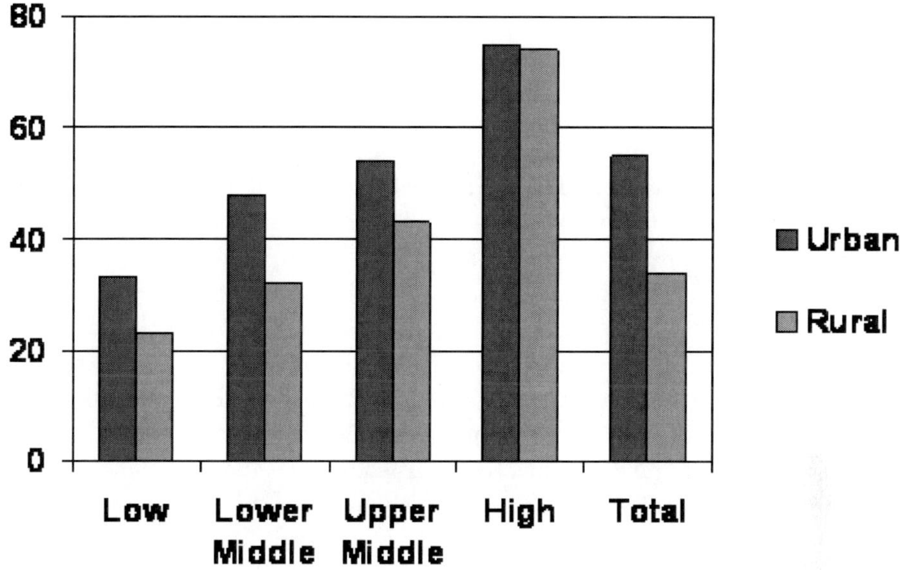

Figure 2.8. Percentage of 65-74-year-olds in low-, middle- and high income countries who received health care related to problems with mouth and teeth, by urbanization [26,27] - The World Health Survey.

2.3. Oral Health Services

Treatment of oral disease is extremely costly, the fourth most expensive disease to treat in most high income countries. Traditional curative dental care is a significant economic burden on many high income countries where 5-10% of public health expenditure relates to oral health [30, 31]. Over the past years, savings in dental expenditures have been noted for high income countries which have invested in preventive oral care and where positive trends are observed in terms of reduction in the prevalence of oral disease. In high income countries, the burden of oral disease has been tackled through establishment of advanced oral health systems which primarily offer curative services to patients. Most systems are based on demand for care as oral health care is provided by private dental practitioners to patients, with or without third-party payment schemes. Some countries, including those of Scandinavia and the United Kingdom, have organized public health services, particularly providing oral health care to children and disadvantaged population groups.

Investment in oral health care is little in most low- and middle income countries and availability and accessibility of oral health services are limited. In these countries, resources are primarily allocated to emergency oral care and pain relief and oral health services are generally confined to hospitals in major urban centres. Making financial resources available for treatment of oral disease at the level of cost as found for high-income countries is not realistic and also not necessary at present time. The good news is namely that the majority of oral diseases are avoidable through community-oriented prevention and oral health promotion. Moreover, it is vital for the health of populations that development or adjustment of oral health services will consider orientation of activities towards disease prevention and health promotion.

2.3.1. Population Coverage in Oral Health Care

In Tanzania, a recent study [32] showed that nearly six out of ten adults had suffered from oral pain and/or discomfort during the past year; however, only one quarter of these people sought emergency oral care from oral health facilities. Important reasons for not seeking emergency care were lack of money for the treatment or for the transport to the dental clinic [32]. Self-medication was used as an alternative to using oral health services, particularly by people living in rural areas. Similar results were obtained from Burkina Faso [33] where two thirds of adult people reported pain or discomfort affecting daily life; only one fourth of these people actually attended oral health facilities for care. People of high education were more likely than people without education to use health facilities; moreover, relatively few people living under poor material and housing conditions attended health services is case of pain and oral problems. Self-medication was employed by half the people with oral pain and such practice was most common among people living under poverty.

In a public health perspective, only a few African people have access to oral health services. In a survey undertaken in Tanzania [6], one tenth of adults had seen a dentist within the past year while four out ten adults had never received dental care. Symptoms or oral problems were the principal reasons for attending for care; nine out of ten adults had a tooth extraction at their recent dental visit and they had to pay directly for services. About one tenth of people studied informed that they consulted a person other than a dentist for care of teeth and mouth, mostly the medical doctor, pharmacist, paramedical, naturopath or a healer. The same study [6] covered schoolchildren 6 years and 12 years of age. Eighty percent of the children had never seen a dentist but just a few saw a dentist within the past year. In Burkina Faso, 12-year-old children and adults were included in a survey [7]. The vast majority of children had never seen a dentist and just a few children saw a dentist over the past year, mainly because of oral pain. One tenth of the adults paid a dental visit within the previous year, meanwhile, dental visits were remarkably more frequent among urban than rural residents [7].

Oral epidemiological surveys undertaken in Asia demonstrate a high need for oral health care. With respect to dental caries, the dt or DT components of the caries indices are relatively high indicating an unmet need for dental care. According to reports from China, about one third of 12-year-olds and one fourth of 18-year-olds had seen a dentist less than one year ago [35]. About one tenth of 12-year-old children had never visited a dentist and this was the case with one fifth of 18-year-olds. Poor oral health service was also observed for adult population groups. About one fourth of adults saw a dentist less than one year ago and tooth extraction was the main service offered to people with toothache [36]; cost of dental care was mostly paid by the patients themselves. In Thailand, a survey of 12-year-olds showed that only half the children had seen a dentist within the last year and four in ten children informed that they had a tooth extraction at their last visit [3]. A recent investigation of Lao children aged 12 years [5] showed that only three out of ten children were seen by a dentist within the last 12 months, and two thirds of the visits were due to acute problems. About four in ten children had never been to a dentist. Remarkably, the study indicates a clear social gradient in dental care; two thirds of children living under poverty had never seen a dentist as compared with one fifth of children of higher socio-economic background.

2.3.2. Oral Health Intervention and Common Risk Factors

As indicated in Figure 2.9, there is critical shortage of oral health professionals to meet the needs of all people in low and middle income countries. Therefore, prevention and control of oral disease must be provided by other personnel, such as primary health workers based in local health stations or community dispensaries. Systematic oral disease prevention and oral health promotion will need an effective new organizational platform whereby oral health is incorporated into general health promotion and chronic disease prevention. A core group of modifiable risk factors is common to many chronic diseases and injuries. The four most prominent chronic diseases – cardiovascular diseases, diabetes, cancer and chronic obstructive pulmonary diseases – share major risk factors with oral diseases. The preventable risk factors are related to lifestyles. For example, dietary habits are significant to the development of chronic diseases and also influence the development of oral disease. Most importantly, excessive amounts and frequent consumption of sugars are the major causes of dental caries and the risk of caries is high if population exposure to fluorides is inappropriate. Proper personal hygiene is crucial in prevention of chronic disease and essential to oral disease prevention as oral cavity bacteria are involved in progression of diseases such as dental caries and periodontal disease. In addition, tobacco use has been estimated to account for over 90% of cancers in the oral cavity, and it is associated with aggravated periodontal breakdown, poorer standards of oral hygiene and thus premature tooth loss. Moreover, the oral cancer risk increases when tobacco is used in combination with alcohol or betel and areca nut.

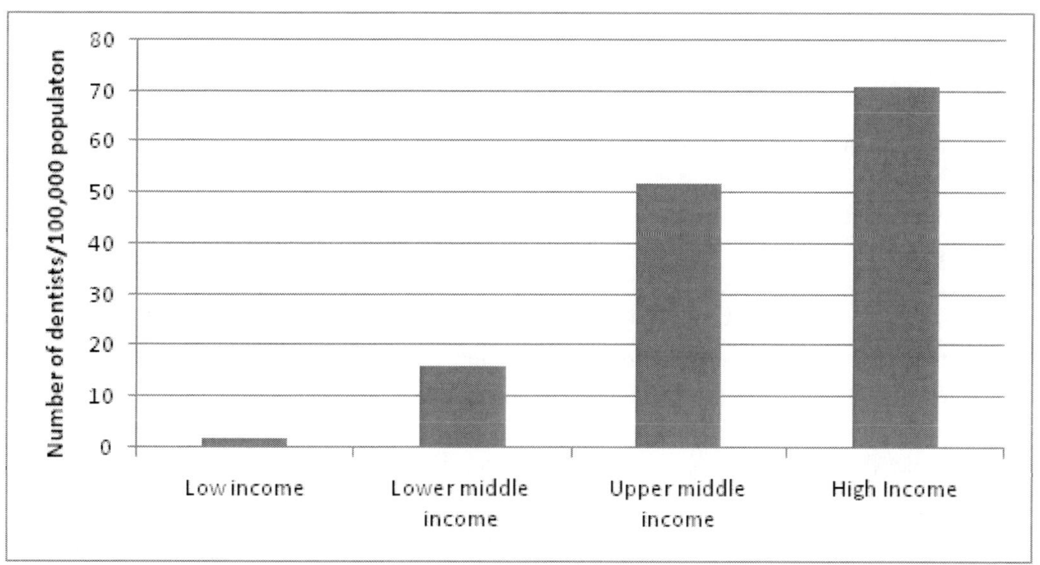

Figure 2.9. Number of dentists per 100,000 population in low-, middle- and high income countries [13].

Many general disease conditions have manifestations that increase the risk of oral disease which, in turn, is a risk factor for a number of general health conditions. Severe periodontal disease, for example, is associated in a two-way relationship with diabetes mellitus and has been considered the sixth complication of diabetes [34]. HIV/AIDS manifests in the oral cavity as well as in relation to general health. Thus, the incorporation of oral health into general health programmes established at community or national levels is the most promising approach to the achievement of better health and quality of life. Figure 2.10 illustrates how the common risk factors approach applies to oral health promotion and disease prevention.

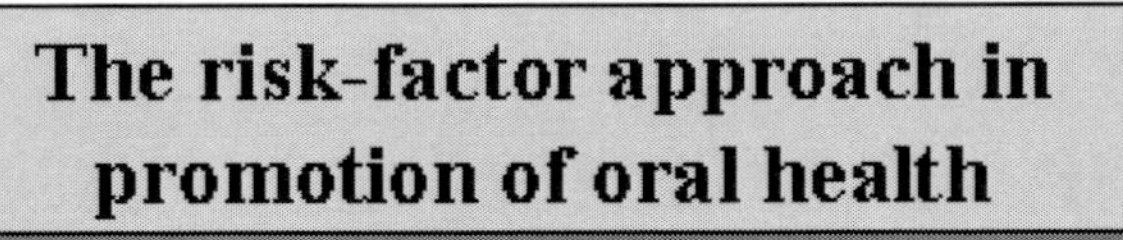

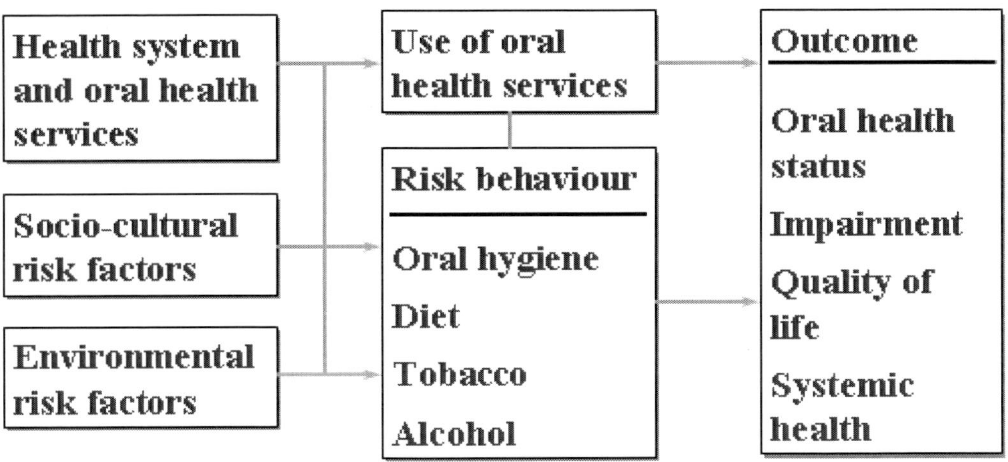

Figure 2.10. Conceptual model on risk factors approach for improving oral health of the population [37].

2.3.3. WHO Policies for Oral Health for All

The WHO Global Oral Health Programme formulated in 2003 the principal approaches and strategies for countries to adopt for the improvement of oral health worldwide [37]. The policy gives special emphasis to work for better health of the poor and disadvantaged population groups in countries. Meeting the oral health needs is particularly critical as regards to the poor people of low- and middle income countries. Meanwhile, most of these countries have no official health policies and health budgets which incorporate oral health. Thus, national capacity building for promoting oral health and disease prevention is highly necessary and the strengthening of health systems including primary oral health care is essential. The World Health Assembly (Geneva, May 2007) confirmed the approaches of the WHO Global Oral Health Programme by its Resolution 60.17 on "Oral health: action plan for promotion and integrated disease prevention" [38, 39]. The Resolution urges Member States to develop or adjust national policies for oral health as mentioned in the following:

To adopt measures to ensure that oral health is incorporated into policies for the integrated prevention of chronic non-communicable diseases and communicable diseases

To take measures to ensure that evidence-based oral health approaches are used

To consider mechanisms to provide essential oral health care and to incorporate oral health within the framework of primary health care, and to promote availability and accessibility of oral health services that should be directed towards disease prevention and health promotion for poor and disadvantaged populations

To consider the development and implementation of fluoridation programmes, giving priority to equitable strategies such as automatic administration of fluoride through water, milk, and salt, and to provision of affordable fluoride toothpaste

To take steps to ensure that prevention of oral cancer is an integral part of national cancer-control programmes, and that oral health professionals or primary health workers with relevant training are involved in detection, early diagnosis and treatment

To ensure the prevention of oral disease associated with HIV/AIDS and the promotion of oral health and quality of life for people living with HIV, involving oral health professionals or primary health workers

To develop and implement oral health promotion for school children as part of activities in health-promoting schools

To scale up capacity to produce oral health personnel, providing for equitable distribution of personnel to the primary-care level

To develop and implement, in countries affected by noma, national programmes to control the disease within national programmes for the integrated management of childhood illness and for the reduction of malnutrition and poverty

To incorporate an oral health information system into national health surveillance plans

To strengthen operational oral health research and use evidence-based oral health promotion and disease prevention

To address human resources and workforce planning for oral health as part of every national plan for health

To increase the budgetary provisions that are dedicated to the prevention and control of oral and craniofacial diseases and conditions

To strengthen partnerships among stakeholders in support of national oral health programmes

In 2008, the *WHO Commission on Social Determinants in Health* launched a report [40] which concerns the challenges related to closing the gap in health between rich and poor. The keys to eliminate the social inequalities in health and health care – between countries and within countries- relate to improving the standard of living among the poor and disadvantaged people, ensuring healthy environments, establishing the necessary conditions for adoption of healthy lifestyles, and to strengthening the access to health services that are financially fair and which possibly will provide for essential primary health care. Tackling the social determinants in oral health remains a huge challenge to all countries around the globe. At the 7th Global Conference on Health Promotion, co-hosted by WHO and the Ministry of Health, Kenya, 2009, discussed the gap in implemention of evidence-based health promotion. Country experiences on community oriented interventions are available and these may serve as important models for improving the health of the poor and disadvantaged population groups.

References

[1]   Petersen P.E. (2008). Oral health (pp 677-685) I: Heggenhougen K, Quah S (eds) *International Encyclopaedia of Public Health*, Vol 4.

[2]   Kwan S, Petersen P.E. (2003) Oral health promotion: an essential element of a Health Promoting School. WHO Information Series on School Health. Document 11. Geneva: WHO.

[3]   Petersen P.E., Hoerup N, Poomviset N, Watanapa A. (2001) Oral health status and oral health behaviour of urban and rural schoolchildren. *Int. Dent. J.*;51:95-102.

[4]   Jiang H, Petersen P.E., Peng B, Tai B, Bian Z. (2005) Self-assessed dental health, oral health practices, and general health behaviors in Chinese urban adolescents. *Acta Odontol. Scand.*; 63:343-352.

[5]   Jürgensen N, Petersen P.E. (2009) Oral health and the impact of socio-behavioural factors in a cross sectional survey of 12-year old schoolchildren in Laos. *BMC Oral Health*; 9:29.

[6]   Petersen P.E, Nyandindi U, Kikiwilu E.N, Mabelya L. (2002) Oral health status and oral health behaviour of schoolchildren, teachers and adults in Tanzania. *WHO Technical Report*. WHO: Geneva.

[7]   Varenne B., Petersen P.E., Seydou O. (2006) Oral health behaviour of children and adults in urban and rural areas of Burkina Faso, Africa. *Int. Dent. J.;* 56:61-70.

[8]   Varenne B., Petersen P.E., Fournet F., Msellati P, Gary J, Ouattara S, Harang M and Salem G. (2006) Illness-related behaviour and utilization of oral health services among adult city-dwellers in Burkina Faso: evidence from a household survey. *BMC Health Services Research,* 6:164.

[9]   Bratthall D., Petersen P.E., Stjernswärd J.R., Brown J. (2006) Oral and craniofacial diseases and disorders (chapter 38). In: Disease control priorities in developing countries. Jamison DT, Breman JG, Measham AR, et al., editors. New York: World Bank Health and Oxford University Press. pp. 723-736.

[10] Harris R., Pine C. (eds). (2007) Community Oral Health. 2nd edition. Berlin: Quintessence,.

[11] Petersen P.E. (2005) Sociobehavioural risk factors in dental caries - international perspectives. *Community Dent. Oral. Epidemiol.*; 33: 274-279.

[12] World Health Organization. (1997) Oral health surveys - Basic Methods (4th Edition). Geneva: WHO.

[13] World Health Organization. (2004) Global Oral Health Data Bank. Geneva: WHO.

[14] World Health Organization. (2003) Diet, nutrition and the prevention of chronic diseases. *Tech. Rep. Series* 916. Geneva: WHO.

[15] Petersen P.E. (2004) Improvement of oral health in Africa in the 21st century – the role of the WHO Global Oral Health Programme. *Developing Dent.*;5: 9-20.

[16] Liu M., Zhu L., Petersen P.E., Zhang B.X. (2007) Changing use and knowledge of fluoride toothpaste by schoolchildren, parents and schoolteachers in Beijing, China. *Int. Dent. J.*;57: 187-194.

[17] Petersen P.E., Ogawa H. (2005) Strengthening the prevention of periodontal disease: The WHO approach. *J. Periodontol.*; 76: 2187-2193.

[18] Stewart B.W., Kleihues P. (2003) World Cancer Report. Lyon: WHO International Agency for Research on Cancer.

[19] Petersen P.E. (2009) Oral cancer prevention and control – The approach of the World Health Organization. *Oral Oncology*;45:454-560.

[20] UNAIDS. (2008) Report on the global HIV/AIDS epidemic 2008. Geneva: UNAIDS.

[21] Coogan M., Greenspan J., Challacombe S.J. (2005) Oral lesions in infection with human immunodeficiency virus. *Bull World Health Organ*; 83: 700-706.

[22] Fabian F.M., Kahabuka F.K., Petersen P.E., Shubi F.M., Jürgensen N. (2009) Oral manifestations among people living with HIV/AIDS in Tanzania. *Int. Dent. J.*; 59: 187-91.

[23] Kahabuka F.K. Fabian F, Petersen P.E, Nguvumali H. (2007) Awareness of HIV AIDS and its oral manifestations among people living with HIV in Dar-es-Salaam, Tanzania. *African Journal of AIDS research*; 6:91-95.

[24] Enwonwu C.O. (1995) Noma: a neglected scourge of children in sub-Saharan Africa. *Bull World Health Organ*; 73: 541-545.

[25] Andreasen J.O., Andreasen F.M. Dental trauma. In: Pine C, editor. (2002) Community Oral Health. London: Elsvier Science Limited.

[26] T.Bedirhan Üstün, Somnath Chatterji, Abdelhay Mechbal, Christopher J.L.Murray, WHS Collaborating Groups. (2003) The World Health Surveys. In: Christopher J.L.Murray, David B.Evans, editors. Health Systems Performance Assessment. *World Health Organization*;. p. 797-808.

[27] Petersen P.E. (2009) The World Health Survey- The global burden of oral disease. Geneva: WHO.

[28] Chen M., Andersen R.M., Barmes D.E., Leclerq M-H., Lyttle S.C. (1997) Comparing oral health systems. A Second International Collaborative Study. Geneva: WHO.

[29] Petersen P.E., Kjöller M., Christensen L.B., Krustrup U. (2004) Changing dentate status of adults, use of dental health services, and achievement of national dental health goals in Denmark by the year 2000. *J. Public Health Dent.*; 64: 127-35.

[30] Widström E., Eaton K.A. (2004) Oral health care systems in the extended European Union. *Oral Health Prev. Dent.*; 2: 155-94.

[31] US Department of Health. (1998) Health Care Financing Administration. National health expenditures,. Washington: Health Care Financing Administration. Available from http://www.nidr.nih.gov/sgr/sgrohweb/toc.htm.

[32] Kikwilu E.N., Masalu J.R., Kahabuka F.K., Senkoro A.R. (2008) Prevalence of oral pain and barriers to use of emergency oral care facilities among adult Tanzanians. *BMC Oral Health*;8:28.

[33] Varenne B., Msellati P., Zoungrana C., Fournet F., Salem G. (2005) Reasons for attending dental care services in Ouagadougou, Burkina Faso. *Bull WHO Org*;83:650-655.

[34] Petersen P.E., Ueda H. (2006) Oral Health in Ageing Societies: Integration of Oral Health and General Health. Report of a meeting convened at the WHO Centre for Health Development in Kobe, Japan, 1-3 June 2005. Geneva: World Health Organization.

[35] Zhu L., Petersen P.E., Wang H.Y., Bian J.Y., Zhang B.X. (2003) Oral health knowledge, attitudes and behaviour of children and adolesents in China. *Int. Dent. J.;* 53:289-298.

[36] Zhu L., Petersen P.E., Wang H.Y., Bian J.Y., Zhang B.X. (2005) Oral health knowledge, attitudes and behaviour of adults in China. *Int. Dent. J.;* 55; 231-241.

[37] Petersen P.E. (2003) The World Oral Health Report 2003: Continuous improvement of oral health in the 21st century – the approach of the WHO Global Oral Health Programme. *Community Dent. Oral Epidemiol.*; 31 (Suppl 1): 3-24

[38] Petersen P.E. (2008) World Health Organization global policy for improvement of oral health - World Health Assembly 2007. *Int. Dent. J.*; 58: 115-21.

[39] Petersen P.E. (2009) Global policy for improvement of oral health in the 21st century - implications to oral health research of World Health Assembly 2007, World Health Organization. *Community Dent. Oral Epidemiol.*; 37: 1-8.

[40] World Health Organization. (2008) Closing the gab in generation- health equity through action on the social determinants of health. Geneva: WHO Commission on Social Determinants of Health.

In: Oral Health Care for Socially Disadvantaged Communities   ISBN: 978-1-62948-287-3
Editors: F.K. Kahabuka, E.N. Kikwilu and I. Anderson © 2013 Nova Science Publishers, Inc.

Chapter III

Management of Dental Caries in Socially Disadvantaged Communities[*]

Jo Frencken[1] and Soraya Leal[2]
[1] College of Dental Sciences, Radboud University Nijmegen
[2] School of Health Science, University of Brasília

3.1. Introduction

'Dental caries is a localized chemical dissolution of a tooth surface resulting from metabolic events taking place in a biofilm (dental plaque) covering the affected area. These metabolic events are the *carious process*. The interaction between the microbial deposits and the hard tissues of the teeth may result in the *carious lesion* that is the sign or symptom of the process' (Fejerskov and Kidd, 2008a). The lesion is influenced by demineralising factors such as sugar-containing diets, by oral hygiene levels and by remineralising factors like the presence of fluoride and saliva.

In principle, dental caries can manifest itself in all individuals at any age. In the mouths of most individuals, a fine balance exists between demineralising and remineralising factors. However, dental caries becomes a health problem if the balance is distorted towards demineralisation over a sufficiently long period. The first visible result of this imbalance is the development of a whitish area in the enamel surface; followed, after continuous demineralisation, by the development of a tooth cavity. In the absence of restorative care, the caries process may cause infection of the pulp complex and subsequently, of bone tissue. However, at any stage in the process, the imbalance towards demineralisation can be halted. An extensive de[1]scription of the onset and development of the dental caries process and its sequels can be found in the textbook on the management of dental caries edited by Fejerskov and Kidd (2008b).

In high-income countries, the prevalence and severity of dental caries in children and adolescents has declined tremendously since the early sixties (Whelton, 2004). During the

---

[*] The co-authors own the copyrights to this chapter.

same period, the percentage of people retaining their natural teeth into old age has increased substantially. T²he decline of dental caries in these countries can be ascribed, amongst other factors, to adequate plaque control through the use of fluoride toothpaste; regular fluoride application and application of other caries control agents; general public awareness of the advantages of having healthy natural teeth; increased and diversified dental personnel; increased dental facilities, allowing increased access to care, and well-functioning public and private health insurance systems. In addition, large-scale restoration of cavitated teeth has allowed these teeth to continue functioning for a long time. This was achieved through the development of adequate restorative materials and systems, and their application by well-trained operators that the national budgets could afford.

In line with Fejerskov and Kidd (2008), the authors of this chapter have opted for the use of 'caries control' rather than 'caries preventive' measures. The reason is that the caries process (metabolism) in the biofim is considered a natural event that cannot, therefore, be prevented and only carious lesion formation and its progression can be controlled.

Overall, the history over the last half-century in high-income countries has shown that carious lesion development can be controlled and cavitated teeth can be restored and continue to be functional into old age (Hugoson et al, 2008). It has also shown that this type of healthcare involves high expenditure on dental personnel and equipment that only a relatively few countries worldwide can afford. Most middle- and low-income countries certainly cannot afford to provide such healthcare systems for their child populations (Yee and Sheiham, 2002).

This chapter describes and discusses caries control and restorative treatments in the context of healthcare systems in countries and communities characterised by limited dental personnel resources, inadequate finances and limited healthcare facilities, materials and equipment. The authors are aware that these countries and communities differ in many ways and that great disparities exist between communities and oral healthcare services within such countries. This chapter concludes with recommendations regarding caries control and restorative treatment options that are considered appropriate for use in socially disadvantaged communities worldwide.

3.1.1. Salient Features of Dental Caries in Socially Disadvantaged Communities

The level of caries experience amongst 12-year-olds in middle- and low-income countries has been fairly stable at a mean DMFT score of 2 since the early nineteen-eighties. There are, however, indications that the level of caries experience in these countries is slightly on the increase (Peterson 2008a). In the 35-44-year age group, some countries in Latin America show high mean DMFT scores ($\geq$ 14 teeth affected), while caries experience in this age group in African and Asian countries is usually much lower (Peterson, 2008a).

The most appalling feature related to dental caries in these countries is that restored cavitated dentine lesions are almost non-existent. This is shown by the high proportion of the D-component of the DMFT index (93%) and the very low M- and F- components amongst 12-year-olds in low-income countries (Figure 3.1). The D-component of 80% for the lower-

and middle-income countries is also very high. A similar situation can be depicted for adults, with the difference that more teeth have been lost due to the end result of the caries process. Dental carious lesions in people in these countries are mainly treated by extraction of cavitated teeth.

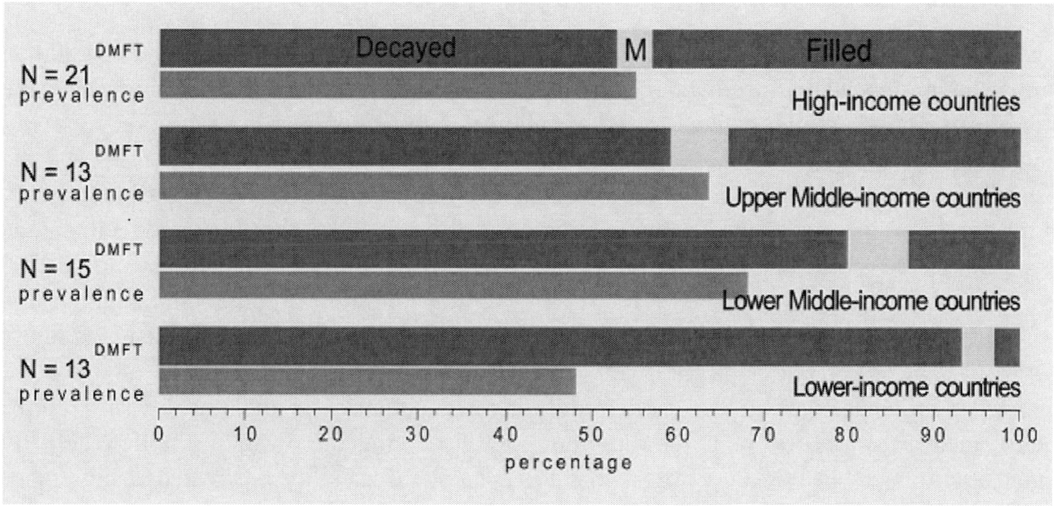

Figure 3.1. Prevalence of dental caries and of DMF components for 12-year olds by income groups. N= number of countries that provided results.

3.1.2. Consequences of Untreated Cavitated Lesions in Children

The unavailability of caries control measures including restorative care in communities in middle- and low-income countries can have serious consequences, especially for children. A study from the Philippines revealed that almost all carious cavities in 6- and 12-year-olds remained untreated and that 40% of these cavities were accompanied by infection of the pulp, abscesses, fistulas and/or infected root remnants (Monse et al, 2010). These conditions can pose a serious threat to children's general health, due to the risk of developing systemic sepsis, osteomyelitis and infection of the neck and the floor of the mouth. Furthermore, toothache may alter children's eating and sleeping habits, which can affect their growth negatively (Miller et al, 1982).

Untreated carious cavities in children have also been associated with protein-energy malnutrition (Alvarez, 1995; Psoter et al, 2005) and stunted growth (Alvarez et al, 1988), and early childhood caries has been associated with lower body-weight and reduced body-length (Ayhan, 1996). Subsequently, extracting cavitated primary teeth in 5- to 6-year-old children promoted weight gain (Body Mass Index) and possibly growth over a 7 months period (Malek et al, 2009). Untreated carious cavities have an impact not only on the physical condition of children; their cognitive development may also become impaired. In a survey of native-American schoolchildren, one third admitted to missing school because of dental pain (Chen et al, 1997), and 70% of children in the Western Cape, South Africa, had missed school because of toothache (Naidoo et al, 2001). The effect of chronic dental pain in children is not a supposition: affected children are unable to focus or complete school assignments, which affects their school performance negatively (Schechter, 2000).

3.1.3. Possible Reasons for the Low Level of Oral Care

There are a few reasons that may explain why palliative caries control and restorative care is lacking in socially disadvantaged communities. Firstly, in many such communities the ratio of operating dental personnel to the population numbers is low. Furthermore, access to health facilities is not always easy because they may be far from some communities and the cost of transport to their locations may be relatively unaffordable (Hobdell, 2007). In many middle- and low-income countries, the population is also not aware that cavitated teeth can be restored and, therefore, do not seek assistance when a painful cavitated tooth can still be restored. Dental practitioners are not always helpful in informing the public about the possibility that a cavitated tooth can be restored, as has been reported from Tanzania recently (Kikwilu et al, 2010). Perhaps the main reason for the very high percentage of untreated cavitated dentine lesions in low- and middle-income countries is the low level of caries control measures and oral health promotional activities, together with the notion held by dental practitioners in these countries, that tooth cavities can only be treated using rotary dental equipment. The equipment frequently fails or is unavailable, which does not contribute to assisting the provision of good oral health care to the public. This situation is frequently present in public oral health services.

Private oral health services in low- and middle-income countries are usually better equipped and dental practitioners are able to serve their clients accordingly. However, they also might experience equipment dysfunctions, maintenance problems and the irregular supply of electricity. These situations vary from country to country. Obviously, reliance on a care system faced with these problems will result in inadequate provision of service to the public.

It is a fact that most people in socially disadvantaged communities end up having an extraction as the treatment for a painful tooth, regardless of whether this tooth could be repaired or was beyond repair. The need for repair or extraction can to a large extent be avoided. This chapter to discusses ways of controlling carious lesion development and treating cavitated dentine lesions, taking into account the circumstances often prevalent in socially disadvantaged communities.

3.2. Caries Control Measures

Until about four decades ago, the caries management concept developed by GV Black, in 1891, was commonly applied throughout the world. Development of both Black's cavity design and the dental nomenclature system (Wilwerding, 2001) was based on the restorative materials available and the dentistry knowledge acquired by then. Notwithstanding the extended cavity designs, Black knew that enamel carious lesions could be controlled through plaque control (Black, 1908).

Since the mid-fifties, new restorative materials with good adhesive properties have been launched and the caries process has become better understood. These developments have paved the way for the emergence of a modern concept of dentistry, departing from the outdated manner of managing carious lesions that is still currently being practiced by many. This concept, termed Minimum Intervention Dentistry (MI), can be defined as a philosophy of oral care that offers the practitioner the maximum possibility of preserving healthy tooth structures (White and Eakle, 2000). MI integrates early disease detection, caries control measures and remineralisation, followed by minimally invasive operative approaches to repair irreversible damage caused by the ongoing caries process (Mickenautsch, 2005).

In light of the current understanding about dental caries and its progression, and taking into account the public oral health scenario in most socially disadvantaged communities (limited personnel and finance resources), a wholly credible assumption is that the best strategy for managing dental caries is to intervene before it can be detected clinically. Disorganization of the biofilm, so that it cannot become cariogenic, is considered the most effective measure to achieve this. And if this can be done by individuals themselves, they contain the power to keep their dentition free from carious lesion development, which is one of the fundamentals of the minimal intervention dentistry concept. This strategy essentially requires measures related to oral health promotion and caries control but, in cases where tooth cavitation is already present, professionals have to assist providing treatments based on minimally invasive operative approaches.

In the remainder of this section the suitability of a number of caries control measures for use in deprived communities are discussed.

3.2.1. Sugar Substitutes and Diet Counseling

Fermentable carbohydrates play an important role in the caries process, as they are an excellent substrate for cariogenic bacteria in the biofilm. Sugar intake was previously assumed to be linearly related to caries incidence. However, "the fluoride era" seems to have interfered in this relationship. A systematic review attempted to answer the question as to whether *in the modern age of extensive fluoride exposure, individuals with a high level of sugar intake, measured either as a total amount or as a high frequency of consumption, experience greater caries severity relative to those with a lower level of sugar intake.* The review concluded that the relationship between sugar intake and caries is much weaker in the modern age of fluoride exposure than it used to be (Burt and Pai, 2001). However, controlling sugar and other fermentable carbohydrate consumption is still an important strategy for carious lesion control, particularly for populations at high caries risk, and/or in the absence of fluoride.

Noncariogenic sweeteners and sugar substitutes have an important role to play in reducing sugar intake. The sugar substitutes most commonly used in dentistry are xylitol and sorbitol. They belong to the sugar alcohol or polyol non-fermentable family. Xylitol is as sweet as sucrose (Lindely et al, 1976), and sweeter than sorbitol. However, sorbitol is cheaper than xylitol which is, nevertheless, being extensively used in sugar-free products (Ly et al, 2006). Both sugar alcohols are frequently added to gums, candies, chocolates, mints, energy bars, oral hygiene and health products. However, the most relevant information from clinical trials is derived from studies that aimed to assess the effectiveness of xylitol chewing gums.

In general, the evidence suggests that sugar-free chewing gum, used immediately after meals, reduces carious lesion progression. Additionally, long-term use of non-sucrose chewing gums has a beneficial effect on plaque pH (Campus et al, 2009). Saliva stimulation, the lack of sucrose and the inability of bacteria to metabolize polyols into acid are factors that contribute to this effect (Mickenautsch et al, 2007). It is important to highlight that dose and frequency of the sugar-free "product" are both extremely important in relation to obtaining good results.

It has been suggested that the use of chewing gum containing protective substances, especially xylitol, can reduce tooth decay and should be considered a strategy for carious lesion control in schools (Ly et al, 2008a). In this regard, it was shown that caries control programs for school children, based on the provision of xylitol gummy bear snacks, are feasible and can be implemented with good compliance from both children and parents (Ly et al, 2008b). According to Zero (2008), sugar substitutes should be recommended as part of an overall carious lesion control strategy for high caries risk individuals in developing countries but, in light of the available evidence regarding the effectiveness of topical fluoride, would not be the first-line choice with regard to caries control measures.

It has been stated that food products containing xylitol are available commercially and have the potential to be widely accessible to consumers (Lynch and Milgrom, 2003). This may be true for high-income countries but is it also true in financially disadvantaged communities? If sugar-free chewing gum is available, it should be used in conjunction with fluoride toothpaste, particularly by those at high caries risk in well-controlled schemes.

However, is it realistic to expect large quantities of products containing sugar substitutes to be available in socially deprived communities? People in these communities very commonly have access to refined sugars and consume them in large quantities. Therefore, the best caries control advice regarding children is to restrict their intake of sugar-containing food products to 5 times per day (Kalsbeek and Verrips, 1994).

3.2.2. Fluoride Agents

The presence of fluoride at the tooth surface is an important factor in the control of carious lesion progression (Groeneveld, 1985). Fluoride can be provided systemically (via water, milk or salt) or administered through topically applied agents (toothpaste, gel, varnish or mouthwash). In addition, a certain level of fluoride can be found naturally in the environment (water and food) or can be artificially added to industrialized products (such as infant formulas and beverages). The widespread use of fluoride sources has contributed to a decline in caries experience but also to an increase in the prevalence of dental fluorosis (Alvarez et al, 2009).

3.2.2.1. Water, Milk and Salt Fluoridation

Water fluoridation has been named the most important oral health measure for managing dental caries, both in developed and in developing countries (Narvai et al, 2006; Pizzo et al, 2007). In terms of public oral health, water fluoridation is a way of making fluoride accessible to an entire community without requiring individuals to change their behavior in order to obtain the benefits of fluoridation (ADA, 2005). However, what many view as a positive method is criticized by others, who affirm that individuals, in this circumstance, are not allowed to avoid fluoride consumption (Cohen and Locker, 2001).

The current literature shows that artificially fluoridating water is beneficial in reducing carious lesion progression (National and Medical Council Research, 2007). The safety and efficacy of fluoridation in drinking water has been assessed, mainly in child populations (McDonagh et al, 2000) and the results can be summarized as follows: fluoride in drinking water is associated with an increased proportion of children without dentine carious lesions and with a reduction in the number of teeth affected by dentine carious lesions; a dose-dependent relationship with dental fluorosis is present.

However, fluoride is not only important in reducing dentine carious lesion progression in children: adults also benefit from fluoridated water schemes, as shown by the 27% reduction of dentine carious lesion development, according to a systematic review (Griffin et al, 2007). Moreover, it has been suggested that suppressing inequalities in the distribution of dental caries experience requires an expanded access to fluoridated tap water (Peres et al, 2006) and that water fluoridation still remains the best strategy for combating dental caries in many societies (Kumar, 2008).

Alternatively, fluoridation of salt and milk has been proposed in cases where exposure to fluoridated water is technically not feasible or culturally not accepted (Petersen, 2004). However, how effective are these two fluoride vehicles?

Information available from good quality studies regarding the caries control effect of milk fluoridation is scarce. The Cochrane Collaboration review (Yeung et al, 2005) concluded that there is insufficient evidence to show the effectiveness of fluoridated milk in controlling tooth decay. However, the few studies included in the systematic review suggested that it has a beneficial effect for school children, mainly in the permanent dentition.

Salt fluoridation is another option for systemic fluoride supplementation. In contrast to fluoridated tap water, it allows the consumer free choice regarding fluoride consumption. It is been largely used in some Latin American countries, including Colombia, Costa Rica, Mexico and Jamaica. However, controversy exists regarding the effectiveness of salt fluoridation (Ellwood et al, 2008). One systematic review that aimed to analyze salt fluoridation efficacy favored salt fluoridation against no exposure to other source of fluoride (Yeangopal et al, 2010). However, the poor quality of papers included in the systematic review made it impossible to calculate the effect of salt fluoridation on DMFT decrease. For that reason, further high quality studies are still needed to confirm salt fluoridation efficacy in caries prevention (Yeung, 2011). Apparently, in Mexico technical problems resulted in large varieties of fluoride concentration in table salt, from 0 ppm to 485 ppm (Hernandez-Guerrero et al, 2008). Moreover, evaluation of the implementation of the fluoridated salt program in Mexico concluded that it greatly increased the risk of fluorosis (Vallejos-Sánchez et al, 2006). Absence of evidence about its effectiveness, and technical problems in its implementation, call for caution when salt fluoridation is considered appropriate for improving the oral health in a community.

It must be stressed that, independently of the source of fluoride administration (water, salt or milk), dietary fluoride consumption and the fluoride level of drinking water must be taken into account before a systemic method of fluoridation application is implemented (Rodrigues et al, 2009). Overexposure to fluoride may easily result in the development of dental fluorosis (Alvarez et al, 2009). As an example, fluoride concentrations in juices, bottled water, nectars and carbonated drinks available in Mexico City were shown to vary from 0.07 to 1.42 ppm

(Jiminez-Farfan et al, 2004). The availability of different sources of fluoride is a potential risk factor for the development of dental fluorosis.

3.2.2.2. Self- and Professionally Applied Fluoride Agents

Initially, the dental community was of the opinion that fluoride's most important effect was related to its systemic action only, mainly when ingested during tooth development in the child's early stages of life. However, today it is accepted that its predominant benefit is derived from its topical application (Fejerskov et al, 1981). Using topical fluoride daily maintains a constant level of fluoride in dental plaque, thereby reducing bacterial ability to produce acid (Welin-Neilands and Svensater, 2007) and contributing to diminishing demineralization while enhancing remineralization. The scheme of topical fluoride application is presented in Table 3.1.

Table 3.1. Fluoride vehicles by application

Self-applied	Professionally applied
Fluoride-containing toothpaste	Varnish
Mouthrinses	Gel
	Foam

Fluoridated toothpaste use is the most widespread method for maintaining a constant level of fluoride in the oral cavity and it is considered one of the major factors related to the decline of caries prevalence in high-income countries (Petterson and Brathall, 1996; Carvalho et al, 2001). Due to its advantages, one of WHO's action plans for promoting and integrating oral disease prevention focuses on the establishment of national plans to advocate the adoption of fluoride toothpaste (Petersen, 2008b). Nevertheless, significant inequities in the affordability of fluoride-containing toothpaste were demonstrated when high-income nations were compared with middle and low-income countries. It was strongly recommended that all efforts should be done to make fluoride toothpaste affordable and available in poorer communities (Goldman et al, 2008). Not only is toothpaste not always available; having a personal toothbrush is also not a usual reality in many socially disadvantaged communities. Shidara et al (2007) investigated the oral health status of a group of schoolchildren from Cambodia and noted that only 44.2% of them owned a toothbrush.

The unavailability of a toothbrush and fluoride toothpaste may be due to ignorance on the part of community members, to other financial priorities of the family or to the high cost of these commodities and may differ from family to family. However, if cost is an issue, governments might consider reducing taxation on these products.

Professional application of fluorides requires the patient to call in at a dental clinic or health centre regularly. This will reduce the importance of these types of fluoride vehicles at population basis in socially disadvantaged communities. Usually, professionally applied fluorides are indicated for patients who are at high risk of carious lesion development and for special patients; like those receiving orthodontic treatment or experiencing decreased salivary flow (Hawkins et al, 2003). It is a very good strategy for controlling carious lesions in private dental practices and in clinics in affluent areas in low- and middle-income countries. It can also be applied in community health programs, as currently implemented in some Brazilian cities through the Family Health Program (Almeida and Ferreira, 2008). In this program, dentists in a group of health professionals participate in visiting families in their homes, and children at public schools in socially disadvantaged communities, providing oral health promotion and caries control measures like fluoride gel application.

A series of Cochrane reviews on self- and professionally applied fluoride agents have been published during the last years. The main results have been summarized by Marinho (2008). More than 130 clinical trials were evaluated regarding the use of fluoride toothpaste, mouthwashes, gels and varnish. These showed that each of the four fluoride agents is able to reduce the incidence of dentine carious lesions, irrespective of whether other fluoride vehicles are used. However, it was observed that when compared to children using fluoride toothpaste only, children who received professionally applied fluoride in addition to toothpaste benefitted from an additional reduction in the incidence of dentine carious lesions. The combination of tooth brushing and fluoride toothpaste, moreover, not only disturbs the biofilm and supplies fluoride ions to the tooth environment but it also has a positive impact on the gingival health through the removal of plaque during tooth brushing.

Would it be possible, considering the information presented above, to answer the question as to whether the best modality of fluoride therapy for socially disadvantaged communities can be determined? The answer, unfortunately, is no. The most appropriate fluoride vehicle for use in those communities is dependent on many community-related aspects. Questions of importance include:

- Are fluoride agents available in the country?
- What is known about logistical aspects in terms of technology and expertise needed for adding and controlling fluoride to water systems, salt, milk and/or toothpaste?
- Does the population that requires protection have access to a piped water system?
- If water fluoridation is not feasible for such population, what costs would be involved in adopting other fluoride agents for mass fluoridation?
- What legal aspects would be involved in the introduction of fluoride agents?

These uncertainties highlight the necessity of establishing policies that are specially developed for each community and take into consideration its specific particularities. Moreover, the support of international dental organizations is essential if fluoride is to be made affordable for everyone. Policymakers, politicians and dentists should be mindful that in general, populations groups most affected by oral health problems are those with the highest poverty rates and the lowest education levels (Timis and Danila, 2005).

Other factors that determine the most appropriate fluoride vehicle are population-related. Does everyone need to be exposed to the same amount of fluoride? Again, caution is required. Caries risk facing individuals or sub-populations should be determined before decisions are made about what the most suitable fluoride scheme would be. In general, fluoride seems not to prevent most of the new carious lesions in low risk populations (Batchelor and Sheiham, 2006). For these populations, mass fluoridation might not be a good preventive option. Therefore, if a choice has to be made regarding fluoride vehicle viability for socially disadvantaged communities, fluoride toothpaste would need to be selected as a first choice.

3.2.3. Chlorhexidine Agent

Carious lesion development control would benefit from reduction of the action of microorganisms in the biofilm through use of therapeutic agents. One such agent is chlorhexidine. It is a chemotherapeutic agent that is able to kill certain oral microorganism and subsequently, to affect biofilm formation.

There is evidence that chlorhexidine is most effective in people who have been highly colonized by streptococcus mutans. Nevertheless, despite intensive chlorhexidine treatment, re-colonization at the tooth surface always occurs (Emilson, 1994). Whelton and O'Mullane (2001) assessed the effectiveness of a combination of chlorhexidine and other agents on carious lesion control. They concluded that theoretically, the use of chlorhexidine in high-risk caries individuals with high levels of streptococcus mutans in saliva has a sound foundation. Amorim et al, (2008) studied the effect of a 4-week alternated application of chlorhexidine and fluoride varnishes on the presence of plaque and on white spot lesion remineralisation in primary teeth. After 3 months, the combination of the two agents was more effective than the sole use of either application. The effectiveness of professionally applied chlorhexidine varnish alone, with a longer application interval of 6 months, was studied (Du et al, 2006). In contrast with a placebo varnish, the chlorhexidine varnish was found to have reduced the incidence of dental carious lesions in primary molars by 37% after 2 years.

However, a subsequent review indicated that clinical evidence regarding the effectiveness of chlorhexidine gel and varnish was inconclusive and that the use of chlorhexidine rinses for carious lesion control should not be recommended because evidence of their effectiveness was lacking (Autio-Gold, 2008). This view was supported by a systematic review aimed at determining the carious lesion inhibiting effect of chlorhexidine varnishes on the permanent dentition of children, adolescents and young adults. Chlorhexidine varnish showed a moderate caries-inhibiting effect when applied every 3 to 4 months but this had diminished 2 years after the last application. Studies that test chlorhexidine effectiveness with longer application intervals are required (Zhang et al, 2006).

The overall conclusion about chlorhexidine as a carious lesion control agent is that evidence of its effectiveness in mouth rinses, gels and varnishes products is lacking. Chlorhexidine varnish can be considered an option for individuals at high caries risk who have high bacteria counts but are chlorhexidine-containing products useful in disadvantaged communities? In order for chlorhexidine to be effective, it needs to be applied frequently. This requires the presence of a dental professional. Would this treatment protocol be suitable for use in a disadvantaged community? This is unlikely. In agreement with Autio-Gold, (2008), we suggest that on the basis of current knowledge regarding chlorhexidine-containing products, carious lesion control measures such as the use of fluoride-containing products, diet counseling and oral hygiene practices are to be preferred.

3.2.4. Silver Diamine Fluoride Agent

In Japan, in the early seventies, a new product for carious lesion management was developed. Called silver diamine fluoride (SDF), this is a combination of silver nitrate and sodium fluoride - $Ag(NH_3)_2F$. It has been suggested that SDF applied to carious lesions inhibits carious lesion progression by its interaction with bacteria. An additional interaction with tooth structures also occurs (Rosenblatt et al, 2009).

However, very few studies assessing the effect of SDF as a caries control agent have been conducted. Braga et al (2008) investigated the effect of SDF in arresting enamel carious lesions in pits and fissures of permanent molars up to 30 months. The results were no different from those achieved by plaque control through tooth brushing and the use of glass-ionomer sealant; two approaches that are largely used for enamel carious lesion management.

Because of the absence of evidence, it is not recommend to use SDF as a caries control agent in socially disadvantaged communities. Its use in cavitated dentine lesions will be discussed later.

3.2.5. Casein Phosphopeptide-Amophfous Calcium Phosphate

A series of investigations conducted at the University of Melbourne in the 80's showed that the casein phosphopeptides (CPP), the casein protein found in milk, contain a sequence of amino acids that have an impressive ability to stabilize calcium and phosphate and keep them in a soluble amorphous state (Reynolds, 1998). The combination of calcium and phosphate usually results in insoluble crystals. However, in CPP both calcium and phosphate remain in an ionic form that can diffuse into demineralized enamel structure, explaining the CPP-ACP nanocomplex preventive- effect.

The CPP-ACP based products are marketed in two different forms: a chewing gum and as a prophylactic dental paste with and without fluoride incorporation. Its effectiveness is still being investigated but, results from in-situ and in-vivo studies tend to indicate that CPP-ACP has a short-term remineralization effect and a promising caries control effect for long-term clinical use (Yengopal and Mickenautsch, 2009). It has been suggested that products with associated CPP-ACP and fluoride may be superior to fluoride-alone products in lowering the caries risk of people (Reynolds et al, 2008).

CPP-ACP can be considered a very promising carious lesion control agent. It is self-applied, no side effects have been reported and the results from in-vitro and in-situ studies indicate a substantial caries-inhibiting effect. Unfortunately, the number of in-vivo studies are low.

What about the costs and availability of products containing CPP-ACP, in disadvantaged communities? At present, there is a lack of information about the cost-effectiveness of CPP ACP. Furthermore, its use as the basis of a caries control program in a large sample (public oral health) has not been tested. Until more relevant information is available, basing preventive oral health schemes in socially disadvantaged communities on the use of CPP-ACP would not be wise. Fluoride-containing products, particularly fluoride toothpaste, should be the preferable carious lesion control agent.

3.2.6. Ozone

The relationship between microorganisms and dental carious lesion development has been discussed earlier in this chapter. Attempts have been made to control initiation and progression of carious lesions by means of antimicrobial agents. It was concluded that the use of chlorhexidine in disadvantaged communities should not be recommended. The search for appropriate new products is ongoing. Recently, ozone gas was proposed as an antimicrobial agent that could be used in managing the process of carious lesion development.

Ozone, the tri-atomic state of di-oxigen, is naturally produced in the presence of light or by different industrial processes. In dentistry, ozone is claimed to have a sterilizing effect, killing cariogenic bacteria and subsequently leading to carious lesion arrestment (Brazzelli et al, 2006). Three systematic reviews about the topic have been produced and the conclusions are presented below.

More than 40 papers and abstracts until 2003 were identified by the Cochrane collaboration review but owing to the high risk of bias, only 3 studies were included in the analyses. The conclusion was that there was no reliable evidence that the application of ozone gas to the surface of cavitated teeth stops or reverses carious lesions (Rickard et al, 2004). In 2006, not only the effectiveness of HealOzone® (Kavo Inc.), the most used ozone delivery system in dentistry, was assessed but also its cost-effectiveness (Brazzelli et al, 2006). According to the authors, HealOzone® is not a cost-effective addition to treatments that are already available for carious lesion management. The latest published systematic review endorsed what had already been shown by the two previous ones. In vitro studies suggest that ozone has a good potential to be used in dentistry but in vivo trials were not able to confirm the laboratory results (Azarpazhooh and Limeback, 2008).

As the effectiveness of Ozone is still being investigated, its use in oral health is not recommended for disadvantaged communities, or for the general population.

3.2.7. Pits and Fissure Sealants

It is common knowledge that in permanent dentitions, carious lesion development manifests itself first in pits and fissures of first molars (Carvalho et al, 1989). This site is particularly vulnerable to carious lesion development during, and just after, tooth eruption (Carvalho et al., 1989; Powell, 1998). The morphology of pits and fissures has been reported to be one of the main caries risk factors (Disney et al., 1992), with molars being more frequently affected than premolars (Feigal, 2002). Modifying the morphology of patent pits and fissures into a smooth, easy to clean, surface is therefore a logical measure for preventing carious lesion development. This is achieved by sealing these carious lesion-susceptible pits and fissures. Not only is use of a sealant effective as a carious lesion preventive measure, it is also effective in curing non-cavitated enamel carious lesions in pits and fissures, according to the outcome of a systematic review (Griffin et al, 2008).

Obviously the first line of action is prevention of carious lesion development in erupting pits and fissures. This can be achieved by using a toothbrush and fluoride toothpaste to remove or disturb the biofilm, (Carvalho et al, 1992). In doing so, parents, caretakers and/or children will be in charge of their own caries control action (see Chapter 2). Application of a glass-ionomer sealant has also been shown to control carious lesion development in erupting teeth over a period of 5 years (Tayfour et al, 2003).

The remainder of this section covers both prevention and treatment of visible enamel carious lesions through the placement of a sealant, in management of the caries process in pits and fissures.

3.2.7.1. Resin-Based and Polyalkenoic-Based Sealant Materials

Basically two families of dental materials are used to seal pits and fissures: resin composites and glass-ionomer cements. It is generally accepted that resin composite sealants are retained longer than glass-ionomer sealants (Simonsen, 2002; Locker et al, 2003). This may largely be due to a focus on the low-viscosity type of glass-ionomer, developed decades ago to flow as easily into pits and fissures as resin-based sealant material does. The outcome was obvious: in most cases, within a short time, the low-viscosity glass-ionomer had almost completely disappeared from the pits and fissures. This seemingly inferior result prompted dental practitioners to opt for resin-based sealant materials.

However, which of the two types of sealant is more able to prevent carious lesion development is less clear. Two systematic reviews comparing the carious lesion preventive effect of resin composite and low- and medium-viscosity glass-ionomer sealants were, however, unable to provide evidence that either of these materials was superior to the other (Beiruti et al, 2006b; Yengopal et al, 2009). This finding is in line with the conclusion of a critical review by Simonson (1996), who concluded that 'the caries preventive effect between resin composite and glass-ionomer sealants is equivocal'.

3.2.7.2. ART Sealants

Many dental practitioners have been taught that resin-based material should be used as the sealant material of choice. These dental practitioners may find themselves in an ethical dilemma, working in a field situation where a resin-based material cannot be used because there is no electricity. A cordless handpiece and burs may provide a solution if electricity for recharging batteries is available at their base. However, as current evidence shows that low- and medium-viscosity glass-ionomer sealants are as good as resin-based sealants in managing carious lesion development in pits and fissures, the use of glass-ionomer material is a real option and, therefore, deserves further discussion.

Glass-ionomers, in hand mixed powder-liquid form, do not require electricity or running water for use as sealants and in restoration. This feature is an important aspect of the caries management concept called Atraumatic Restorative Treatment (ART). This concept was developed in Tanzania in the mid-eighties, initially to provide preventive and restorative care to disadvantaged communities worldwide (Frencken et al, 1996). However, ART is currently also being practised in high-income countries such as the USA (Seale and Casamassimo, 2003), UK (Burke et al, 2005) and Netherlands (Bulut and Sharif, 2004). ART is characterized by the fact that only hand instruments in combination with adhesive dental materials are being used to produce sealants and restorations. Electricity and running water are not required. Therefore, managing carious lesion development through sealing caries-prone pits and fissures and restoring cavities with minimum openings of 1 mm or more can be performed outside the dental clinics, in schools, homes or the open fields. Use of the ART approach for managing dental carious lesion development can increase access to basic care for many population groups currently deprived of such care in low- and middle-income countries.

Initially, ART used medium-viscosity glass-ionomers as sealant materials but high-viscosity glass-ionomers succeeded these in the mid-nineties. A 9-month study demonstrated that the retention rates of high-viscosity glass-ionomer sealants, applied using the press-finger technique (ART sealants), was higher than those of low-viscosity glass ionomer sealants, applied without finger pressure (Weerheijm et al, 1996). Table 3.2 shows the step-by-step process of placing an ART sealant. More recently, a few longer-term studies have been published, reporting on the retention and caries preventive effect of ART sealants. Using the weighted mean to reflect the number of sealants of the individual studies until June 2005 in the final outcome, a meta-analysis was carried out to assess the survival of ART sealants, (van 't Hof et al, 2006). The analysis showed a weighted mean survival rate of fully and partially retained high-viscosity glass-ionomer ART sealants after 1, 2 and 3 years, of 90%, 82% and 72%, respectively (van't Hof et al, 2006). These relatively high retention rates resulted in a weighted mean annual failure rate (completely lost high-viscosity glass-ionomer ART sealants) in permanent teeth of 9.3% over the first 3 years. The carious lesion preventive effect of high-viscosity glass-ionomer ART sealants appears to be very high. The weighted mean annual caries incidence rate in previously sealed pits and fissures was 1% over the first 3 years (van't Hof et al, 2006).

**Table 3.2. Step-by-step description of the process of placing an ART sealant
(Frencken and Wolke, 2010)**

1.	Isolate the tooth with cotton wool rolls. Keep the treatment area free from saliva.
2.	Gently remove plaque and food debris from the deepest parts of the pits and fissures with an explorer.
3.	Wash the pits and fissures, using wet cotton wool pellets.
4.	Apply enamel conditioner to the pits and fissures according to the manufacturer's instruction. Condition for the specified time.
5.	Immediately wash the pits and fissures, using wet cotton wool pellets to clean off the conditioner. Wash 2-3 times.
6.	Dry the pits and fissures with cotton wool pellets. Do not use the 3-way syringe. The enamel surface should not be completely dry.
7.	Mix the glass-ionomer and apply it in all pits and fissures with the round end of the ART applier/carver instrument or shake the encapsulated glass-ionomer in a suitable mixing machine and extrude the mixture into all pits and fissures.
8.	Rub a small amount of petroleum jelly onto the gloved index finger.
9.	Press the glass-ionomer mixture into the pits and fissures with the index finger (press-finger technique). Then, remove the finger sideways after 10 -15 seconds.
10.	Remove visible excess of the mixture with the carver or a large excavator.
11.	Check the bite using the articulation paper and adjust until comfortable.
12.	Remove the petroleum jelly top surface with the carver or a large excavator when the mixture is partly set.
13.	Apply a new layer of petroleum jelly.
14.	Remove the cotton wool rolls.
15.	Ask the patient not to eat for at least one hour.

3.2.7.3. ART Sealants and Resin Composite Sealants over Time

Toward the end of 2009, the only comparative study covering ART and resin composite sealants was carried out amongst children with a mean age of 7.8 years with a low- to medium caries risk profile (Beiruti et al, 2006a). No resealing was performed, as one of the aims of the study was to mimic the real situation present in many disadvantaged communities with little or no access to dental care. It was assumed that if organised school oral health services were to start in these communities, considering the number of children needing care and the low number of dental personnel available to provide it, the long-term effect of a one-time application of sealants should be assessed. The authors found that the carious lesion preventive effect of high-viscosity glass-ionomer ART sealants was between 3.1 and 4.5 times higher than that of resin composite sealants after 3 to 5 years. This information is important, as the logical choice for the dental operator would be to use the sealant that has showed the longest carious lesion preventive effect. Another result was that about 60% of sealants of both materials had completely disappeared after 3 years.

What could be the reason for the carious lesion preventive action of glass-ionomer sealants after the material had disappeared? Torppa-Saarinen and Seppå (1990) investigated the pits and fissures of low-viscosity glass-ionomer-sealed occlusal surfaces of second molars and premolars that had been clinically scored as having partial or total loss of sealant under stereomicroscope and SEM after 4 months. In most cases, glass-ionomer material was still present in the bottom of the fissures. The authors assumed that this finding was part of the reason why glass-ionomer sealants have prevented carious lesion development even after they appear to be lost. This assumption is in agreement with the conclusion reached in studies conducted by other researchers (Mejàre and Mjör, 1990; Övrebö and Raadal, 1990; Williams et al, 1996).

Further evidence, from a case study that describes the fate of 2 high-viscosity glass-ionomer ART sealants after 12 and 13 years, has been presented by Frencken and Wolke (2010). The clinical situation of these sealants at baseline and in subsequent years is presented in Figure 3.2. Figure 3.3 shows colour and SEM photographs of fully sealed pits and fissures and of pits and fissures whose sealant material after 12 years was clinically diagnosed as having disappeared (B1 and D3) although on the SEM photographs it was clearly present. Note the tight adhesion of the glass-ionomer to enamel (C2). This clinical case shows that remnants, most likely of high-viscosity glass-ionomer sealant material, are retained in the deeper parts of pits and fissures that appear clinically to be free of sealant material (D3). This material appears, therefore, able to exercise its carious lesion preventive effect over a long period.

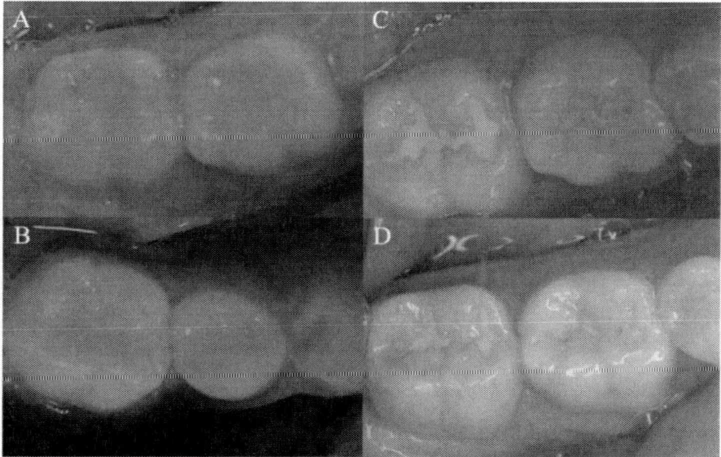

Figure 3.2. ART high-viscosity glass-ionomer (FUJI IX) sealant in teeth 4.6 and 4.7 over time. A) sealant in tooth 4.6 at start; B) sealant tooth 46 after 1 year and in tooth 47 soon after placement; C) sealant in tooth 4.6 after 5 years and in tooth 47 after 4 years; D) sealant in tooth 46 after 13 years and in tooth 47 after 12 years.

These remnants are probably present because glass-ionomer fractures cohesively, in contrast to resin-based materials, which tend to fracture adhesively (Papacchini et al, 2005). A cohesive fracture indicates a strong bond of the material to enamel. As a result, the deeper parts of the pits and fissures remain covered with glass-ionomer material to various degrees. An adhesive fracture would re-expose the pits and fissures to the oral environment; a situation that should be avoided when prevention of carious lesion development is the goal.

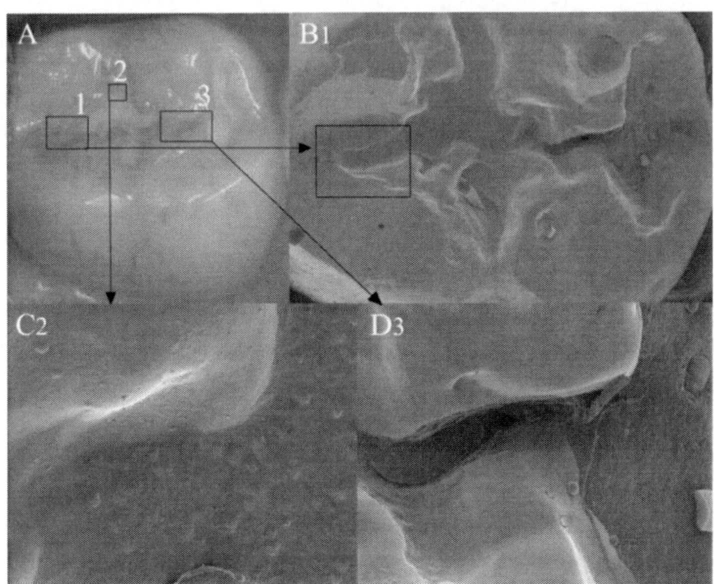

Figure 3.3. A) High-viscosity glass-ionomer (Fuji IX) sealant in tooth 47 after 12 years. The distal fissure appears to be clinically free of glass-ionomer material. B1) On the SEM image (12x), glass-ionomer material is clearly visible till the end of the distal fissure. C2) Good adhesion of high-viscosity glass-ionomer to enamel (SEM: 100x). D3) Glass-ionomer material present in the fissure connecting the central with the mesial pit (SEM: 100x). The glass-ionomer sealant was clinically not visible in the fissure.

In conclusion, the outcome of the systematic reviews by Beiruti et al, (2006b) and Yengopal et al, (2009), and that of the sealant comparative study referred to above (Beiruti et al, (2006a), indicate that glass-ionomers, particularly high-viscosity glass-ionomer, should be the material of choice for sealing caries-susceptible pits and fissures in field situations in disadvantaged communities. Obviously, dental practitioners should be well trained in handling and understanding the chemistry of glass-ionomer and in placing the sealants according to protocol. In general, high-viscosity glass-ionomer ART sealants are indicated for use alongside light-cured resin composite sealants when used in a dental practice setting. The fact that sealants are indicated means that the dentition is at risk of developing carious lesions. This calls for oral health information and in particular, for proper plaque control measures in conjunction with the placement of sealants.

3.2.7.4. Conclusion: Caries Control Agents

Considering the evidence regarding the appropriateness, effectiveness and availability of carious lesion control measures for use in disadvantaged communities, it can be concluded that sealants, particularly high-viscosity glass-ionomer ART sealants, are suitable in caries high-risk individuals, as they have a high preventive effect and can be placed without using expensive and complicated dental equipment, both by dentists and by dental therapists. For daily management of carious lesions, fluoride toothpaste and a toothbrush is the most suitable combination. Individuals at caries risk will further benefit from reduced sugar intake and other fluoride vehicles that are available. Thus, the first step in a program aimed at improving oral health in disadvantaged communities, should be to ensure the availability of toothbrushes and affordable fluoride toothpaste, as well as quality high-viscosity glass-ionomers. These recommendations complement those on oral health promotion presented in Chapter 2.

Table 3.3. Summary of caries control measures and their usefulness in socially disadvantaged communities

FLUORIDE AGENTS	
	Discussion
Water Fluoridation	Evidence showing its beneficial effect on delaying carious lesion progression. Can be a good caries control measure in communities where piped water is available and expertise/technology for its implementation exists
Milk Fluoridation	Insufficient evidence to show its effectiveness. However, it has potential to be used in school preventive-based programs.
Salt Fluoridation	Absence of evidence of its effectiveness and it seems to present technical problems in its implementation. Not recommended.
Toothpaste	Considered the main factor related to the decline of caries prevalence and incidence in high-income countries. It is the preferred vehicle for fluoride administration worldwide. However, the issue of affordability in disadvantaged communities should be addressed
Mouthrinse	Evidence showing that supervised use of fluoride mouthwashes is effective for caries reduction in children.
Varnish*	Evidence of being effective when applied professionally 2 to 4 times a year. Recommended as a last line of action.
Gel*	Evidence of fluoride gel caries inhibiting effect in children when applied few times a year. Recommended as a last line of action
*Professionally applied. Recommended for populations at caries high-risk	
NON-FLUORIDE AGENTS	
Sugar substitutes	Dietary counseling is strongly recommended for high caries risk groups and those who are not exposed to fluoride. The use of sugar-free chewing-gum can be introduced as part of caries control programs for school children. Restrict sugar intake in children to 5 times/day
Chlorhexidine	Lack of evidence. The varnish may have a carious lesion control effect in high caries risk individuals. Not recommended.
Silver Diamine Fluoride	Lack of evidence. Not recommended
Casein phosphopeptide-amorphous calcium phosphate	Good evidence derived from in vitro and in-situ studies but requires more clinical trials to prove its effectiveness. Product might not be accessible in many socially disadvantaged communities. Is more expensive than fluoride toothpaste. Not recommended yet
Ozone	Lack of evidence regarding its effectiveness. Not recommended
Sealants	Very suitable, particularly high-viscosity glass-ionomer ART sealants. Quality glass-ionomers are not always available

3.3. Management of Cavitated
Dentine Carious Lesion

3.3.1. Introduction

As explained earlier in this chapter, epidemiological studies have revealed that most cavitated dentine carious lesions in people living in disadvantaged communities are left unrestored. Reasons for this situation were also presented. Most of these communities have poor access to oral healthcare facilities and most of the oral health facilities lack equipment or are ill-equipped. Furthermore, they lack regular and proper maintenance required in providing restorative care. If such a situation exists for years, people in such communities get used to extraction as the only remedy for alleviating pain derived from a cavitated tooth. Waiting for the construction of dental facilities equipped with well-functioning dental units is no option for improving the situation. It is expensive and often heads of oral health departments have earmarked funds for improving dental facilities in their annual government budget, only to find that their superiors have used those funds for other, more pressing, purposes.

The health burden from cavitated dentine lesions, with or without dental pain, in communities in middle- and low-income countries should not be ignored (Kikwilu et al, 2008). How might such teeth be treated using available resources? The following section discusses various treatment options available to the dental practitioner for treating cavitated dentine lesions in general and their suitability for use, particularly in disadvantaged communities.

3.3.2. Treatment Options

Considering the current delivery of oral health services in many middle- and low income countries, pain relief through extraction of the badly cavitated tooth is a well-proven treatment which is available in many disadvantaged communities in these countries. This manner of providing palliative care is an essential option and should be a corner stone in basic oral healthcare packages (Frencken et al, 2002). Treating toothache merely by advocating caries control measures and oral health promotion actions, as suggested by Varenne et al, (2004), ignores the people in pain. However, the pain from reversible pulpitis can also be alleviated through restoration of the cavitated tooth. Table 3.4 presents an overview of the common options available for treating cavitated teeth.

Conventional, air- and sono abrasion, laser and ozone treatments rely heavily on special equipment, which must be maintained and requires electricity and running water. In general, they are an expensive, inappropriate management for cavitated teeth in many socially disadvantaged communities. Technical innovations, such as rechargeable hand-pieces, may make conventional restorative care possible in certain communities. The chemomechanical caries removal gel and the use of stepwise excavation treatment are useful, in principle, but have no additional benefit over cavity excavation using hand instruments only (ART) (Nadanovski et al, 2001; Topaloglu-Ak et al, 2009). Therefore, their application will not be discussed further. This leaves the Hall, ART, Silver Diamine Fluoride (SDF) and the ultra-conservative therapy of cavity cleaning with fluoride toothpaste as potentially suitable approaches for managing teeth with obvious cavities, in socially disadvantaged communities. These therapies are discussed in the following sections.

Table 3.4. Management options for treating cavitated teeth in disadvantaged communities

Management options	Discussion
Conventional	Requires electrically-driven equipment and rotary instruments. Electricity and running water are not always available, nor is maintenance care. Purchasing cost is high. Using a rechargeable hand piece would be an option in certain communities
Air- and sonoabrasion	Requires electrically-driven equipment and rotary instruments. Electricity and running water are not always available, nor is maintenance care. Purchasing cost is very high. Not recommended
Lazer therapy	As above, not recommended.
Ozone therapy	As above. No evidence that it is effective. Ozone should not be considered an alternative to current treatment methods in dental practices. Not recommended
Chemo-mechanical carious tissue removal	Uses hand instruments and a gel. In principle useful. Product is difficult to get and expensive. No evidence that the use of the chemo-mechanical gel provides an added benefit to the carious lesion removal by hand instruments only. Therefore, treatment becomes significantly more costly. Not recommended
Stepwise excavation of carious tissues	Sometimes rotary instruments are needed. In principle useful, but there is a great risk that people will not return for a second appointment. Has been made less useful in recent years by the success of one-time conventional excavation of carious lesions, using hand instruments only
Hall technique	Uses prefabricated metal crowns cemented over unprepared cavitated primary molars without removing carious tissues or needing local anesthesia. Initial short-term results are promising. May become useful
Atraumatic Restorative Treatment (ART)	Uses hand instruments only, in conjunction with an adhesive restorative material. No electricity and running water is needed. Can be applied anywhere; in the dental clinic and in outreach situations without the use of local anesthesia. Has proven effective in single-surface cavities in primary and permanent teeth. Is no different from comparable amalgam restorations in single-surface cavities in permanent and primary teeth. More cost-effective than comparable amalgam restorations Recommended
Application of 38% silver diamine fluoride (SDF)	Uncomplicated application method for arresting active cavitated lesions, primarily in deciduous teeth. Evidence of its effectiveness is low. Not recommended
Cleaning accessible tooth cavities with a toothbrush and fluoride toothpaste	This is a feasible option, particularly for use in primary teeth if no treatment other than plaque control through tooth brushing with fluoride toothpaste is available. Should be carefully encouraged

3.3.3. Treatment of Small Dentine Carious Lesions

The systematic review by Griffin et al, (2008) concluded that sealing in enamel carious lesions is effective in stopping carious lesion progression. This conclusion is supported by the systematic review of Oong et al, (2008), who concluded that sealants reduced the number of bacteria in carious lesions in most of the included studies. As discussed in 3.2.7, application of a sealant is an effective way of preventing dentine lesion development in pits and fissures. What about using a sealant as a therapeutic measure by placing it over a small, cavitated dentine lesion in pits and fissures? This is a legitimate question, considering the nearly total absence of rotary dental equipment in many communities in middle- and low-income countries. Would a sealant, most probably of glass-ionomer material, be able to prevent dentine carious lesions in pits and fissures from progressing further?

Evidence was produced by a clinical trial in which medium-sized cavities in occlusal surfaces were treated with a sealant-restoration, without removal of soft infected dentine. The study showed a success rate of 86% after 10 years (Mertz-Fairhurst et al, 1998). Since then, discussions have been held in the literature and in congresses about the need to remove all infected dentine from tooth cavities in order to stop carious lesion progression. The slogan 'The Seal is the Deal' was born (Van Amerongen et al, 2008). Would this slogan be applicable for treating small dentine carious lesions in pits and fissures without using instruments for the enamel and dentine? A few studies related to this issue have been published.

In the late seventies, Mertz-Fairhurst et al, (1979a,b) showed that sealing over small dentine lesions in pits and fissures stopped carious lesion progression. She based this finding on the assessment of lesion depth and bacterial counts, and on radiographic and clinical examination. Years later, small dentine lesions (<0.9mm orifice) in youngsters with an average age of 14 years were sealed with medium-viscosity glass-ionomer ART sealants. After 3 years these sealants had prevented dentine lesion progression in 87.4% of the cases in this low-caries risk group, which was a significantly higher percentage than for small dentine lesions that were left untreated (RR=0.30; CL= 0.12-0.72) (Frencken et al, 1998). In a medium caries risk group of 7-year-olds, dentine lesion progression was halted in 68.2% of small dentine lesions that were sealed over with resin composite and high-viscosity glass-ionomers after 5 years (Beiruti et al, 2006a).

Although not so common in clinics with fully functional dental equipment, sealing over small dentine lesions seems to be a realistic therapy for reducing the progression of dentine carious lesions and should, therefore, be considered in situations where restorative therapy is not possible.

3.3.4. Restorative Therapies for Obvious Tooth Cavities

3.3.4.1. Hall Technique

The Hall technique is a relatively novel treatment developed for managing small to moderate carious lesions in primary molar teeth. Carious tissue is not removed and a preformed metal crown is cemented into place without tooth preparation, and without the use of local anesthesia. The protocol for the provision of the Hall Technique Preformed Metal Crowns (Hall PMC) includes the following major steps (Innes et al, 2006).

- Select the size of PMC that covers all cusps and that gives a feeling of 'spring-back' when placed up to, but not through, the contact points.
- After removing only debris from the tooth cavity, the latter is rinsed and dried.

- The dried PMC is filled with glass-ionomer luting cement and placed evenly over the tooth.
- The child is instructed to bite down firmly until the crown is pushed down over the tooth. Separating the cavitated tooth, using orthodontic separators, two to three days before the appointment, is sometimes required.
- Excess of glass-ionomer is then removed and after-treatment, instruction is provided.

The placement of the Hall PMC results in an open bite of up to 2.5mm, which seems to disappear within weeks (Innes et al, 2007). The majority of dentists, children and their parents in the study area in Scotland preferred the Hall PMC to the conventional restorative treatment (Innes et al, 2007). As this treatment is rather new, the level of evidence is low. However, considering the few instruments and materials required to produce the Hall PMC and the absence of the need for special and expensive equipment, it may become very suitable for use in communities in middle- and low-income countries. An illustrated manual on the Hall Technique, with practical advice on providing Hall PMCs is available for free downloading (Innes et al 2009). An example of a Hall PMC restoration over time is presented in figure 3.4.

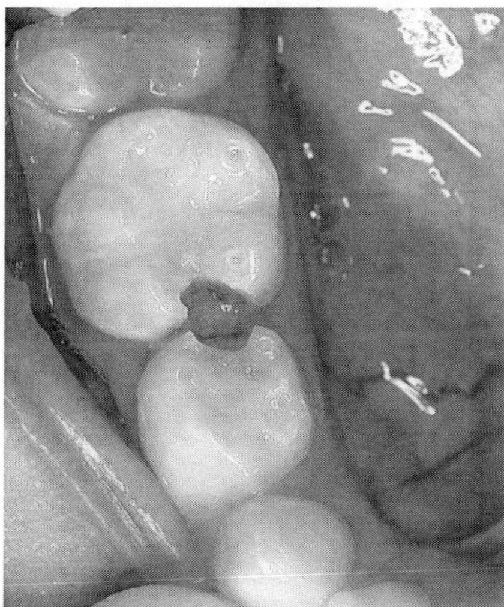

(a) Cavitated lesion in 1st and 2nd primary molar

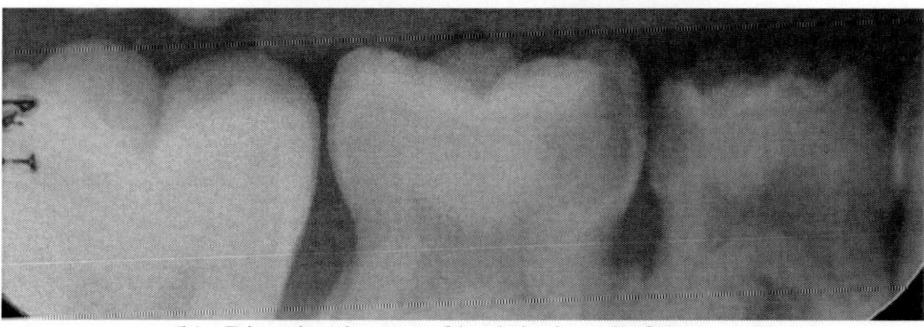

(b) Bitewing image of both lesions before treatment

Figure 3.4. (Continued).

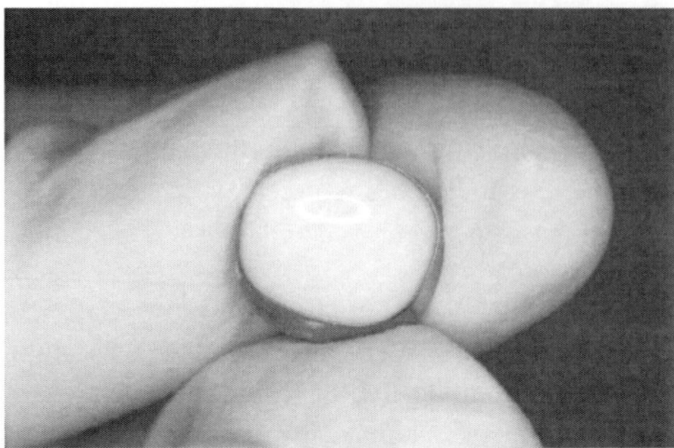

A preformed metal crown filled with glass-ionomer cement prior to placing it over a 2nd primary molar

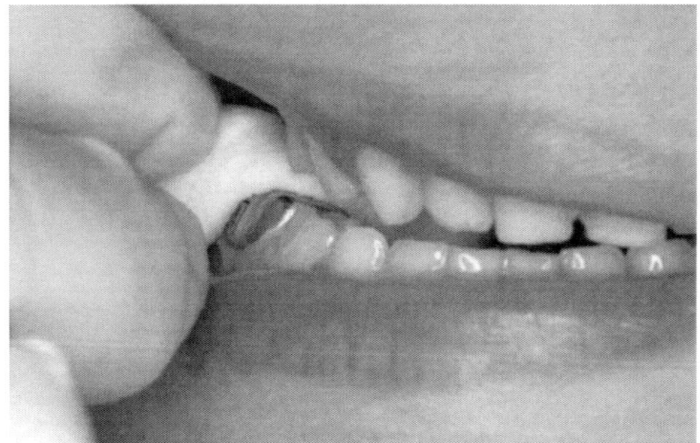

Preformed metal crown bitten into place

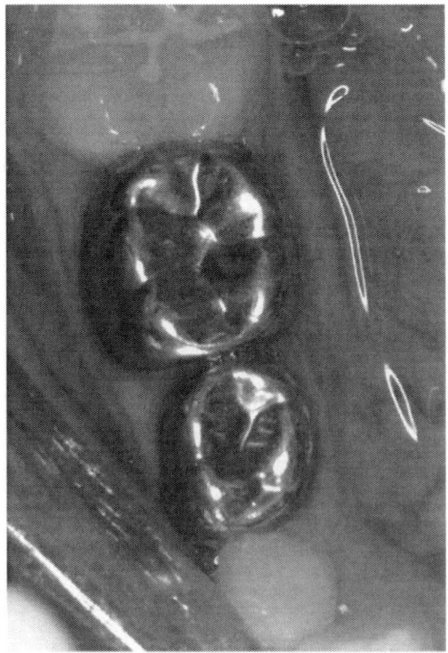

The two preformed metal crowns after 2.5 years (same patient as shown in a and b)

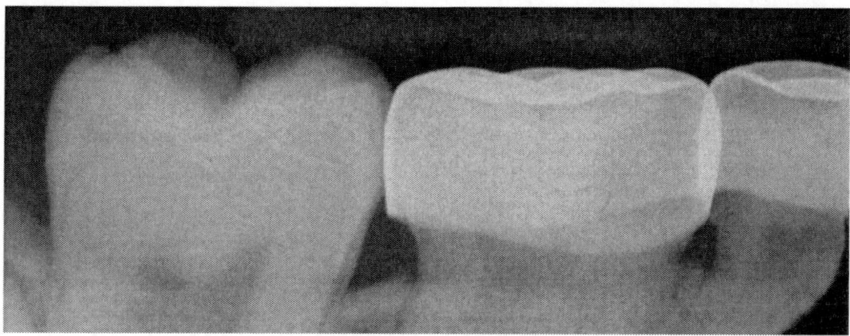

Figure 3.4. Hall technique. A) cavitated lesion in 1st and 2nd primary molar; b) bitewing image of both lesions before treatment; c) a preformed metal crown filled with glass-ionomer cement prior to placing it over a 2nd primary molar; d) preformed metal crown bitten into place; e) the two preformed metal crowns after 2.5 years (same patient as shown in a and b); f) bitewing image after 2.5 years.

3.3.4.2. Atraumatic Restorative Treatment (ART) Approach

ART is a minimally invasive approach that can be used both to prevent carious lesion formation and to stop its further progression. It consists of two components: sealing of caries-prone pits and fissures (ART sealants) and restoration of cavitated dentin lesions with sealant-restorations (ART restoration) (Frencken and Holmgren, 1999). The process involved in placing an ART sealant has been presented in Table 3.2. An ART restoration involves the removal of soft, completely demineralised carious tooth tissue with hand instruments. This is followed by restoration of the cavity with an adhesive dental material that simultaneously seals any remaining pits and fissures that remain at risk. A local anaesthetic is rarely needed. The protocol for producing ART restorations is presented in Table 3.5.

ART was initially developed in Tanzania in the mid-eighties, in response to the need to find a method of preserving decayed teeth in people of all ages, both in developing countries and in disadvantaged communities.

Many researchers from many countries have investigated different aspects of ART. Salient findings from these studies can be summarised as follows (Frencken, 2010):

- Survival rates of single-surface ART restorations using high-viscosity glass-ionomers in primary and permanent posterior teeth are high and meet the specifications of the American Dental Association (ADA) for quality restorations (van 't Hof et al, 2006);
- Survival rates of multiple-surface ART restorations using high-viscosity glass-ionomers in primary posterior teeth do not meet the ADA specifications (van 't Hof et al, 2006);
- Survival rates of single-surface ART restorations in permanent posterior teeth, using high-viscosity glass-ionomers, do not differ significantly from comparable traditional restorations using amalgam (Frencken et al, 2004; Mickenautsch et al, 2010);
- Survival rates of single-and multiple-surface ART restorations, using high-viscosity glass-ionomers, in primary posterior teeth do not differ significantly from comparable traditional restorations using composite (Eden et al, 2006; Ersin et al, 2006) and compomer (Louw et al, 2002);

- Pain felt during treatment was lower in child populations treated restoratively with ART using high-viscosity glass-ionomers, than when traditional restorative procedures were used (Rahimtoola et al, 2000; Honkala et al 2003; Schriks et al, 2003; Abreu et al, 2009). Even ART without local anaesthesia was better accepted than traditional treatment with local anaesthesia (van Bochoven et al, 2006).
- Studies developed to measure dental anxiety contained methodological errors that made it impossible to confirm the hypothesis that ART is less dental anxiety provoking than conventional treatments (Leal et al, 2009).
- Initial wear rates of ART restorations using high-viscosity glass-ionomers are low (Ho et al, 1999; Lo et al, 2001).
- ART restorations using high-viscosity glass-ionomers were more cost-effective after 2 years than comparable amalgam restorations (PAHO, 2006).

These outcomes show that the ART approach using high-viscosity glass-ionomers produces quality restorations in single-surface cavities in primary and permanent posterior teeth, which are the cavities most prevalent in most countries. The ART approach saves teeth that otherwise would have to be extracted and prevents carious lesion development. Examples of how to produce ART restorations are presented in Figures 3.5a-f and on ART restoration over time, in Figures 3.6a-d.

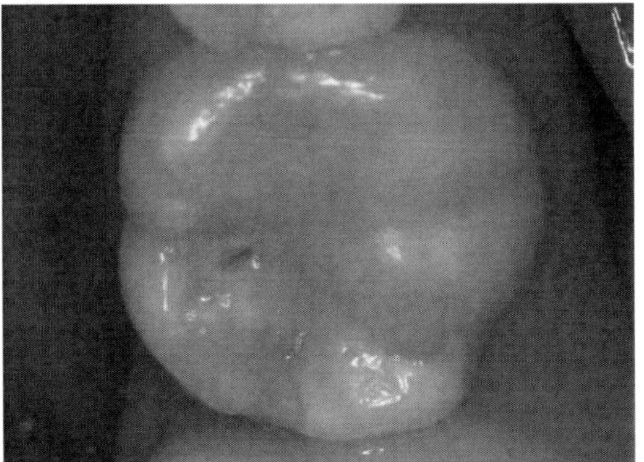

Cavitated dentine lesion in a second primary molar

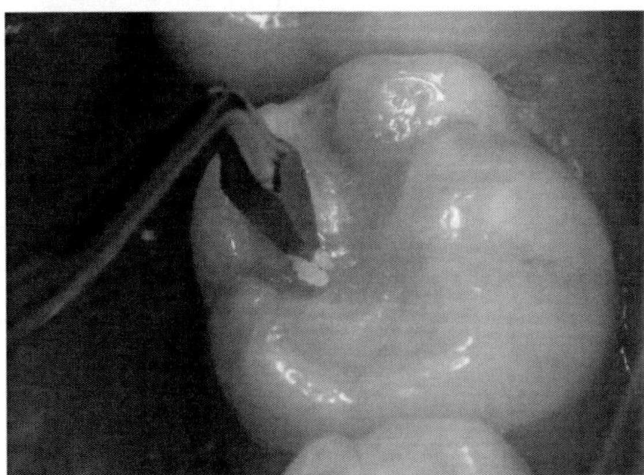

Gaining access to the cavitated dentine lesion using the ART enamel access cutter (EAC)

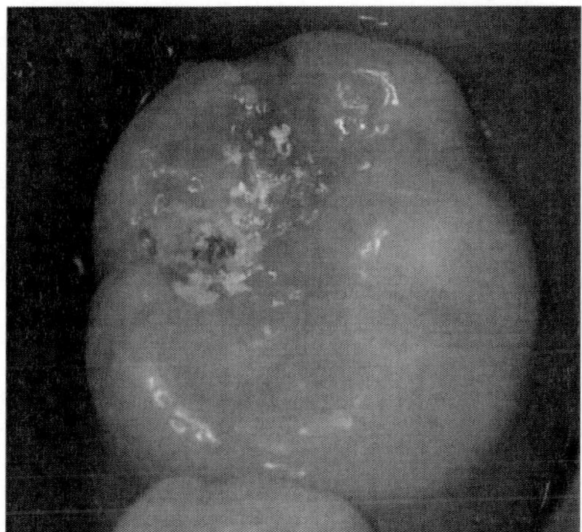

Crumbled enamel after use of EAC

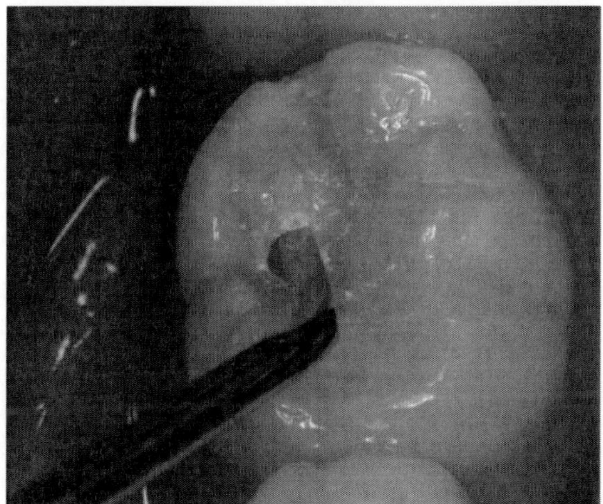

Entrance is widened with a hatchet to allow a small-size excavator to enter the cavity

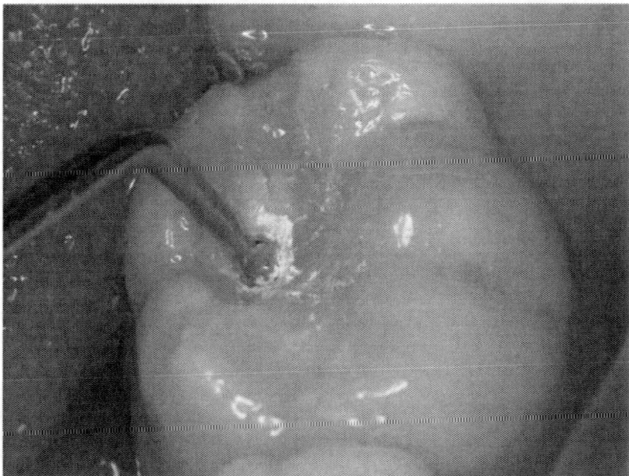

A small-size excavator is used to remove infected dentine with scooping movements

Figure 3.5. (Continued).

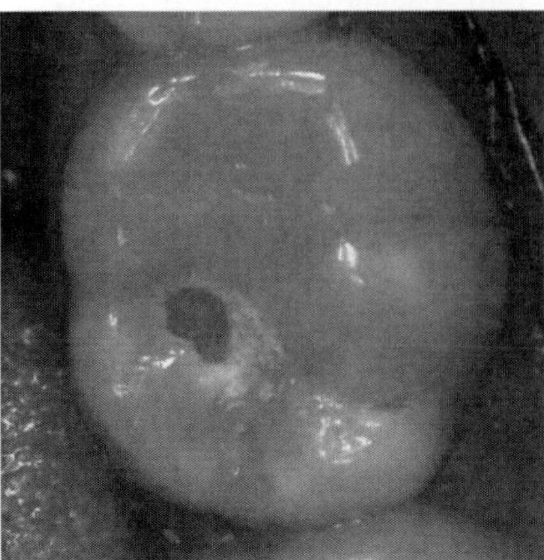

Cavity is clean and ready to be conditioned and then filled with a high-viscosity glass-ionomer

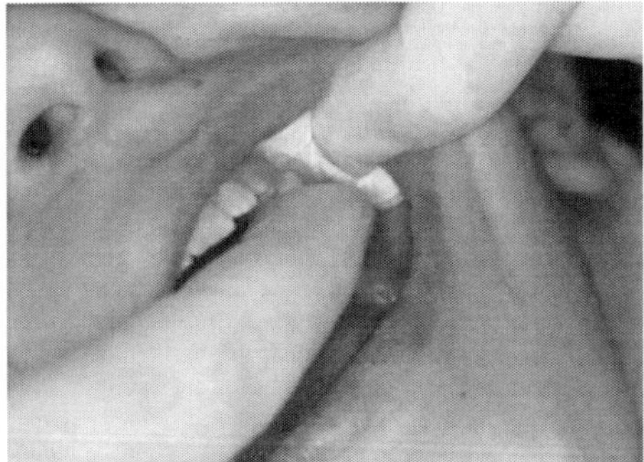

Coat index finger with petroleum jelly and then press firmly (press-finger technique) over glass-ionomer

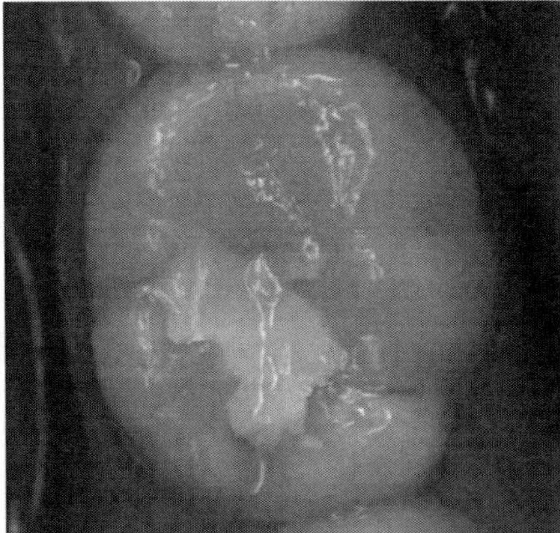

Completed ART restoration, the cavity is filled and pits and fissures are sealed in one restoration

Figure 3.5. The placement of an ART restoration step-by-step. a) Cavitated dentine lesion in a second primary molar; b) Gaining access to the cavitated dentine lesion using the ART enamel access cutter (EAC); c) crumbled enamel after use of EAC; d) Entrance is widened with a hatchet to allow a small-size excavator to enter the cavity; e) a small-size excavator is used to remove infected dentine with scooping movements; f) cavity is clean and ready to be conditioned and then filled with a high-viscosity glass-ionomer; g) coat index finger with petroleum jelly and then press firmly (press-finger technique) over glass-ionomer; h) completed ART restoration, the cavity is filled and pits and fissures are sealed in one restoration.

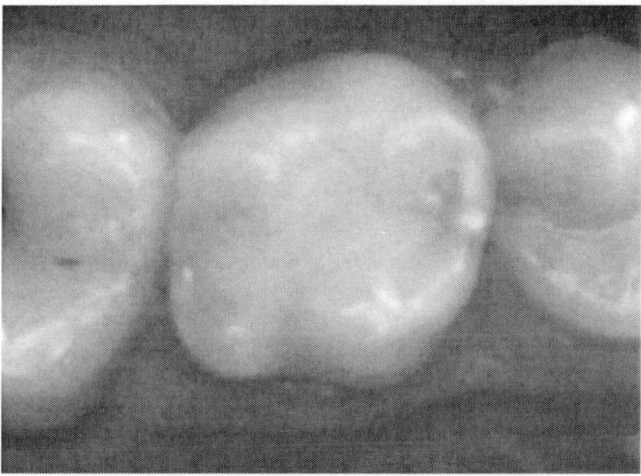

ART restoration in occlusal surface of a primary tooth after 3 years

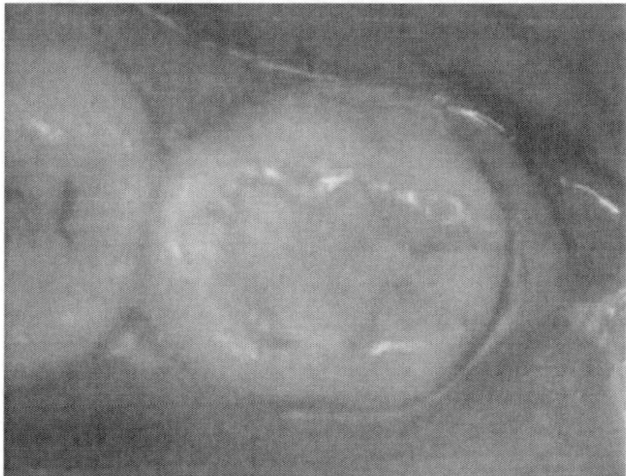

ART restoration in the distal-occlusal surface and a sealant in the pits and fissures of a
primary molar after 4 years

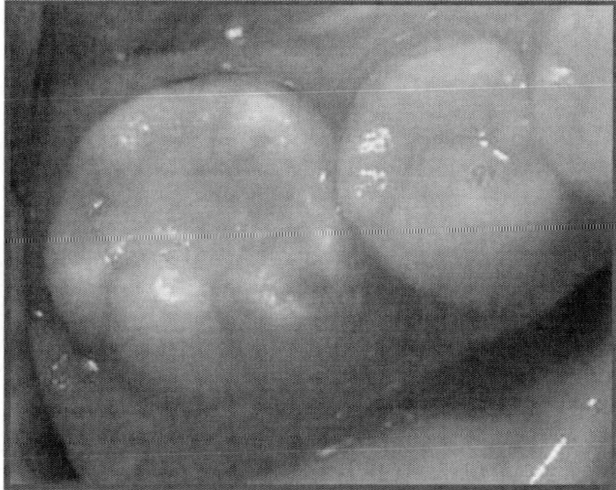

ART restoration in the occlusal surface of a permanent molar after 2 years

Figure 3.6. (Continued).

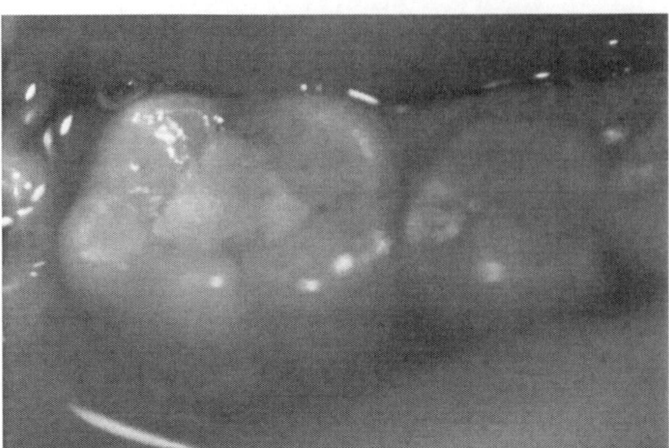

ART restoration in the occlusal surface of a permanent molar after 6.3 years

Figure 3.6. Survival of ART restorations over time. a) in occlusal surface of a primary tooth after 3 years; b) restoration in the distal-occlusal surface and a sealant in the pits and fissures of a primary molar after 4 years; c) in the occlusal surface of a permanent molar after 2 years; d) in the occlusal surface of a permanent molar after 6.3 years.

Table 3.5. Protocol for producing ART restorations

1.	Isolate the tooth with cotton wool rolls. Keep the treatment area free from saliva.
2.	With an explorer, gently remove plaque and food debris from the deepest parts of the available pits and fissures.
3.	Wash the pits and fissures, using wet cotton wool pellets.
4.	Assess the extent of the carious lesion.
5.	Enlarge the entrance of the cavity if it is found to be too small, using an Enamel Access Cutter or dental hatchet.
6.	Break only very thin enamel that might fracture when the restoration is in place, using hatchet.
7.	Remove the carious dentine with hand excavators in a scooping movement, starting at the dentin-enamel junction and ending at the floor of the cavity. Leaving a little infected dentine behind is permitted if it is difficult to remove or if the child becomes impatient.
8.	Clean the cavity with a wet cotton pellet(s) followed by a dry one.
9.	Ensure that the fissures which run into the cavity are free from debris. Remove debris with a sharp probe.
10.	Ensure that the enamel that forms the cavity opening is free from demineralisation (as far as possible).
11.	Place 2 drops of liquid on the mixing pad. The first one, positioned in the corner of the pad, usually contains air bubbles and is, therefore, used, for conditioning. Without releasing pressure, move the bottle to the centre of the pad and place a second drop there. This one should not contain air bubbles and will be used for mixing.
12.	Condition the cavity and adjacent pits and fissures with diluted (15-20%) polyacrylic acid by passing a moist cotton pellet, dipped in the conditioner, around the dentine and enamel in the cavity for some 10 -15 seconds.
13.	Ensure that the pellet touches the cavity walls. This is not always easy in small cavities. Use pellets appropriate to the size of the cavity. A disposable brush can also be used.
14.	Wash with a wet cotton pellet(s) for some 5 seconds. Repeating this is necessary
15.	Dry with cotton pellet(s) (do not use the air syringe). The cavity will look shiny. Keep this situation uncontaminated by saliva and/or blood.
16.	Ensure proper isolation. Perhaps replace cotton rolls.
17	Mix the GIC according to the manufacturer's instructions. Only accept a properly mixed GIC; no runny or dry mixture is acceptable.

18.	Insert the GIC material into the cavity with the applier/carver instrument. Push the GIC into the corner(s) of the cavity (in case of an enamel overhang) with the round end of the medium excavator. Insert a second portion of GIC and press it into place with the round end of the large excavator. Fill the adjacent pits and fissures but DONOT overfill much, as the excess has to be removed.
19.	Rub some petroleum jelly over your index finger (very thin layer), place the finger over the tooth surface and press for 20 seconds.
20.	Remove the visible GIC excess with the carver end of the applier/carver instrument.
21.	Check the occlusion with articulation paper.
22.	Wait until the material has set a bit and then adjust the bite with a medium-sized excavator and/or carver instrument.
23.	Remove petroleum jelly-covered top layer of the GIC with a large excavator and/or carver instrument. Ensure a smooth GIC-onto-enamel junction. Use the round end of the small and/or large excavator to achieve this.
24.	Protect the restoration with a thin layer of petroleum jelly again.
25.	Remove the cotton wool rolls.
26.	Ask the patient not to eat for at least one hour.

3.3.4.2.1. Introducing ART into Public Oral Healthcare Service Systems

Research over two decades has shown the potential of ART sealants and of ART restorations with glass-ionomer cement. Many dental practitioners in many low- and middle-income countries are using ART; for example, between 2002 and the end of 2006, the Dental Department in the Ministry of Health of Mexico trained 810 dentists in ART and caries prevention. This appears to have resulted in a 400 percent increase in ART restorations provided by the public oral health services during this period. However, it was discovered in 2008 that just over 55% of the dentists strictly followed the ART approach. Thus the increase in ART restorations was overestimated (Hermosillo et al, 2009). Evaluation of other aspects of the introduction of the ART approach in the oral health service system in Mexico, such as the quality of ART restorations, is underway.

Introducing a novel treatment concept is rarely a smooth process. At the turn of this century, when it became clear that the ART approach was no ephemeron, (oral) health authorities in a province in South Africa decided to incorporate ART into the provincial public health services, as the level of restorative care had been low for many years. All the 21 dentists in two regions attended a 3-day ART training course, after which they were requested to treat patients restoratively using ART. No further support was provided. The recorded clinical procedures of 11 of the 21 dentists were available from the beginning until 5 years after the ART training (Mickenautsch and Frencken, 2009). Analysis showed that the predominant mode of treating cavitated dentine lesions over the 5-year period remained extraction but positive influences of the ART introduction were noticed. Of the total number of restorations placed in primary teeth, the proportion of ART restorations increased from zero to 81% at year 1 and remained high during the following 4 years (73% at year 5 after training). Of the total number of restorations in permanent teeth, the mean percentage of ART restorations increased significantly from zero to 24% at year 1 and to 43% at year 5 (Figure 3.7). The main factor that hindered proper adoption of ART by these dentists was the unavailability of sufficient dental instruments and glass-ionomers for producing ART restorations.

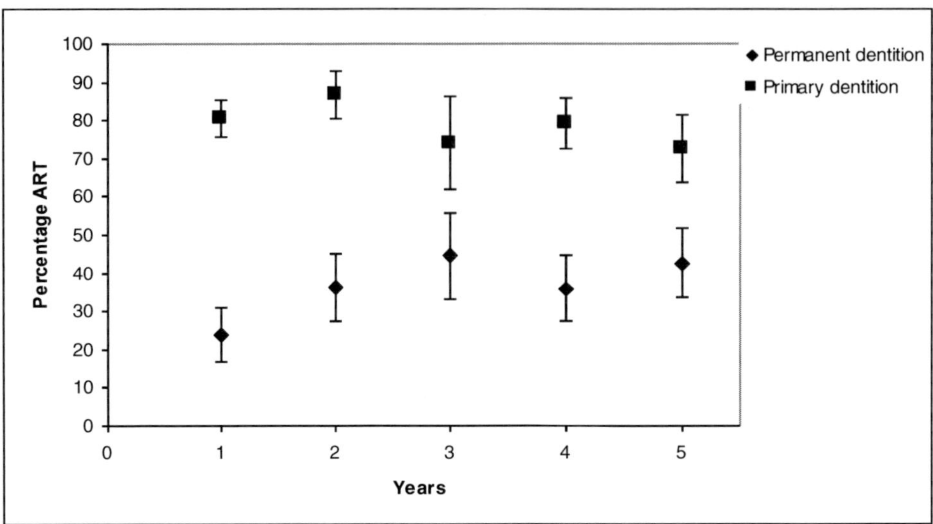

Figure 3.7. Percentages of ART restoration (%ART) and Standard Error (SE) for the primary and permanent dentition by year of investigation.

The introduction of ART into the public oral healthcare service system of Tanzania benefitted from the experiences obtained in South Africa. The training course was extended to 7 days and before public dental personnel were trained in ART and caries prevention, investigations into potential barriers causing the lack of restorative care in the public oral health services were carried out among patients (Kikwilu et al, 2009a) and public dental personnel (Kikwilu et al, 2010). In addition, dental practitioners were interviewed about their attitudes and intentions regarding use of the ART approach (Kikwilu et al, 2009b). The findings of these studies were discussed with the participating dental personnel during the first days of the ART course. During the 31-month period following the ART course, ART restorations using high-viscosity glass-ionomers accounted for between 4% and 13% of the total number of procedures in these 13 public dental clinics (Figure 3.8). However, the percentage of ART restorations relative to the total number of restorations placed, at the 31-month period after ART training, was 89 percent (Kikwilu et al, 2009c). Many of the teeth treated by ART during this follow-up period would have been extracted had the approach not been introduced to the resident dentists and dental therapists. As in South Africa, the availability of glass-ionomer and hand instruments was the main factor that had inhibited the full adoption of ART by the public oral health service system of Tanzania after 31 months (Kikwilu et al, 2009d).

Ruiz and Frencken (2009) conducted a pilot investigation into the level of introduction of ART in public health services in Latin American countries. It was concluded that more training courses on ART needed to be organised and that sufficient high-viscosity glass-ionomer and ART instruments needed to be made available in order to assure proper implementation and adoption of ART in these countries.

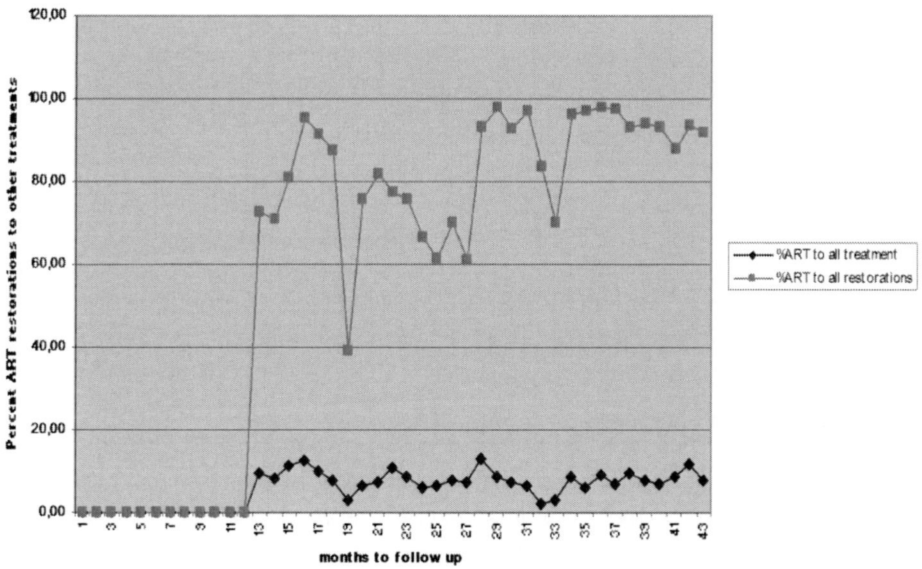

Figure 3.8. Effectiveness of introduction of ART restorations in treatment profiles of 13 government dental clinics in Tanzania (2004–2008). Pre-ART training (0–11-months); post-ART training (12–43-months to follow up).

On the basis of 20 years of research it can be concluded that the ART approach is an appropriate therapy for managing cavitated dentine lesions in single tooth surfaces in primary and permanent teeth. Its success in multiple-surface cavities in deciduous teeth needs to be improved. Available data on multiple-surface cavities in permanent teeth is scarce (Holmgren and Figueiredo, 2009). Sufficiently large supplies of high-viscosity glass-ionomer and hand instruments need to be available when the ART approach is introduced in communities in middle- and low-income countries. For further information, the reader is referred to the chapter on the ART approach in the textbook on caries management (Frencken and van Amerongen, 2008). Obviously, in order to produce quality ART sealants and ART restorations, dental practitioners have to participate in well-organised training courses of sufficient duration.

3.3.5. Non-Restorative Therapies

The principle aim in the provision of restorative care for cavitated deciduous teeth comprises pain reduction, proper plaque control facilitation, stopping the caries process and assisting undisturbed eruption of permanent teeth. The first two treatment options focus on restoring the cavity in order to achieve this aim. However, considering current evidence that the main etiological factor for carious lesion development is the cariogenic plaque, the question remains as to whether restoring a cavity is always necessary. Would removing the etiological factor regularly be sufficient? Factors that influence this decision in deciduous teeth include the size, shape and cleansability of the cavity, the age of the child, the possibility for providing restorative care and the predicted survival results of restorations using conventional restorative materials in deciduous teeth, which vary in multiple-surface cavities (Hickel et al, 2005). The following two cases exemplify situations relevant to decisions regarding appropriate treatment. A 3-4-year-old child with sizable, non-pulpally involved, tooth cavities whose teeth need to function for another 6-7 years, may be better off having these teeth restored and accepting that the restorations have to be repaired on the way until the teeth exfoliate naturally. However, the same situation in a 6-7-year-old child with only 3-4 years to go before the tooth will exfoliate, may call for an alternative approach. What will happen to such a mutilated tooth if it is not restored but kept plaque-free? Will it be able to exfoliate naturally or will it need to be extracted early, perhaps causing insufficient space for permanent teeth to erupt normally? Two retrospective studies from the United Kingdom have provided some answers. Tickle et al, (2002) reported that 84% of untreated cavitated deciduous teeth exfoliated without any symptoms, whilst only 16% had been extracted due to pain or sepsis. The other study, by Levine et al, (2002), reported that 12% of untreated cavitated deciduous teeth had been extracted because of pain and 4% became painful and were treated, whereas 84% exfoliated normally despite the presence of cavities which were not restored. It appears from the foregoing that the large majority of untreated cavitated lesions in deciduous teeth have a high chance of exfoliating naturally, without symptoms. The study outcomes were obtained without specific interventions geared to keep these tooth cavities free from cariogenic plaque in the Tickle study, whereas in the Levine study, management consisted of regular reinforcement of simple dietary and tooth-brushing advice. It can be argued that, in the two UK-studies, if supervised plaque control measures had taken place, the numbers of untreated cavitated teeth that would have exfoliated normally, would have been higher than those observed.

May we then conclude that the probability for an increased chance of exfoliation of mutilated, non-pulpally involved but non-restored teeth is dependent on the level of cariogenic plaque in the cavity? This plaque level, in turn, is dependent upon the level of cleanliness of the cavitated teeth, achieved with or without the help of plaque-reducing agents. In the following paragraphs the effectiveness of two non-restorative therapies is discussed.

3.3.5.1. Cavity Cleaning with Fluoride Toothpaste

As cariogenic plaque is considered the main etiological factor in the development of carious lesions, managing the presence of dental plaque on tooth surfaces is a major caries management measure. Usually, plaque control refers to cleaning sound and restored tooth surfaces. However, in situations in many socially disadvantaged communities where a restoration is not the best option or cannot be provided for obvious reasons referred to earlier, meticulous cleaning accessible tooth cavities definitely will arrest carious lesion progression. This effect has been demonstrated in easily accessible root surface carious lesions. Meticulous plaque control used together with fluoride toothpaste application had changed all active carious lesions from soft, greasy and yellowish, to leathery or hard, darkly discoloured tissue, indicating a gradual transition from active into inactive stages of the carious lesion within a period of 2 - 6 months (Nyvad and Fejerskov, 1986). Therefore, cleaning dentine lesions in teeth with fluoride toothpaste and a suitable toothbrush may be a viable option in caries management. However, this option requires investigation.

This measure could be particularly suitable in deciduous teeth. The cavity, however, must be accessible to the toothbrush and the child needs to apply a different brushing regime from that used for cleaning non-cavitated tooth surfaces. This means that only sizable cavities, perhaps those that have a low prognosis of surviving long after being restored, would need to be selected as cavities suited to cleaning. For such mutilated teeth the ultimate goal is for the tooth to exfoliate symptomless, so preventing malalignment of the permanent premolar, rather than for it to be a fully functioning unit for chewing food. The tooth acts as a space maintainer.

Evidence other than the outcomes of the retrospective studies by Tickle et al, (2002) and Levine et al, (2002) from the UK, is not yet available. As prospective studies have not been carried out, currently caution should be taken when this strategy is implemented (Kidd et al, 2008).

3.3.5.2. Silver Diamine Fluoride (SDF) Application

Silver Diamine Fluoride, $Ag(NH_3)_2F$, is a black staining liquid that, if applied on the walls and floor of an active cavitated dentine lesion, is able to kill microorganisms in the infected dentine and to inhibit plaque formation (Rosenblatt et al, 2009). It was developed in the nineteen-sixties. SDF can easily be applied in a tooth cavity without the need for excavation of soft infected dentine by dental practitioners and trained dental auxiliary personnel. This aspect would make the application of SDF a suitable treatment approach for use in disadvantaged communities.

Only a few studies have been conducted, mainly in deciduous dentition, in which the application of SDF has been researched clinically. A systematic review (Rosenblatt et al, 2009) identified two quality studies and one additional quality study has subsequently been published (Yee et al, 2009). Important information pertaining to these three studies is presented in Table 3.6.

Table 3.6. Main characteristics of 3 studies into the effectiveness of 38% SDF.
(X = mean; N = number

	Baseline information						Outcome	
Authors	Country	Age (yrs)	Duration (yrs)	38% SDF frequency	Caries experience	X. active dentine lesions	Arrested carious surfaces	N. new dentine lesions
Chu et al, 2002	China	4	2.5	1/1 yr	dmfs = 5	4.3	100%	0.47
Llodra et al, 2005	Cuba	6.3	3	1/0.5 yr	dmfs = 3.7	3.3	77%	0.3
Yee et al, 2009	Nepal	5	2	1/2 yrs	dmft = 4.5	6.6	31%	4.1

Carious lesion activity was distinctly higher in the Nepalese children than in children of the two other studies. While arrestment of carious lesion activity was reported in all three studies, the proportion of teeth benefiting from arrested carious lesion activity after 2 years was markedly lower in the Nepalese children than in children of the two other studies. They also had a significantly higher number of new dentine lesions after 2 years than the Chinese and Cuban children did. The Nepalese study group result did not differ from that of the control group, who received tooth brushing instruction only. The aim of the Nepal research was to assess the effectiveness of a one-time application of 38% SDF as a carious lesion-arresting agent, because repeated application was considered impractical and unaffordable for local communities in middle- and low-income countries (Yee et al, 2009). This research was very appropriate, considering the low number of dental personnel and the rudimentary organization and financing of (oral) health services in communities in many middle- and low-income countries.

In summary; the results of these three studies indicate that 38% SDF may be effective in arresting active cavitated dentine lesions in deciduous teeth and that the magnitude of its effect is dependent upon the initial caries activity of the children who receive the agent and upon the frequency of its application. On the basis of these few studies, it appears that 38% SDF may be effective in inhibiting carious lesion progression in deciduous teeth in low- to medium caries risk children when applied at least once per year, whereas high caries risk children require more frequent applications; perhaps once per 6 months. Obviously, available evidence is currently insufficient as a basis for advocating widespread use of SDF as a therapy for treating cavitated carious lesions in children and in adults from disadvantaged communities. Therefore, the notion that SDF application meets the criteria of the WHO Millennium Goals, as reported by Rosenblatt et al, (2009), is too optimistic and cannot be concluded from the evidence currently available. Furthermore, it can be argued that application of SDF without support through proper plaque control cannot yield the desired effect of people becoming self-responsible for their oral health.

The blackening of tooth cavities, due to the silver particles in the agent, is a noticeable side effect but it was not considered problematic by parents and children in the Nepalese study.

The children in the China study, however, did not like the metallic taste. Elimination of the staining effect is currently under investigation; not in conjunction with SDF however, but for silver fluoride as the carious lesion-arresting agent. Applying potassium iodide over silver fluoride produces a white silver iodide product which may be generally accepted by the population. However, this new agent is still under *in vitro* investigation (Knight et al, 2009).

In conclusion; SDF is currently not recommended for treating cavitated lesions, as evidence for its efficacy is not available.

3.3.6. Summary

Because functional dental facilities are few or absent and levels of access to oral care, manpower and finances are low, in many disadvantaged communities in low- and middle-income countries, oral care based on complicated dental equipment is largely inappropriate. Remaining appropriate options are the ART approach and perhaps, the Hall Technique in primary teeth, as suitable treatments for cavitated dentine lesions. Both treatments have their strengths and weaknesses, and dental practitioners need to be aware of these. They need to ensure continuous professional education and training on oral health matters. Most importantly; people in disadvantaged communities should be educated about the necessity to regularly remove or disturb the biofilm on their teeth, including that within cavities. They should be responsible about controlling the caries process instead of waiting for dental professionals to restore cavities.

3.4. Recommendation: An Oral Health Care Package

In 2002, the WHO Collaborating Centre of the Radboud University Nijmegen in the Netherlands published a monograph on a Basic Package of Oral Care (BPOC) for use in deprived communities (Frencken et al, 2002). The package has palliative, preventive, promotional and a restorative components based on the best evidence available at that time. The components are Oral Urgent Treatment (OUT), Affordable Fluoride Toothpaste (AFT) and Atraumatic Restorative Treatment (ART). OUT implies pain relief through medication, extraction or restoration of badly decayed teeth. AFT relates to daily preventive measures of plaque control and fluoride application involving the use of fluoride toothpaste and the toothbrush. Preventive care for caries risk individuals and restorative care for all are achieved through ART sealants and ART restorations, respectively. These three components should be implemented in tandem with Oral Health Promotion (OHP) activities, cross-infection control and good programme governance.

In most low- and middle income countries, pain relief through extraction (OUT) and affordable fluoride toothpaste (AFT) are, to a certain extent, available to the population. The ART and oral health promotion (OHP) components of the BPOC are usually missing. The introduction and adoption of ART in the oral health services makes a basic comprehensive oral health care programme available to the population through the residential dental practitioners in these countries. Introduction of OHP is a matter for consideration by governments and health institutions to develop in order to make the public aware of healthy lifestyles and create healthy environments. However, obviously the primary need of people, wherever in the world, is to be free of toothache. The second is to have their cavities treated. Meeting these creates a condition for change and adoption of healthy lifestyles and gives the individual a second start.

Adoption of BPOC may improve the oral health of people in disadvantaged communities, as recently reported in Cambodia (Chher et al, 2009). It seems that the Achilles heel of the package is the need for regular availability of affordable fluoride toothpaste, tooth brushes and quality high-viscosity glass-ionomers. Eight years after its launch, the BPOC is still considered the most appropriate, cost-effective and evidence-based comprehensive oral health care package for use in low- and middle-income countries. Other, more complicated and expensive caries management treatments can be introduced according to local circumstances. There is however, a need to investigate the introduction, adoption and effectiveness of BPOC in different communities.

References

Abreu D., Leal S.C., Frencken J.E. (2009) Self–report of pain by children treated according to the Atraumatic Restorative Treatment and the Conventional Restorative Treatment - a pilot study. *J. Clin. Paed Dent.*; 34: 149–154.

Almeida G.C., Ferreira M.A. (2008) Oral health in the context of the Family Health Program: preventive practices targeting individual and public health. *Cad Saúde Pública*; 24: 2131-2140.

Alvarez J.A., Rezende K.M.P.C., Marocho S.M.S., Alves F.B.T., Celiberti P., Ciamponi A.L. (2009) Dental fluorosis: exposure, prevention and management. *Med. Oral. Patol. Oral. Cir. Bucal*; 14: E103-107.

Alvarez J.O. (1995) Nutrition, tooth development and dental caries. *Am. J. Clin. Nutr.*; 61: 410-416.

Alvarez J.O., Lewis C.A., Saman C, Caceda J, Montalvo J, Figueroa M.L., Izquierdo J, Caravedo L, Navia J.M. (1988) Chronic malnutrition dental caries, and tooth exfoliation in Peruvian children aged 3-9 years. *Am. J. Clin. Nutr.*; 48: 368-372.

American Dental Association. (2005) Fluoridation facts [Online]. [cited 2009 Oct]. Available from: URL http://www.ada.org/public/topics/fluoride/facts/ fluoridation_facts.pdf.

Amorim R.G., Leal S.C., Bezerra A.C., Amorim F.P., Toledo O.A. (2008) Association of chlorhexidine and fluoride for plaque control and white spot lesion remineralization in primary dentition. *Int. J. Paediatr. Dent.*; 18: 446-451.

Australia. (2007) A Systematic review of the efficacy and safety of fluoridation. Part A: review of methodology and results. Canberra: National and Medical Council Research;.

Autio-Gold J. (2008) The role of chlorhexidine in caries prevention. *Oper. Dent.*; 33: 710-716.

Azarpazhooh A., Limeback H. (2008) The application of ozone in dentistry: a systematic review of the literature. *J. Dent.;* 36: 104-116.

Ayhan H., Suskan E., Yildirim S. (1996) The effect of nursing or rampant caries on height, body weight and head circumference. *J. Clin. Pediatr. Dent.*; 20: 209-212.

Batchelor P.A., Sheiham A. (2006) The distribution of burden of dental caries in schoolchildren: a critique review of the high risk prevention strategy for populations. BMC Oral Health; 6:1

Beiruti N., Frencken J.E., van 't Hof M.A., Taifour D., van Palenstein Helderman W.H. (2006[a]) Caries-preventive effect of a one-time application of composite resin and glass-ionomer sealants after 5 years. *Caries Res.*; 40: 52-59.

Beiruti N., Frencken J.E., van 't Hof M.A., van Palenstein Helderman W.H. (2006[b]) Caries preventive effect of resin-based and glass ionomer sealants over time: A systematic review. *Community Dent. Oral Epidemiol.*; 34: 403-409.

Black G.V. (1908) A work on operative dentistry. Chicago: The medical-dental publishing Co; p 110-116.

Braga M.M., Mendes F.M., De Benedetto M.S., Imparato J.C. (2009) Effect of silver diammine fluoride on incipient caries lesions in erupting permanent first molars: a pilot study. *J. Dent. Child*; 76: 28-33.

Brazzelli M., McKenzie L., Fielding S., Fraser C., Clarckson J., Kilonzo M., Waugh N. (2006) Systematic review of the effectiveness and cost-effectiveness of HealOzone for the treatment of occlusal pit/fissure caries and root caries. Health Technol Assess; 10:16.

Bulut T., Sharif S. (2004) Atraumatic Restorative Treatment in Nederland. MSc Dissertation. Nijmegen: College of Dental Sciences.

Burke FJ, McHugh S, Shaw L, Hosy MT, MacPerson L, Delargy S, Dopheide B. (2005) UK dentists' attitudes and behaviour towards Atraumatic Restorative Treatment for primary teeth. *Br. Dent. J.*; 199: 365-369.

Burt B.A., Pai S. (2001) Sugar consumption and caries risk: A systematic review. *J. Den. Educ.*; 65: 1017-1023.

Campus G., Cagetti M.G., Sacco G., Solinas G., Mastroberardino S., Lingstrom P. (2009) Six month of daily high-dose xylitol in high risk schoolchildren: a randomized clinical trial on plaque pH and salivary mutans streptococci. *Caries Res*; 43: 455-461.

Carvalho J.C., Ekstrand K.R., Thylstrup A. (1989) Dental plaque and caries on occlusal surfaces of first permanent molar in relation to stage of eruption. *J. Dent. Res*; 68:773-779.

Carvalho J.C., Thylstrup A., Ekstrand K.R. (1992) Results after 3 years of non-operative occlusal caries treatment of erupting permanent first molars. *Community Dent. Oral Epidemiol.*; 20:187-192.

Carvalho J.C., Nieuwenhuysen J.P., D'Hoore W. (2001) The decline in dental caries among Belgian children between 1983 and 1998. *Community Dent. Oral Epidemiol.*;29: 55-61.

Chen M.S., Andersen R.M., Barmes D.E., Leclercq M.H., Lyttle C.S. (1997) Comparing oral health care systems: a second international collaborative study. Geneva: World Health Organization.

Cohen H., Locker D. (2001) The science and ethics of water fluoridation. *J. Can. Dent. Assoc.;* 67: 578-580.

Chher T., Hak S., Courtel F., Durward C. (2009) Improving the provision of the Basic Package of Oral Care (BPOC) in Cambodia. *Int. Dent. J.*; 59: 47-52.

Chu C.H., Lo E.C., Lin H.C. (2002) Effectiveness of silver diamine fluoride and sodium fluoride varnish in arresting dentin caries in Chinese pre-school children. *J. Dent. Res*; 81:767-70.

Disney J.A., Graves R.C., Stamm J.W., Bohannan H.M., Abernathy J.R., Zack D.D. (1992) The University of North Carolina Caries Risk Assessment study: further developments in caries risk prediction. *Community Dent. Oral Epidemiol.*; 20: 64-75.

Du M.Q., Tai B.J., Jiang H., Lo E.C.M., Fan M.W., Bian Z. (2006) A two-year randomized clinical trial of chlorhexidine varnish on dental caries in Chinese preschool children. *J. Dent. Res*; 85: 557-559.

Eden E., Topaloglu-Ak A., Frencken J.E., van 't Hof M.A. (2006) Two-year survival of composite ART and traditional restorations. *Am. J. Dent.*; 19:359-363.

Ellwood R. Fejerskov O., Cury J.A., Clarkson B. (2008) Fluorides in caries control. In: Fejerskov O. and Kidd E. (eds). Dental caries. The disease and its clinical management. Oxford: Blackwell Munksgaard Ltd; p. 308

Emilson C.G. (1994) Potential efficacy of chlorhexidine against mutans streptococci and human dental caries. *J. Dent. Res*; 73: 682-691.

Ersin N.K., Candan U., Aykut A., Oncag O., Eronat C., Kose T. (2006) A clinical evaluation of resin-based composite and glass ionomer cement restorations placed in primary teeth using the ART approach. *J. Am. Dent. Assoc.*; 137:1529-1536.

Feigal RJ: (2002) The use of pits and fissure sealants. *Pediatr. Dent.*; 24: 415-422.

Fejerskov O., Thylstrup A., Larsen MJ. (1981) Rational use of fluorides in caries prevention. A concept based on possible cariostatic mechanisms. *Acta Odont. Scand.*; 39: 241-249.

Fejerskov O., Kidd E.A.M. (2008[a]) Preface: an Editors'guide to reading the book. In: Fejerskov O and Kidd E (eds). Dental caries; the disease and its management. Oxford: Blackwell Munksgaard Ltd;. pp xiii.

Fejerskov O., Nyvad B., Kidd E.A.M. (2008[b]) Pathology of dental caries. In: Fejerskov O and Kidd E (eds). Dental caries; the disease and its management. Oxford: Blackwell Munksgaard Ltd; pp.19-48.

Frencken J.E., Pilot T., Songpaisan Y., Phantumvanit P. (1996) Atraumatic Restorative Treatment (ART): rationale, technique and development. *J. Public Health Dent.*; 56: 135-140.

Frencken J.E., Makoni F., Sithole W.D., Hackenitz E. (1998) Three-year survival of one-surface ART restorations and glass-ionomer sealants in a school oral health programme in Zimbabwe. *Caries Res.*; 32:119-126.

Frencken J.E., Holmgren C.J. (1999) Atraumatic Restorative Treatment for dental caries. Nijmegen: Benda Drukkers.

Frencken J.E., Holmgren C.J., van Palenstein Helderman W.H. (2002) Basic package of oral care. WHO Collaborating Centre for Oral Health Care Planning and Future Scenarios, Nijmegen, the Netherlands.

Frencken J.E., van 't Hof M.A., van Amerongen W.E., Holmgren C.J. (2004) Effectiveness of single-surface ART restorations in the permanent dentition: A meta-analysis. *J. Dent. Res*; 83:120-123.

Frencken J.E., van Amerongen. The Atraumatic Restorative Treatment (ART) approach to manage dental caries. In: Fejerskov O and Kidd E (eds). (2008) Dental caries; the disease and its management. Oxford: Blackwell Munksgaard Ltd.

Frencken J.E., Wolke J. (2010) Clinical and SEM assessment of ART high-viscosity glass-ionomer sealants after 8-13 years in 4 teeth. *J. Dent.*; 38: 59-64.

Frencken J.E. (2010) The ART approach using glass-ionomers in relation to oral health. *Dent Mater*; 26: 1-6.

Goldman A.S., Yee R., Holmgren C.J., Benzian H. (2008) Global affordability of fluoride toothpaste. *Global Health*; 4:7. doi:10.1186/1744-8603-4-7.

Griffin S.O., Regnier E., Griffin P.M., Huntley V. (2007) Effectiveness of fluoride in preventing caries in adults. *J. Dent. Res*; 86: 410-415.

Griffin S.O., Oong E., Kohn W., Vidakovic B., Gooch B.F.; CDC Dental Sealant Systematic Review Work Group, Bader J., Clarkson J., Fontana M.R, Meyer D.M., Rozier R.G., Weintraub J.A., Zero D.T. (2008) The effectiveness of sealants in managing caries lesions. *J. Dent. Res;* 87:169-174.

Groeneveld A. (1985) Longitudinal study of prevalence of enamel lesions in a fluoridated and non-fluoridated area. *Community Dent. Oral. Epidemiol.*;13:159-63.

Hawkins R., Locker D., Noble J., Kay J. (2003) Prevention. Part 7: professionally applied topical fluorides for caries prevention. *Brit. Dent. J*; 195: 313-317.

Hellwig E., Lennon A.M. (2004) Systemic versus topical fluoride. *Caries Research*; 38: 258-262.

Hermosillo H.V., Quintero E.L., Guerrero D.N., Suarez D.S.D., Hernandez A.M., Holmgren C.J. (2009) The implementation and preliminary evaluation of an Atraumatic Restorative Treatment (ART) strategy in Mexico − A country example. *J. Appl. Oral. Sci*;17 Suppl:114-21.

Hernández-Guerrero J.C., de la Fuente-Hernández J., Jiménez-Farfán M.D., Ledesma-Montes C., Castañeda-Castaneira E., Molina-Frechero N., Jacinto-Alemán L.F., Juárez-Lopez L.A., Moreno-Altamirano A. (2008) Fluoride content in table salt distributed in Mexico City, Mexico. *J. Public Health Dent.*; 68:242-245.

Hickel R., Kaaden C., Paschos E., Buerkle V., García-Godoy F., Manhart J. (2005) Longevity of occlusally-stressed restorations in posterior primary teeth. *Am. J. Dent.*;18:198-211.

Ho T.F.T., Smales R.J., Fang D.K.S. (1999) A 2-year clinical study of two glass ionomer cements used in the atraumatic restorative treatment (ART) technique. *Community Dent. Oral Epidemiol.*; 27:195-201.

Hobdell M.H. (2007) Poverty, moral health and human development: Contemporary issues affecting the provision of primary oral health care. *J. Am. Dent. Assoc.*; 138:1433-1436.

Honkala E., Behbehani J., Ibricevic H., Kerosuo E., Al-Jame G. (2003) The atraumatic restorative treatment (ART) approach to restoring primary teeth in a standard dental clinic. *Int. J. Paediat. Dent.* 13:172-179.

Holmgren C.J., Figueiredo M.C. (2009) Two decades of ART - Improving on success through further research. *J. Appl. Oral. Sci.*: 17 Suppl: 122-133.

Hugoson A., Koch G. (2008) Thirty year trends in the prevalence and distribution of dental caries in Swedish adults (1973-2003). *Swed. Dent. J.*; 32: 57-67.

Innes N.P., Evans D.J., Stirrups D.R. (2007) The Hall Technique: a randomized controlled clinical trial of a novel method of managing carious primary molars in general dental practice: acceptability of the technique and outcomes at 23 months. *BMC Oral Health*; 20: 7-18.

Innes N. Evans D.J.P. (2009) The Hall Technique. A child-centred approach to managing the carious primary molar - A Users Manual. http://www.scottishdental.org/resources/HallTechnique.htm.

Jimenez-Farfan M.D., Hernandez-Guerrero J.C., Loyola-Rodriguez J.P., Ledesma-Montes C. (2004) Fluoride content in bottled waters, juices and carbonated soft drinks in Mexico City, Mexico. *Int. J. Paediatr. Dent.*; 14: 260-266.

Kalsbeek H., Verrips G.H. (1994) Consumption of sweet snacks and caries experience of primary school children. *Caries Res.*;28(6):477-83.

Kidd E.A.M., van Amerongen J.P., van Amerongen W.E. The role of operative treatment in caries control. In: Fejerskov O and Kidd E (eds). (2008) Dental caries; the disease and its management. Oxford: Blackwell Munksgaard Ltd; p 363.

Kikwilu E.N., Masalu J.R., Kahabuka F.K., Senkoro A.R. (2008) Prevalence of oral pain and barriers to use of emergency oral care facilities among adult Tanzanians. *BMC Oral Health*; 29:8-28.

Kikwilu E.N., Frencken J.E., Mulder J., Masalu J.R. (2009[a]) Barriers to restorative care as perceived by dental patients attending government hospitals in Tanzania. *Community Dent. Oral Epidemiol.*; 37:35-44.

Kikwilu E.N., Frencken J.E., Mulder J., Masalu J.R. (2009[b]) Dental practitioners' attitudes, subjective norms and intentions to practise Atraumatic Restorative Treatment (ART) in Tanzania. *J. Appl. Oral Sci.*; 17: 97-102.

Kikwilu E.N., Frencken J.E., Mulder J. (2009[c]) Impact of the Atraumatic Restorative Treatment (ART) on the treatment profile in government dental clinics in Tanzania. *BMC Oral Health*; 9: 14.

Kikwilu E.N., Frencken J.E., Mulder J. (2009[d]) Barriers to the adoption of ART as perceived by dental practitioners in government dental clinics, in Tanzania. *J. Appl. Oral Sci.*;17: 408-413.

Kikwilu E.N., Frencken J.E., Mulder J., Masalu J.R. (2010) Barriers to restorative care as perceived by dental practitioners in Tanzania. *Community Dent Health*; 27(1):23-28.

Knight G.M., McIntyre J.M., Craig G.G., Mulyani, Zilm P.S., Gully N.J. Inability to form a biofilm of Streptococcus mutans on silver fluoride- and potassium iodide-treated demineralized dentin. *Quintessence Int.* 2009; 40:155-61.

Kumar J. (2008) Is water fluoridation still necessary? *Adv Dent Res*; 20: 8-12.

Leal S.C., Abreu D.M.M., Frencken J.E. (2009) Dental anxiety and pain related to ART. *J. Appl. Oral Sci.* 17 Suppl:84-88.

Levine R.S., Pitts N.B., Nutgent Z.J.l. (2002) The fate of 1,587 unrestored carious deciduous teeth: a retrospective general dental practice based study from northern England. *Brit. Dent. J.;* 193: 99-103.

Lindely M.G., Birch G.G., Khan R. (1976) Sweetness of sucrose and xylitol. Structural considerations. *J. Sci. Food Agric.*; 27:140-144.

Llodra J.C., Rodriguez A., Ferrer B., Menardia V., Ramos T., Morato M. (2005) Efficacy of silver diamine fluoride for caries reduction in primary teeth and first permanent molars of schoolchildren: 36-month clinical trial. *J. Dent. Res*; 84:721-724.

Lo E.C.M., Luo Y., Fan M.W., Wei S.H.Y. (2001) Clinical investigation of two glass-ionomer restoratives used with the Atraumatic Restorative Treatment approach in China: Two-years results. *Caries Res.*; 35:458-463.

Locker D., Jokovic A., Kay E.J. (2003) Prevention. Part 8: The use of pit and fissure sealants in preventing caries in the permanent dentition of children. *Br. Dent. J.;* 195: 375-378.

Louw A.J., Sarvan I., Chikte U.M.E., Honkala E. (2002) One-year evaluation of atraumatic restorative treatment and minimum intervention techniques on primary teeth. *S. Afr. Dent. J.*; 57: 366-371.

Ly K.A., Milgrom P., Rothen M. (2006) Xylitol, sweeteners and dental caries. *Pediatr Dent*; 28: 154-163.

Ly K.A., Milgrom P., Rothen M. (2008[a]) The potential of dental protective chewing gum in oral interventions. *J Am Dent Assoc*; 139:553-563.

Ly A., Riedy C.A., Milgrom P., Rothen M., Roberts M.C., Zhou L. (2008[b]) Xylitol gummy bear snacks: a school-based randomized clinical trial. *BMC Oral Health*; 8:20.

Lynch H., Milgrom P. (2003) Xylitol and dental caries: an overview for clinicians. *J. Calif Dent Assoc*; 31: 205-209.

Marinho V.C.C. (2008) Evidence-based effectiveness of topical fluoride. *Adv. Dent. Res.*; 3:7.

McDonagh MS, Whitining PF, Wilson PM, Sutton AJ, Chestnutt I, Cooper J, Misso K, Bradley M, Treasure E, Kleijnen J. (2000) Systematic review on water fluoridation. *BMJ*; 321: 855-859.

Mejàre I., Mjör I.A. (1990) Glass ionomer and resin-based fissure sealants: a clinical study. *Scand. J. Dent. Res*; 98: 345-350.

Mertz-Fairhurst E.J., Schuster G.S., Williams J.E., Fairhurst C.W. (1979[a]) Clinical progress of sealed and unsealed caries. Part I: Depth changes and bacterial counts. *J. Prosthet. Dent*, 42: 521-526.

Mertz-Fairhurst E.J., Schuster G.S., Williams J.E., Fairhurst C.W. (1979[b]) Clinical progress of sealed and unsealed caries. Part II: Standardized radiographs and clinical observations. *J. Prosthet. Dent.*; 42: 633-637.

Mertz-Fairhurst E.J., Curtis J.W. Jr., Ergle J.W., Rueggeberg F.A., Adair S.M. (1998) Ultraconservative and cariostatic sealed restorations: results at year 10. *J. Am. Dent. Assoc.*; 129: 55-66.

Malek M.T., Wright C.M., Kay E.J. (2009) Childhood growth and dental caries. *Community Dent Health*; 26:38-42.

Mickenaustch S. (2005) An introduction to Minimum Intervention Dentistry. *Singapore Dent J*; 27: 1-6.

Mickenautsch S., Frencken J.E., van't Hof M.A. (2007) Atraumatic Restorative Treatment and dental anxiety in outpatients attending public oral health clinics in South Africa. *J. Public Health Dent.*; 67:79-84.

Mickenaustch S., Leal S.C., Yengopal V., Bezerra A.C., Cruvinel V. (2007) Sugar free chewing gum and dental caries: a systematic review. *J. Appl. Oral. Sci.*; 15:83-88.

Mickenautsch S., Frencken J.E. (2009) Utilization of the Atraumatic Restorative Treatment (ART) approach in a selected group of public oral health operators in South Africa 5 years after training. *BMC Oral Health*; 9: 10.

Mickenautsch S., Yengopal V., Banerjee A. (2010) Atraumatic restorative treatment versus amalgam restoration longevity: a systematic review. *Clin. Oral Investig.* 14:233-240.

Miller E., Vaughan-Williams R., Furlong R., Harrison L. (1982) Dental caries and children's weights. *J. Epidemiol. Community Health*; 36:49-52.

Monse B., Heinrich-Weltzien R., Benzian H., Holmgren C., van Palenstein Helderman W.H. (2010) PUFA – An index of clinical consequences of untreated dental caries. *Community Dent. Oral Epidemiol.*; 38: 77–82.

Naidoo S., Chikte U.M.E., Sheiham A. (2001) Prevalence and impact of pain in 8 year olds in the Western Cape. *S. Afric. Dent. J.*; 56: 701-705.

Nadanovsky P., Cohen Carneiro F., Souza de Mello F. (2001) Removal of caries using only hand instruments: a comparison of mechanical and chemo-mechanical methods. *Caries Res*; 35: 384-9.

Narvai P.C., Frazão P., Roncalli G.A., Antunes J.L.F. (2006) Dental caries in Brazil: decline, polarization, inequality and social exclusion. *Rev. Panan Salud Publica*; 19: 385-393.

Nyvad B., Fejerskov O. (1986) Active root surface caries converted into inactive caries as a response to oral hygiene. *Scand. J. Dent. Res*; 94:281-284.

Oong E.M., Griffin S.O., Kohn W.G., Gooch B.F., Caufield P.W. (2008) The effect of dental sealants on bacteria levels in caries lesions: a review of the evidence. *J. Am. Dent. Assoc.*;139:271-278.

Övrebö R.S., Raadal M. (1990) Microleakage in fissures sealed with resin or glass ionomer cement. *Scand. J. Dent. Res.*; 98: 66-69.

PAHO. (2006) Oral health of low income children. Procedures for Atraumatic Restorative Treatment. Final Report. Washington: Pan American Health Organization.

Papacchini F., Goracci C., Sadek F.T., Monticelli F., Garcia-Godoy F., Ferrari M. (2005) Microtensile bond strength to ground enamel by glass-ionomers, resin-modified glass-ionomers, and resin composites used as pit and fissure sealants. *J. Dent.*; 33: 459-467.

Pizzo G., Piscopo M.R., Pizzo I., Giuliana G. (2007) Community water fluoridation and caries prevention: a critical review. *Clin. Oral Invest*; 11: 189-193.

Peres M.A., Antunes J.L.F., Peres K.G. (2006) Is water fluoridation effective in reducing inequalities in dental caries distribution in developing countries? Recent findings from Brazil. *Soc. and Prev. Med.*; 51: 302-310.

Petersen P.E. (2004) Effective use of fluorides for the prevention of dental caries in the 21st century: the WHO approach. *Community Dent. Oral Epidemiol.*; 32: 319-321.

Petersen P.E. (2008[a]) Oral Health. In: Heggenhougen K Quah S (eds), International Encyclopidia of Public Health, vol4. San Diego: Academic Press; p 677-685.

Petersen P.E. (2008[b]) World Health Organization global policy for improvement of oral health- World Health Assembly 2007. *Inter. Dent J.*; 58:115-121.

Petersson G.H., Bratthall D. (1996) The caries decline: a review of reviews. *Eur. J. Oral Sci.*;104: 436-443.

Powell L.V: (1998) Caries prediction: a review of the literature. *Community Dent. Oral Epidemiol.*; 26: 361-371.

Psoter W.J., Reid B.C., Katz R.V. (2005) Malnutrition and dental caries: A review of the literature. *Caries Res.*; 39: 441-447.

Rahimtoola S., van Amerongen E., Maher R., Groen H. (2000) Pain related to different ways of minimal intervention in the treatment of small caries lesions. *J. Dent. Child*; 67:123-127.

Rickard G.D., Richardson R.J., Johnson T.M., McColl D.C., Hooper L. (2004) Ozone therapy for the treatment of dental caries. Cochrane Database of Systematic Reviews, Issue 3. Art. No.: CD004153. DOI: 10.1002/14651858.CD004153.pub2

Reynolds E.C. (1998) Anticariogenic complexes of amorphous calcium phosphate stabilized by casein phosphopeptides: a review. *Spec Care Dentist*; 18: 8-16.

Reynolds E.C., Cai F., Cochrane N.J., Shen P., Walker G.D., Morgan M.V., Reynolds C. (2008) Fluoride and casein phosphopeptide-amorphous Calcium phosphate. *J. Dent. Res.*, 87: 344-348.

Rodrigues M.H., Leite A.L., Arana A., Villena R.S., Forte F.D., Sampaio F.C., Buzalaf M.A. (2009) Dietary fluoride intake by children receiving different sources of systemic fluoride. *J. Dent. Res.*; 88: 142-145.

Rosenblatt A., Stamford T.C.M., Niederman R. (2009) Silver diammine fluoride: a caries silver fluoride bullet. *J. Dent. Res;* 88:116-125.

Ruiz O., Frencken J.E. (2009) ART integration in oral health care systems in Latin American countries as perceived by directors of oral health. *J. Appl. Oral Sci.*; 17 Suppl:106-113.

Schechter N. (2000) The impact of acute and chronic dental pain on child development. *J Southeastern Soc Pediatric Dent*; 6:16.

Schriks M.C.M., van Amerongen W.E. (2003) Atraumatic perspective of ART. Psychological and physiological aspects of treatment with and without rotary instruments. *Community Dent. Oral Epidemiol.*; 31:15-20.

Seale N.S., Casamassimo P.S. (2003) Access to dental care for children in the United States. A survey of general practitioners. *J. Am. Dent Assoc.*; 134:1630-1640.

Shidara E.K., McGlothlin J.D., Kobayashi S. (2007) A vicious cycle in the oral health status of schoolchildren in a primary school in rural Cambodia. *Int. J. Dent Hyg*; 5: 165-173.

Simonsen R.J. (1996) Glass ionomer as fissure sealant – a critical review. *J. Public Health Dent*; 56:146-149.

Simonsen R.J. (2002) Pit and fissure sealants: review of the literature. *Pediatr. Dent.*; 24: 393-414.

Tayfour D., Frencken J.E., van't Hof M.A., Beiruti N., Truin G.J. (2003) Effects of glass ionomer sealants in newly erupted first molars after 5 years: a pilot study. *Community Dent. Oral Epidemiol.*.; 31:314-319.

Tickle M., Milsom K., King D., Kearney-Mitchell P., Blinkhorn A. (2002) The fate of the carious primary teeth of children who regularly attend the general dental service. *Brit. Dent J.*; 192: 219-223.

Timis T., Danila I. (2005) Socioeconomic status and oral health. *J. Prevent Med.*; 13: 116-121.

Topaloglu-Ak A., Eden E., Frencken J.E. (2007) Perceived dental anxiety among schoolchildren treated for dental caries in primary molars through three caries removal approaches. *J. App. Oral. Sci.*; 15: 235-240.

Torppa-Saarinen E., Seppå L. (1990) Short-term retention of glass-ionomer fissure sealants. *Proc. Finn. Dent. Soc.*; 86: 83-88.

Vallejos-Sánchez A.A., Medina-Solís C.E., Casanova-Rosado J.F., Maupomé G., Minaya-Sánchez M., Pérez-Olivares S. (2006) Dental fluorosis in cohorts born before, during, and after the national salt fluoridation program in a community in Mexico. *Acta Odontol. Scand.*; 64: 209-213.

van Amerongen J.P., van Amerongen W.E., Watson T.F., Opdam N.J.M., Roeters F.J.M., Bittermann D., Kidd E.A.M. (2008) Restoring the tooth: 'the seal is the deal'. In: Fejerskov O. and Kidd E. (eds). Dental caries; the disease and its management. Oxford: Blackwell Munksgaard Ltd; p 385.

van Bochove J.A., van Amerongen W.E. (2006) The influence of restorative treatment approaches and the use of local anaesthesia, on the children's discomfort. *Eur. Arch. Ped. Dent.*; 7:11-16.

van 't Hof M.A., Frencken J.E., van Palenstein Helderman W.H., Holmgren C.J. (2006) The ART approach for managing dental caries: A meta-analysis. *Int. Dent. J.;* 56:345-351.

Varenne B., Petersen P.E, Ouattara S. (2004) Oral health status of children and adults in urban and rural areas of Burkina Faso, Africa. *Int. Dent. J.;* 54: 83-89.

Weerheijm K.L., Kreulen C.M., Gruythuisen R.J. (1996) Comparison of retentative qualities of two glass-ionomer cements used as fissure sealants. *J. Dent. Child*; 63: 265-267.

Welin-Neilands J., Sevensater G. (2007) Acid tolerance of biofilm cells of streptococcus mutans. *Appl. Environ. Microbiol.*; 73: 5633-5638.

Whelton H., O'Mullane D. (2001) The use of combinations of caries preventive procedures. *J. Dent. Edu;* 65: 1110-1113.

Whelton H. (2004) Overview of the impact of changing global patterns of dental caries experience on caries clinical trials. *J. Dent. Res.*; 83 Spec No C:C29-34.

White J.M., Eakle W.S. (2000) Rationale and treatment approach in minimally invasive dentistry. *J. Am. Dent. Assoc.*; 131: 13S-19S.

Williams B., Laxton L,. Holt R.D., Winter G.B. (1996) Fissure sealants: a 4-year clinical trial comparing an experimental glass polyalkenoate cement with a bis glycidyl methacrylate resin used as fissure sealants. *Br. Dent. J.*; 180: 104-108.

Wilwerding T. (2001). .History of dentistry http://cudental.creigton.edu/htm/ history2001.pdf.

Yee R., Holmgren C., Mulder J., Lama D., Walker D., van Palenstein Helderman W.H. (2009) Efficacy of silver diamine fluoride for Arresting Caries Treatment. *J. Dent. Res* 88: 644-647.

Yee R., Sheiham A. (2002) The burden of restorative dental treatment for children in Third World countries. *Int. Dent. J.*; 52:1-9.

Yengopal V., Mickenaustch S. (2009) Caries preventive effect of casein phosphopeptide-amorphous calcium phosphate (CPP-ACP): a meta-analysis. *Acta Odontol. Scand.*; 21: 1-12.

Yengopal V., Mickenautsch S., Bezerra A.C., Leal S.C. (2009) Caries-preventive effect of glass ionomer and resin-based fissure sealants on permanent teeth: a meta-analysis. *J. Oral. Sci.*; 51:373-382.

Yengopal V., Chitkte U.M., Mickenaustsch S., Oliveira L.B., Bhayat A. (2010) Salt fluoridation: a meta-analysis of its efficacy for caries prevention. *South Afr. Dent. J.;* 65: 60-64, 66-67.

Yeung A., Hitchings J.L., Macfarlane T.V., Threfall A., Tickle M., Glenny A.M. Fluoridated milk for preventing dental caries. Cochrane database for systematic review. In Cochrane Library, Issue 3, Art. No. CD 003876. DOI: 10.1002/14651858.

Yeung C.A. (2011) Efficacy of salt fluoridation. *Evid Based Dent*; 12:17-18.

Zero D. (2008) Are sugar substitutes also anticariogenic? *J. Am. Dent. Assoc.*; 139:9S-10S.

Zhang Q., van Palenstein Helderman W.H., van't Hof M.A., Truin G.J. (2006) Chlorhexidine varnish for preventing dental caries in children, adolescents and young adults: a systematic review. *Eur. J. Oral Sci.;* 114:449-455.

In: Oral Health Care for Socially Disadvantaged Communities   ISBN: 978-1-62948-287-3
Editors: F.K. Kahabuka, E.N. Kikwilu and I. Anderson © 2013 Nova Science Publishers, Inc.

Chapter IV

Gingival and Periodontal Diseases in Socially Disadvantaged Communities

Elifuraha G. Mumghamba[1] and Evelyn G. Wagaiyu[2]
[1] School of Dentistry, Muhimbili University of Health and Allied Sciences
[2] School of Dental Sciences, College of Health Sciences, University of Nairobi

4.1. Introduction

Periodontal diseases (periodontitis) are among the most widespread diseases in mankind (WHO 1978). Periodontal diseases are inflammatory diseases and poly-microbial infections that affect the supporting tissues of the teeth and causes progressive destruction of periodontal ligaments, loss of connective tissues attachment, periodontal pocket formation and alveolar bone loss (Page and Eke 2007, Armitage and Robertson 2009). However, periodontal diseases always start as gingival diseases whereby at a certain unknown time it may advance to overt periodontal disease. Gingival disease itself is defined as an inflammatory condition of the gingival tissues which constitute the superficial supporting structures of the tooth, as opposed to periodontal diseases that affect the deep supporting structures of the tooth. Gingivitis that is associated with dental plaque is the most common form of gingival disease (Aldred and Bartold 1998). It can be modified by local factors, systemic factors, medications and malnutrition. Non-plaque induced gingival lesions are oral manifestations of systemic conditions that produce lesions in the tissues of the periodontium. These diseases like the specific bacterial, viral and fungal infections of the gingiva are rare and mainly seen in lower socioeconomic groups like the underprivileged in developing countries and immunocompromised individuals (Holmstrup 1999).

Periodontitis is defined as an inflammatory disease of the supporting tissues of the teeth caused by specific microorganisms or groups of specific microorganisms resulting in progressive destruction of the periodontal ligament, alveolar bone with pocket formation, recession or both (Lindhe et al. 1999). The destructive changes seen in periodontal diseases are brought about by the interplay between the microbial dental biofilm at the gingival margin and the host response (Page 1998). The extent to which progression will take place depends on the sex, age, race, socioeconomic status, education, psychological symptoms and personality factors, genetic factors, nutritional factors, and systemic condition. All these risk factors and risk indicators have been studied extensively over the years (Albander 2002).

Several varieties of periodontal diseases are recognized today for example aggressive periodontitis, chronic periodontitis, necrotizing ulcerative gingivitis/periodontitis, and periodontitis as a manifestation of systemic diseases (Armitage 1999). Periodontal diseases are viewed as infectious diseases (Slots et al. 1978, Socransky and Haffajee 1997, Mombelli 2003). The relationship between the biofilm and gingivitis has been well documented starting with the experimental gingivitis in man (Loe et al.1965).

Chronic periodontitis, the most frequently occurring form of periodontitis, is an infectious disease resulting in the inflammation of the supporting tissues of the teeth. The inflammatory response seen in chronic periodontitis is initiated by bacterial products, mainly Lipopolysaccharides (LPS) but propagated by the host. The host response provides tissue resistance to bacterial invasion but also initiates mechanisms that contribute to tissue damage. It has become clear that the host derived enzymes known as matrix metalloproteinases (MMPs) as well as changes in osteoclast activity driven by cytokines and prostanoids cause most of the tissue destruction in the periodontium (Offenbacher 1996). Chronic Peridontitis is characterized by high concentrations of MMPs, cytokines and prostanoids in the periodontal tissues whereas the opposite is present in periodontal health (Page 1999).

Chronic periodontitis in the underprivileged will follow the same pattern as any other group where only a fraction of the population suffers from the severe form of the disease (Baelum, 1996). If left untreated, periodontal diseases may result into further destruction of the gingiva, periodontal fibres, alveolar bone and finally tooth loss after a long or short period of time depending on the severity of the specific periodontal disease entity.

After reading this chapter on management of gingival and periodontal diseases in socially disadvantaged communities, the reader will be able to:

1) Describe the current classification of periodontal diseases
2) Explain the risk factors for periodontal diseases
3) Describe the prevalence of Periodontal diseases in different continents
4) Manage periodontal diseases among the socially disadvantaged communities.

4.2. Classification of Periodontal Diseases and Conditions

Classification of Periodontal diseases is a long-standing dilemma. Based on the understanding of the natural history of periodontal diseases (PD), over time different classifications have been proposed and used. Previously Periodontal diseases were earlier considered as a single disease entity whereas today with better understanding of the diseases, it is understood to be more than one entity thus known as periodontal diseases (Armitage 2002). The latest classification of periodontal diseases was internationally developed and accepted as a consensus in 1999 at the International Workshop for the Classification of Periodontal Diseases organized by the American Academy of Periodontology (AAP) (Armitage 1999). The AAP 1999 classification of periodontal diseases (PD) addressed most but not all of the short- comings of the previous classifications for example abolishing the use of age, early- versus adult-onset of PD in the classification, introduced a new category of gingival diseases as well as periodontal abscesses, and addressed the issue of heterogenicity of the rapidly progressing periodontitis, refractory periodontitis and prepubertal periodontitis (Table 4.1). Periodontal diseases can also be on the basis of extent and severity. Extent can be described as "localized" when the sites involved are not more than 30% and termed as generalized when the involved sites exceeds 30%. Severity in terms of the clinical attachment loss (CAL) can be categorized as "slight" when 1-2 mm CAL is observed, moderate where there is up to 3-4 mm CAL and severe in instances where there will be CAL more or equal to 4-5mm.

Table 4.1. Classification of periodontal diseases and conditions

1. Gingival Diseases

1.1 Dental plaque-induced gingival diseases

1.1.1 Gingivitis associated with dental plaque only
    1.1.1.1 Without other local contributing factors
    1.1.1.2 with local contributing factors

1.1.2 Gingival diseases modified by systemic factors
    1.1.2.1 Associated with endocrine system
    1.1.2.1.1 Puberty associated gingivitis
    1.1.2.1.2 Menstrual cycle associated gingivitis
    1.1.2.1.3 Pregnancy associated gingivitis
    1.1.2.1.4 Diabetes mellitus associated gingivitis
    1.1.2.2 Associated with blood dyscrasias
    1.1.2.2.1 Leukaemia associated gingivitis
    1.1.2.2.2 Other

1.1.3 Gingival diseases modified by medications
    1.1.3.1 Drug influenced gingival diseases
    1.1.3.1.1Drug influenced gingival enlargements
    1.1.3.1.2 Drug influenced gingivitis

1.1.4 Gingival diseases modified by malnutrition
    1.1.4.1 Ascobic acid-deficiency gingivitis
    1.1.4.2.Other

1.2 Non-plaque-induced gingival diseases
1.2.1 Gingival diseases of specific bacterial origin
1.2.1.1 *Neisseria gonorrhoea*-associated lesions
1.2.1.2 *Treponema pallidum*-associated lesions
1.2.1.3 Strptococcal species – associated lesion
1.2.1.4 Other

1.2.2 Gingival diseases of viral origin
1.2.2.1 Herpes virus infections
1.2.2.1.1 Primary herpetic gingivostomatitis
1.2.2.1.2 Recurrent oral herpes
1.2.2.1.3 Varicella-zoster infections
1.2.2.2 Other

    1.2.3 Gingival diseases of fungal origin
    1.2.3.1 *Candida*-species infections
1.2.3.1.1 Generalized gingival candidosis
    1.2.3.2 Linear gingival erythema
    1.2.3.3 Histoplasmosis
    1.2.3.4 Other

    1.2.4 Gingival lesions of genetic origin
    1.2.4.1 Hereditary gingival stomatosis
    1.2.4.2 Other

1.2.5 Gingival manifestations of systemic conditions
    1.2.5.1 Mucocutaneous disorders
    1.2.5.1.1 Linchen planus
    1.2.5.1.2 Pemphigoid
    1.2.5.1.3 Pemphigus vulgaris
    1.2.5.1.4 Erythema multiforme
    1.2.5.1.5 Lupus erythmatous
    1.2.5.1.6 Drug induced
    1.2.5.1.7 Other
    1.2.5.2 Allergic reactions
    1.2.5.2.1 Dental restorative materials
    1.2.5.2.1.1 Mercury
    1.2.5.2.1.2 Nickel
    1.2.5.2.1.3 Acrylic
    1.2.5.2.1.4 Other
    1.2.5.2.2 Reactions attributable to
    1.2.5.2.2.1 Toothpaste/dentifrices
    1.2.5.2.2.2 Mouthrinses/mouthwashes
    1.2.5.2.2.3 Chewing gum additives
    1.2.5.2.2.4 Foods and additives
    1.2.5.2.3 Other

1.2.6 Traumatic lesions (factitious, iatrogenic, accidental)
    1.2.6.1 Chemical injury
    1.2.6.2 Physical injury
    1.2.6.3 Thermal injury

    1.2.7 Foreign body necrosis
    1.2.8 Not otherwise specified (NOS)

Table 4.1. (Continued).

2. Chronic Periodontitis
Localized
Generalized

3. Aggressive Periodontitis
Localized
Generalized

4. Periodontitis as a Manifestation of Systemic Diseases
4.1 Associated with haematological disorders
4.1.1 Acquired neutropenia
4.1.2 Leukemias
4.1.3 Other
4.2 Associated with haematological disorders
4.2.1 Familiar and cyclic neutron penia
4.2.2 Down syndrome
4.2.3 Leucocyte adhesion deficiency syndrome
4.2.4 Papillon-Lefevre syndrome
4.2.5 Chediac-Higashi syndrome
4.2.6 Histiocytosis syndrome
4.2.7 Glycogen storage disease
4.2.8 Infantile genetic agranulocytosis
4.2.9 Cohen syndrome
4.2.10 Ehlers-Danlos syndrome (Type IV and VIII)
4.2.11 Hypophosphatasia
4.2.12 Other
4.3 Not otherwise specified (NOS)

5. Necrotizing Periodontal diseases
5.1 Necrotizing ulcerative gingivitis (NUG)
5.2 Necrotizing ulcerative Periodontitis (NUP)

6. Abscesses of the Periodontium
6.1 Gingival abscess
6.2 Periodontal abscess
6.3 Pericoronal abscess

7. Periodontitis Associated with Endodontic Lesions
7.1 Endodontic-periodontal lesion
7.2 Periodontal - Endodontic- lesion
7.3 Combined lesion

8. Developmental or Acquired Deformities and conditions
8.1 Localized tooth related factors that predispose to plaque induced gingival diseases or periodontitis
8.1.1 Tooth anatomic factors
8.1.2 Dental restorations/appliances
8.1.3 Root fractures
8.1.4 Cervical root resorption and cementum tears

8.2 Mucogingival deformities and conditions around the teeth
8.2.1 Gingival /Soft tissue recession
8.2.1.1 Facial and lingual surfaces
8.2.1.2 Interproximal (papillary)
8.2.2 Lack of keratinized gingiva
8.2.3 Decreased vestibular depth
8.2.4 Aberrant frenum/muscle position
8.2.5 Gingival excess
8.2.5.1 Pseudopocket
8.2.5.1 Inconsitent gingival margin
8.2.5.1 Excess gingival display
8.2.6 Abnormal colour

9. Mucogingival deformities and conditions on edentulous ridges occlussal trauma.
9.1 Vertical and /or horizontal
9.2 lack of gingival/keratinized tissue
9.3 Gingival and soft tissue enlargement
9.4 Aberrant frenum/ muscle position
9.5 Decreased vesticular depth
9.6 Abnormal colour

10. Occlusal trauma
10.1 Primary occlusal trauma
10.2 Secondary occlusal trauma

Data source: Armitage GC. Annals of Periodontology 1999; 4:1-6.

Epidemiology of Periodontal Diseases in Socially Disadvantaged Communities

The following section is going to describe the prevalence of periodontal diseases in different continents. However, the reports are made by different researchers using different methodology and therefore caution is needed to interpret such information appropriately.

4.3.1. Global Epidemiology of Periodontal Diseases in Socially Disadvantaged Communities

Occurrence of different forms of periodontal diseases is a global problem (Albandar and Rams 2002). Therefore, proper management of periodontal diseases taking into account all the risk factors is justified. The socially deprived populations, depending on the dictating situation, may include children, elderly people, the poor ones, illiterate or least educated, of low socio-economic status, rural residence and others (Chapter one).

The presence of socially disadvantaged populations (SDP) is a world-wide problem that is exhibited by inequalities in access and utilization of oral health services in different countries in Africa (Lalloo et al. 2004, Okullo et al. 2004, Nunn et al. 2008), Asia (Garcha et al. 2010, Somkotra and Detsomboonrat (2009), Europe (Mamai-Homata et al. 2010, Syrjälä et al. 2010), and United States (Alfaro and Ahluwalia 2010, Wells et al. 2010, Finlayson et al. 2010).

4.3.2. Periodontal Diseases in Socially Disadvantaged communities in Africa

The occurrence of periodontal diseases among the socially disadvantaged communities in Africa show for example that, African tribal ethnicity as compared to afro-Arabs had higher prevalence of periodontal attachment loss and aggressive periodontitis among high school students aged in 13 to 19 years old in Sudan (Elamin et al. 2010). Also the prevalence of periodontal diseases was high among the 12-15 years child population in the underserved regions in Tunisia (Abid 2004). In Tanzania, children aged 7-22 years who were handicapped most of their teeth had gingivitis and calculus and thus necessitated to have scaling and polishing for more than eighty percent of the study participants (Simon et al. 2008). Also another study by Lembariti and coworkers showed that Tanzanian population which was actually deprived of regular dental care had people with high tendency of bleeding on probing (Lembariti et al. 1997). In Kenyan rural population, in general, it has been shown that although many patients have heavy plaque and calculus deposits, minimal destruction of the periodontium occurs and this is mainly recession that takes place (Baelum et al. 1988). In Ethiopian child population who were 12 years and above, periodontal diseases affected more than half of the study subjects, being significantly higher in males, those having 'Injera' as staple diet, and those with poor oral hygiene (Simon et al. 2003). The occurrence of periodontal diseases in child and adult populations in some countries in East, South, and West Africa, have been found to be severe in the rural as compared to the urban population (Mumghamba et al. 1995, Luhanga and Ntabaye 2001, Brindle et al. 2000, Sofola et al. 2003, Varenne et al. 2004). Furthermore, periodontal diseases have been ranked as number two of the causes of tooth loss among the disadvantaged rural population in East and West African populations (Mumghamba and Fabian 2005, Oginni 2005, Esan et al. 2010).

Acute Necrotizing Ulcerative Gingitivitis (ANUG) has been diagnosed among the poor and malnourished population in Nigeria and other developing countries with persistently low socioeconomic status, parasitic infections and poor nutritional status, (Taiwo 1995, 1996, Folayan 2004). The occurrence of ANUG in some populations has shown some seasonal variations for example in South and East Africa (Arendorf et al. 2001, Kaimenyi 1999). The acute necrotizing gingivitis if left untreated may lead to a more serious infectious disease of the oral-facial and other neighboring structures known as noma or cancrum oris. Noma affects mostly children aged 2-16 years particularly in sub-Saharan Africa whereby the key risk factors have been found to include malnutrition, close residential proximity to livestock, deplorable environmental sanitation, poor oral hygiene, poverty and infectious diseases for example measles (Enwonwu et al. 1999). Countries that have been affected by noma include Nigeria, Senegal (Idigbe et al. 1999, Ndiaye 1999).

4.3.3. Periodontal Diseases in Socially Disadvantaged communities in Asia

A survey among adults in a deprived district of Karachi has shown that over half the subjects suffered from poor oral health and that female gender was significantly associated with bleeding gums and periodontitis (Tanwir et al. 2006). A survey of oral health status in Kuwait showed that periodontal diseases are common, affecting the majority of the population and that disadvantaged groups of the population should be given the priority when focusing on national oral health care efforts (Behbehani and Scheutz 2004). In Jordan, the reasons for tooth loss in disadvantaged population were due to periodontal diseases then caries (Sayegh et al. 2004). Among the disadvantaged communities in Indonesia who were deprived of regular dental care, it has been found that main risk markers for periodontal diseases progression, has been age, amount of subgingival calculus and subgingival presence of Aggregatibacter actinomycetemcomitans were identified as (Timmerman et al. 2000).

4.3.4. Periodontal Diseases in Socially Disadvantaged communities in Europe

In disadvantaged communities in South Wales, United Kingdom, periodontal diseases were ranked as second to dental caries in relations to causes of tooth extraction (Richard et al. 2005). A study in the Netherlands, has shown that periodontitis aggregates in families that are deprived from regular dental care (van der Velden et al. 1993). In croatia, the greatest burden of oral diseases such as periodontal diseases were found in the socially marginalized population that included those living in small rural villages and post-war areas that was characterized by poverty, low education and low oral hygine habits (Spalj et al. 2008). In inner district of London in an area that is highly disadvantaged area where immigrants from Bangladeshi were living, it was found that children aged 7-15 years had poorer gingival conditions than the Caucasian citizens (Laher 1990).

4.3.5. Periodontal Diseases in Socially Disadvantaged communities Australia

In Australia, indigenous adults are among the disadvantaged groups and public dental patients had worse periodontal health than their counterparts the non-Indigenous patients (Brennan et al. 2007). Studies on older Australians as one of the disadvantaged communities, have shown that about one third of the dentate persons had a serious periodontal condition, defined as the presence of four or more teeth with at least 5 mm or more of periodontal attachment loss and periodontal pocketing of 4 mm or more at one or more of those teeth (Slade et al. 1993). Therefore, a strategy aimed at closing up the gap in health services provision, involved establishment of sustainable programmes to serve disadvantaged communities in the country (Kruger et al. 2010).

4.3.6. Periodontal Diseases in Socially Disadvantaged communities in America

In America, persons from socially disadvantaged groups that encompassed low level of education, homeless, the unemployed or recent immigrants, were more likely to have advanced periodontal diseases and and subsequently increasing complexity of periodontal treatment needs than their better endowed counterparts (Dye and Vargas 2002, Clarke et al. 1996). Economically and socially disadvantaged older adults in United States were more likely to have untreated periodontal diseases than their equivalents (Dolan and Atchison 1993). Poverty (low-income) and residence in a disadvantaged neighborhood in United States were associated with higher odds (1.8-fold) of severe periodontitis among Caucasians (Borrel et al. 2006). The disadvantaged and poor in United States did not fully benefit from the community water fluoridation programs in terms of reduced tooth decay as well as periodontal diseases as they were living in the underserved areas (Milgrom and Reisine 2000). Coming from a more disadvantaged background was found to be associated with the deterioration of self-perceived oral health status assessed over a period of time among the community-dwelling Canadians aged 50 years (Locker and Jokovic 1997).

4.4. Burden of Gingival and Periodontal Diseases among the Socially Disadvantaged communities

Periodontal diseases have been considered to be among the most important global oral health burdens (Petersen et al. 2005). In the general population, the prevalence of gingivitis particularly, the plaque associated gingivitis in many populations approaches 99%. Worldwide, the burden of severe form of periodontitis that may lead to tooth loss is found in about 5-20% of the adult population (Petersen et al. 2005). Using the Community Periodontal Index of Periodontal Needs (CPITN), (WHO, 1987) that was later limited to Community Periodontal Index (CPI), in Africa, the burden of gingivitis is mostly estimated to be about 80-99%, and that of overt periodontitis ranges from about 1% to 82% where the advanced, severe form of periodontitis did show a very wide range, from less than 1% to about 44%, depending on the age group studied and periodontal diseases diagnosis threshold (Mumghamba 2009). Furthermore, aggressive periodontititis has been reported to be high among males (about 34%) and low in females (about 22%) in one of the East African child population (Albandar 2002).

In Asia for example, among the tea labourers, who have never been exposed to the treatment or prevention of periodontal diseases, it was evident that there are three subpopulations: those who showed no evidence of periodontal diseases progression beyond gingivitis (11%), those who had moderate progression (81%), and those who had rapid progression (8%) of periodontal diseases (Loe et al. 1986). When the ratio of the poor oral health services infra-structure and the oral health personnel among the developing countries where most of the disadvantaged communities live, are compared to developed countries,

1:150,000 compared to 1:2000 (Petersen et al. 2005), it then becomes obvious that much of the problems are left un-attended.

4.4.1. Gingival Diseases

Gingival diseases can be suspected by an individual if blood stain is noted on biting a piece of bread, fruits, sugarcane and even on tooth brushing. This should be considered as an important signal that the gum tissue is having a long standing problem unless the blood stain is arising from a traumatic wound on the gum. Serious issues may be seen as spontaneous gum bleeding in the sense that when one attempts to exert intra-oral suction forces using his/her own masticatory muscles can be able to express some amount of blood oozing from the gingival tissues. Gum bleeding in such a population is sometimes misinterpreted as lack of vitamin C. Such explanation is inappropriate due to the fact that the SDP are most of the time living on naturally available fruits rather than processed foods. It is well known that the accumulation of microbial biofilm at the gingival margin will trigger an inflammatory and immune response of the gingivae leading to gingival inflammation and if treatment is not sort, eventually progress to the development of periodontitis but only in a fraction of the population. Gingivitis and periodontitis are the two major inflammatory conditions affecting the periodontium.

Gingival diseases affect the gingival tissue which is part of the periodontium. However, this disease entity does not involve the underlying deep structures. For example, Necrotizing Ulcerative Gingivitis (NUG) affects the interdental papillae of the gingival tissues causing necrosis (Figure 4.1), if it involves the deep structures then it becomes, "Necrotizing Ulcerative Periodontitis (NUP).

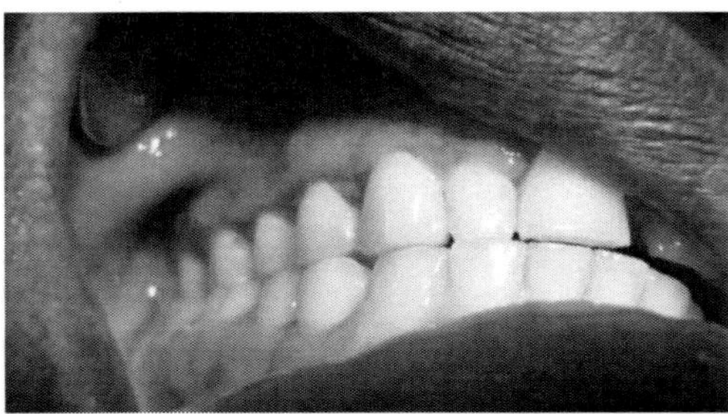

Figure 4.1. Necrotizing Ulcerative Gingivitis (NUG) in its early stage on buccal interdental papilla of teeth no. 13-16 on adult female patient (Courtesy of E.G. Mumghamba).

4.4.2. Periodontal Diseases

Based on clinical and radiological features, there are varieties of periodontal diseases that can be recognized. These include for example the aggressive periodontitis, chronic periodontitis and the periodontitis associated with systemic conditions.

4.4.2.1. Aggressive Periodontitis

Aggressive periodontitis (AP) is a severe type of periodontal disease that is characterized by deep periodontal pocket (5 mm or more) and severe alveolar bone loss (2 mm or more) around the single or multi-rooted tooth mostly in otherwise systemically healthy individuals aged less than 30 years old, although older persons may sometimes be affected. Earlier classification of AP included terminologies such as juvenile periodontitis (Manson and Lehner 1974) and early onset periodontitis.

The alveolar bone loss can be localized in at least two teeth of the permanent dentition, especially first permanent molar and incisors (Figure 4.2). Also it may spread to involve several teeth around all the quadrants (Figure 4.3).

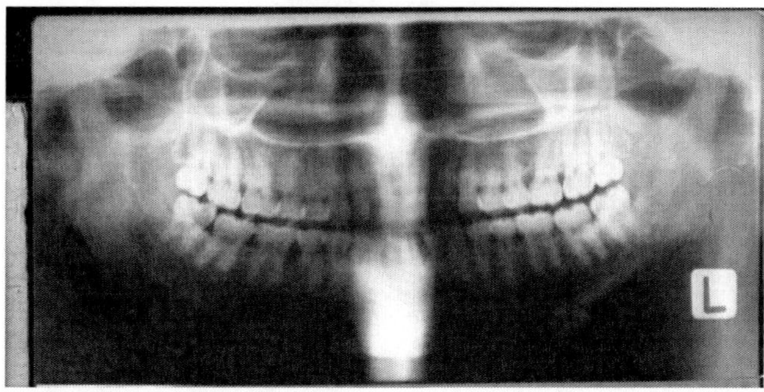

Figure 4.2. Aggressive periodontitis – Localized on 46 and 26 mesial approximal surface (Courtesy of E.G. Mumghamba).

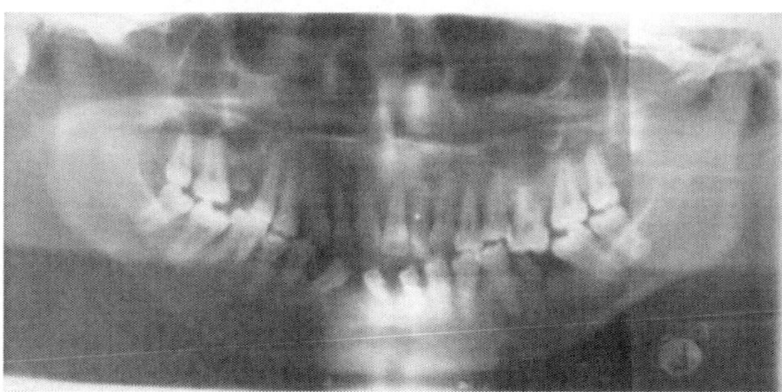

Figure 4.3. Aggressive periodontitis – Generalized type in a 21 years old female (Courtesy of E.G. Mumghamba).

In some other cases the first and second molars may also be involved at different severity (Figure 4.4). In localized aggressive periodontitis (LAP), obvious clinical inflammation is not evident despite the presence of deep periodontal pockets and extensive bone loss. Microbiologically, it has been suggested that this is a result of high number of *Aggregatibacter (formerly Actinobacillus) actinomycetemcomitans* (A.a.) and *Porphyromonas gingivalis* (p.g.).

The onset is sudden and the lesion progresses fast within a short time. The presence of predisposing factors in particular microbial plaque and dental calculus in this case is usually not in abundance.

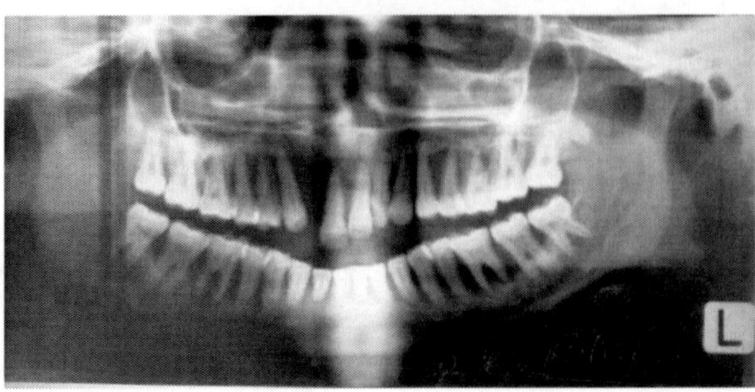

Figure 4.4. Aggressive periodontitis – generalized type in a 20 years old female (Courtecy of E.G. Mumghamba).

Therefore, in examination, it will be found that the amount of plaque and calculus are not commensurate with the deep periodontal pockets and extensive loss of the alveolar bone around the tooth/teeth involved, whereby the age of onset is around puberty (Baer 1971). Other features of LAP include tooth mobility of the mandibular and maxillary incisors as well as first molars, with or without tooth sensitivity and dull pain during mastication (Novak and Novak 2006a). The pathognomonic radiological features of LAP include vertical alveolar bone loss around the first molars and incisors among healthy individuals at or around puberty. Generalized aggressive periodontitis (GAP) affects at least three teeth of the permanent dentition in addition to the first molars as well as incisors. In this case there is severe gingival inflammation, ulceration, gingival bleeding, suppuration, extensive and advanced alveolar bone loss and these individuals may have systemic manifestations as weight loss and mental depression. However, mild forms of GAP are also possible.

Although there is no clear sex predilection in the occurrence of AP, in persons of African descent it has been reported to be more in males than in females, while in Caucasians it is more prevalent among females than in males. In developed countries, the prevalence of AP is less than 1%, whereas in developing countries it has been reported to be as high as 8% in Sri Lanka (Loe et al. 1986) and even shocking figures of up to 29% in Uganda (Albandar et al. 2002). In Kenya, the prelence of aggressive periodontitis among young people was reported as 0.28% in a study carried out in 1992 (Wagaiyu and Wagaiyu, 1992).

4.4.2.2. Chronic Periodontitis

Chronic periodontitis (CP) is defined as "an infectious disease resulting in inflammation within the supporting tissues of the teeth, progressive attachment loss, and alveolar bone loss" (Flemming 1999). Earlier, this disease entity was classified as "adult periodontitis" or "chronic adult periodontitis" (Novak and Novak 2006b). As opposed to aggressive periodontitis, chronic periodontitis is considered to be a slowly progressive disease, and much more prevalent among adults although the chronic form may also be found among young adults as well as in children. Long standing irritation from microbial plaque accumulation and dental calculus accounts for the gradual development of the periodontal diseases into a chronic form. In chronic periodontitis, due to the slow progressive nature, the alveolar bone loss is mainlyof horizontal type, (Figure 4.5 and Figure 4.6) rather than the vertical type of bone loss seen more frequently in aggressive periodontitis.

The characteristic features of CP includes presence of supragingival and subgingival plaque, calculus, gingival bleeding, periodontal pockets, periodontal attachment loss, gingival recession, alveolar bone loss around the teeth, tooth mobility, drifting of teeth, development of a diastema acquired in adult life, and sometimes in severe cases may present with pus discharge.

Pain is not a major feature in CP and therefore many patients are not aware of the problem unless they have experienced other symptoms like gum bleeding during tooth brushing, and fresh blood stains on eating/biting fruits and even slices of bread.

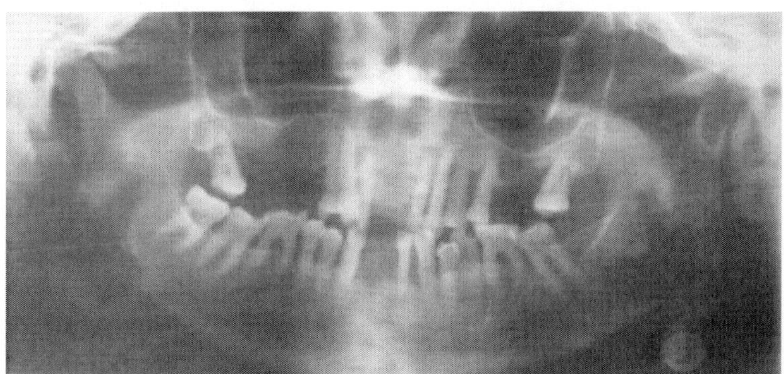

Figure 4.5. Chronic periodontitis –advanced stage with horizontal bone loss and furactional involvement (grade III) in tooth no. 36 and 46 in a 65 years old female (Courtesy of E.G. Mumghamba).

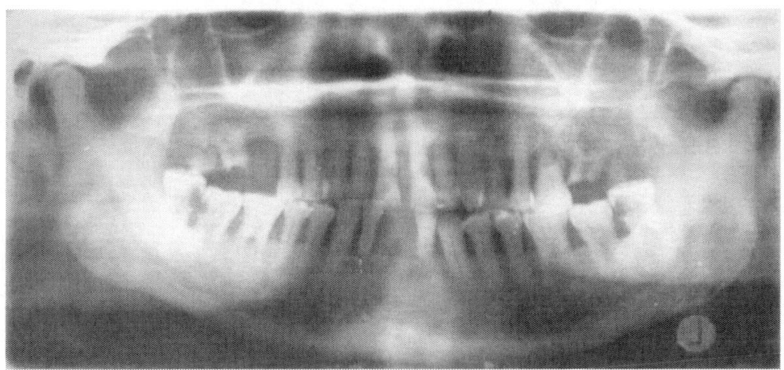

Figure 4.6. Chronic periodontitis with horizontal alveolar bone loss and furcational involvement (grade III) on tooth no. 26 and 46 in a 60 years old male (Courtesy of E.G. Mumghamba).

4.4.2.3. Periodontitis as Associated with Systemic Conditions

Periodontal diseases may be a manifestation of systemic conditions or may have an effect on the occurrence of systemic diseases. Situations where periodontal diseases may be a manifestation of systemic conditions include blood diseases such as leukaemias, and genetic disorders that include Down's syndrome, familiar and cyclic neutropenia, Chediak Higashi syndrome, and Papillon Leferve syndrome (Armitage 1999). Effect of periodontal diseases on systemic conditions may be seen in diabetes mellitus, coronary heart disease (CHD)/arthcrosclerosis, stroke, acute respiratory tract infections and adverse pregnancy outcomes (low birth weight, pre-eclampsia (Mealey and Klokkevold 2006).

4.4.2.4. Bad Mouth Breath

Bad mouth breath (BMB) refers to an unpleasant or fowl smell coming from the mouth during the time of exhalation or breathing out of air. In the general population, BMB is attributed to poor oral hygiene, tongue coating (Figure 4.7) as a result of not cleaning the tongue as well as putrefaction and exudation in tissue pockets in periodontal diseases (Miyazaki et al. 1995, Liu et al. 2006). The bad mouth breath include include other terminologies such as breath malodour, oral malodour, foetor ex ore and halitosis.

The main cause of BMB are volatile sulphur compounds (VSCs) particularly hydrogen sulphide, methylmercaptan, dimethyl-sulphide, and organic acids (Soder et al. 2000) from putrefying oral bacteria. There is also a non-oral human malodour that can arise from diabetes mellitus, kidney and liver diseases (Sanz et al. 2001, Quirynen and Steenberghe 2006). A false type of BMB where there are no gases involved as it is only an imagination is named psychosomatic breath malodor, halitophobia, pseudo-halitosis and cannot be objectively determined (Yaegaki and Coil 2000).

Most of the time an individual having BMB, do not sense it for him/herself unless such problem is disclosed by those who are around. Since it is thought that it is an embarrassment to tell someone that he/she is having BMB, the problem often goes unreported.

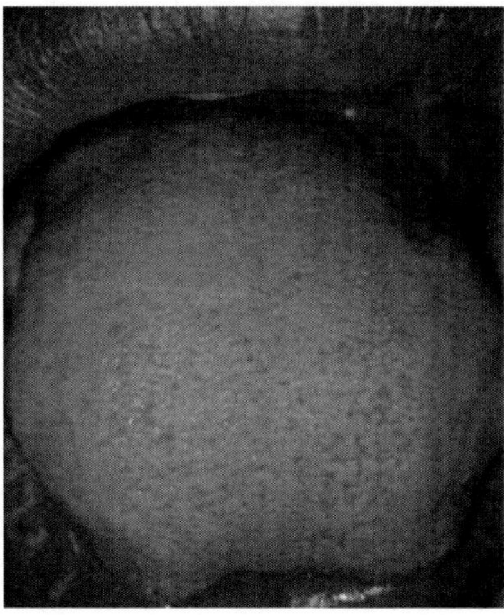

Figure 4.7. Tongue – unclean, yellowish white in colour (Courtesy of E.G. Mumghamba).

Furthermore, BMB is not seen or rather it does not appear to be a public health problem. Given the fact that in SDP poor environment by itself causes bad smell from un-sanitary environment, even if BMB is very prevalent, it may be considered as part and parcel of the polluted environment (Wing et al. 2008, Song et al. 2009).

4.5. The Role of Risk Assessment and Periodontal Disease Management

Risk factors are those correlates that have been confirmed in longitudinal studies whereas risk indicators are those identified in cross-sectional studies. Risk indicators are not always confirmed in longitudinal studies as risk factors (Timmerman and van der Weijden 2006). Some risk factors through various studies have been associated with periodontal diseases development. Assessment of these risk factors may help in clinical decision making and help the patient in understanding the importance of following a satisfactory oral hygiene regimen to minimize the chances of developing the disease. In addition to improving clinical decision making, risk assessment may reduce the need for complex periodontal therapy, improve patient outcomes and ultimately reduce oral health care costs (Page et al. 2003, Cutress et al. 1982). The following are the recognized risk factors for periodontal disease and that will need to be controlled as part of the managemet strategy against the disease.

a) Oral hygiene has been shown to be associated with gingivitis in many cross sectional, longitudinal and experimental studies (Baelum et al. 1986, Baelum et al. 1988, Position paper 1996).

b) Elderly: The older individuals have been shown epidemiologically to have more disease but this is attributed to the cumulative effect of disease over the years rather than an increase in age-related susceptibility (Baelum et al. 2003). Thus it is important to emphasize the importance of maintaining a good oral hygiene regimen through out life.

c) Gender: Males have consistently been found to have more disease than females. This may not be due to increase in susceptibility but more to do with behaviour (US Public Health Service 1979)

d) Socio-economic status has been associated with gingivitis but not periodontitis (Burt et al. 1990) both in developing countries and in industrialized countries it was found that lower socio-economic status was not associated with severity of periodontitis (Baelum et al. 2003).

e) Current disease status has also been associated with an increase in periodontal diseases susceptibility. Higher baseline scores for plaque, calculus and gingivitis has been reported in edentulous persons compared to age-matched dentate individuals. Periodontal attachment loss ≥ 4 mm and educational attainment were also found to be significant risk factors in the regression analysis (Burt et al. 1990).

f) Smoking has been identified by several studies to predispose to the development of Periodontal diseases (Zee 2009)

g) Diabetes has been associated with an increase in periodontal destruction when the glucose control is not well managed (Chávarry et al. 2009).

h) Putative periodontal pathogens: Slots et al. 1986 reported, in a retrospective study, a relationship between the presence of *Actinobacillus actinomycetemcomitans*, *Porphyromonas gingivalis* and *Prevotella intermedia* and progression of periodontal diseases.

The strategy to address these risk factors should follow the common risk factor approach whereby it is emphasized to handle risk factors that are responsible for the occurrence of more than one disease or condition. For example, in dealing with "tobscco smoking" by tobacco cessation programme, one will have addressed also the risk factor for lung cancer. Likewise, dietary counseling for dental diseases would address also the issue of diet in the management of diabetes mellitus that is also related to the occurrence of periodontal diseases.

Dealing with oral hygiene alone, this will have an effect on the occurrence of both periodontal diseases and dental caries. This common risk factor approach seems to be more cost-effective when compared to single risk factor approach.

4.6. Management of Gingival and Periodontal Diseases

Management of all gingival and periodontal diseases have a number of features in common. One, there is a need for proper control of microbial plaque that causes both gingival and periodontal diseases (Loe et al. 1965, Lindhe et al. 1986). Two, control of microbial plaque is followed by scaling and root planning. This is the mechanical removal of dental calculus on tooth surfaces both supra- and sub-gingivally, particularly on the crown, cervical margin and on root surfaces (Pattison and Pattison 2006). The goals of periodontal therapy are to preserve the natural dentition by keeping the periodontium healthy, and also to maintain comfort, aesthetics and function. A healthy periodontium is where there is absence of signs of inflammation like redness, swelling, suppuration and bleeding on probing. The patient should first receive a comprehensive examination which will lead to establishing a diagnosis, prognosis and the development of a treatment plan. The treatment plan is made in the light of the circumstances presented by each individual patient.

The periodontal treatment plan is usually divided into three phases and that are first, the initial or cause-related periodontal therapy; second, Corrective or definitive periodontal therapy; and thirdly, the maintenance or supportive periodontal therapy. The cause related periodontal therapy deals with the control and elimination of the causative agents and that is the control of plaque whereby the issue of oral hygiene is addressed as well as the removal of dental calculus (scaling and root planing) and plaque retentive factors. The corrective phase include treatment procedures that are geared to the correction and establishment of a conducive environment whereby plaque can be controlled adequately by the patient without much impediments, and that encompasses procedures like restorations of carious lesions that interferes with gingingival and periodontal health, and also periodontal surgery. The supportive periodontal therapy ensures that the disease do not reccurr and therefore is a surveillance and vigilant type of treatment.

In the under privileged, the issue of cost of treatment, number of visits and any medication recommended or prescribed will have to be taken into consideration. Additionally, depending on the type of job or business the individual is engaged in, availability to attend clinics may also need to be considered as well as the distance travelled to the services. Some individuals have to travel long distances to access dental clinics and this would affect compliance especially if they are required to attend several times. The issue of cost of transport will also require to be factored-in depending on the patient's socio-economic status.

The following are some major steps of a typical periodontal treatment plan that must be considered in the management of a periodontal patient (Cobb et al. 2003) and the *sequence of major phases* includes:

a)   Address acute periodontal problems and/or pain
b)   Review and update medical and dental histories

c)   Assessment of systemic risk factors and referral for medical consultation as needed
d)   Extraoral examination
e)   Oral cancer evaluation
f)   Assessment of periodontal risk and modifying factors
g)   Periodontal examination to include dental implants
h)   Dental examination to include occlusal relationships and dental implants
i)   Radiographic examination
j)   Establish a definitive diagnosis
k)   Generate a diagnosis-driven periodontal treatment plan and sequence of treatment
l)   Determine required adjunctive restorative, prosthetic, orthodontic, and/or endodontic treatments and sequence
m)   Execute Phase I therapy (anti-infective or nonsurgical therapy) with consideration given to adjunctive use of chemotherapeutic agents
n)   Re-evaluation (assessment) of Phase I therapy
o)   If end-points are not achieved, consider selective retreatment, need for surgical therapy, specialty referral, or use of adjunctive diagnostic aides, like microbial, genetic, and medical laboratory tests.
p)   Determine interval for periodontal maintenance and continued assessment of periodontal status.

However, management of periodontal problems in underprivileged may be limited to basics like; periodontal examination, establishing a diagnosis and prognosis, development of a treatment plan, simple treatment procedures and maintenance care. Tissue regeneration and provision of dental implants to replace extracted teeth form an integral part of periodontal therapy but may not be realistic in the underprivileged. In the underprivileged, outreach programs will form a better form of service to those with no access to health care and also provide education in oral health care matters thus enlighten the population.

Probing evaluations are an important diagnostic tool that can be used to help decide if therapy is needed and to evaluate treatment responses. However, they are flawed diagnostic assessments when predicting disease progression (Greestein 2006). Meta analysis of studies by Cobb 1996, calculated the mean probing depth reduction and gain of clinical attachment that can be achieved with root planing at sites that initially were 4 to 6 mm in depth and 7 mm or greater in depth and reported mean pocket depth reductions of 1.29 mm and 2.16 mm, respectively, and mean gains of clinical attachment of 0.55 mm and 1.29 mm, respectively. In that review, probing depth reduction usually was greater at sites with larger initial probing depths. The decrease in probing depth consisted of two components: gain of clinical attachment and recession. Thus probing depth and clinical attachment gain are useful measures in assessing results of treatment. The treatment that may be feasible and affordable for the underprivileged includes oral hygiene instruction and patient education, scaling and root planning. Maintenance care is recommended but follow up will be an uphill task since majority of the patients may find it difficult or unaffordable to attend regularly. This being due to the distances they may have to travel or the cost of transport.

4.6.1. Cause Related Periodontal Therapy

The management of periodontal diseases have to consider first the cause of the disease and how to eliminate it while altering the environment surrounding the tooth for the purpose of making it conducive to maintaing good periodontal health status. This phase involves informing the patient the status of his/her periodontal condition, motivation of the patient, giving oral hygiene instructions, scaling and root planning,

4.6.1.1. Patient Information

The cause of periodontitis is microbial plaque on tooth surface as well as on the surface of mineralized dental calculus (Figure 4.8 (a-f). It has been reported that in socially disadvantaged communities most people have a lot of plaque seen as soft dental deposits and a lot of dental calculus reported as hard dental deposits (Baelum 1988, Timmerman et al. 2000). These two conditions most of the times do not cause any dental pain or discomfort and therefore many people are unaware of the harmful effects that can arise from long standing accumulation of microbial plaque and calculus. After examination, a periodontal patient needs to be informed of the examination findings in simple terms that are easily understandable.

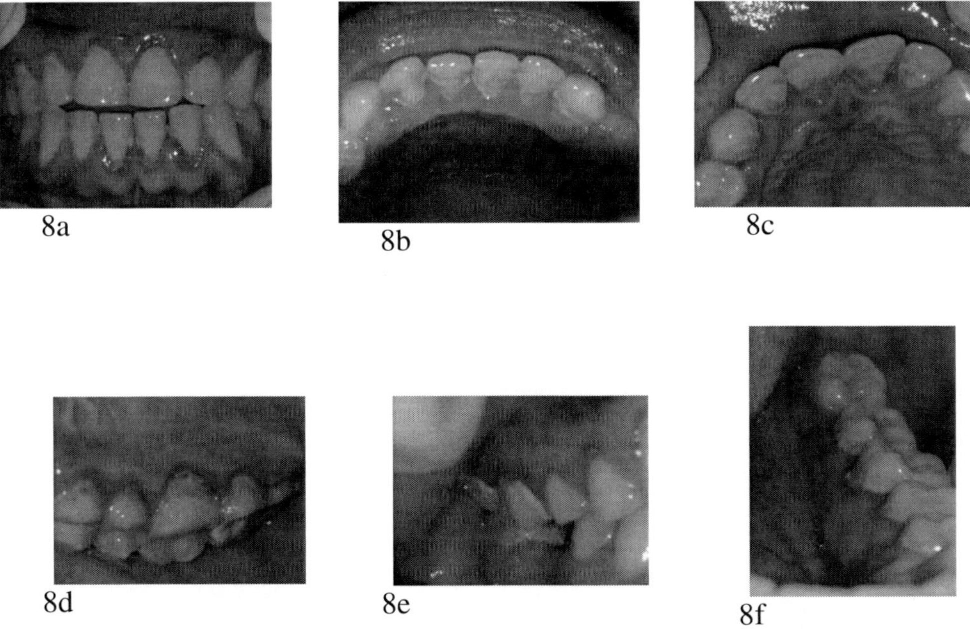

Figure 4.8 (a-f) Calculus deposits: (Courtesy of E.G. Mumghamba). 8a. Upper and lower anterior teeth on labial surfaces, 8b. Calculus deposits on lower anterior teeth on lingual surfaces, 8c. Calculus deposits on upper anterior teeth on palatal surfaces, 8d. Calculus deposits on upper left posterior palatal surfaces, 8e. Calculus deposits on posterior upper and lower right teeth on buccal surfaces, 8f. Calculus deposits on lower left posterior lingual surfaces.

The conditions to be discussed with the patient include the microbial plaque (soft deposits on tooth surfaces), dental calculus (hard deposits) on teeth above, below or both sides of the gingival margin). Easily bleeding gums should be reported to the patient and other findings such as periodontal pocketing, recession of the gums, mobile teeth, tooth decay, root stumps, periapical periodontal lesions, as well as evidence of alveolar bone loss on the radiographs.

4.6.1.2. Patient Motivation

In order to contribute effectively to the management of periodontal diseases, patients need to be motivated to be responsible for their own oral home care. Patients should not depend on the professional for home care. For this to take place the patient needs to be shown the actual problem in their mouth for example using plaque disclosing agent or food colouring material to disclose presence of soft deposits on tooth surfaces. Also the charting system and scores used for all periodontal conditions that are assessed should be explained in simple language and interpreted adequately to the patient for their understanding. Based on these scores, any evidence of improvement based on patients' compliance to professional advice and instructions should be commended for the purpose of encouraging the patient to do much better on that specific item and all other related ones. Deteriorations should also be recorded and discussed carefully for the purpose of further re-instruction without endangering the doctor-patient relationship and in particular the confidence each one has on the other.

4.6.1.3. Oral Hygiene Instruction (OHI)

The patient's understanding on oral hygiene should guide the depth of oral hygiene instruction (OHI) one would give. For example, there might be no need to instruct on change of brushing technique if the level of oral hygiene is within the acceptable standards. However, in socially disadvantaged communities, the individuals are mostly pre-occupied with basic needs and therefore meticulous oral hygiene practices may not be a priority. At this state, clear instructions should be given in relation to the need for daily tooth brushing, preferably brushing twice per day and in particular before going to bed. The effective tooth brushing practice relies upon the design of the toothbrush, the skill of the individual using the tooth brush, and the frequency and duration of use.

The tooth brushing should be done in a systematic manner starting with brushing the lower lingual surfaces from right to left hand side, followed by upper left to the upper right palatal surfaces, and thereafter to maintain this sequence while cleaning all of the buccal, occlusal, and finally the interdental surfaces (Rateitschak et al. 1989).

4.6.1.3.1. Tooth Brushing Methods

There are many tooth brushing methods ((Perry and Beemsterboer 2007) that in principle apply role stokes (Modified Stillman technique), vibratory stokes (Stillman, Charters, and Bass), Circular strokes (Fones technique), Vertical strokes (Leonard technique), and Horizontal stokes (Scrub technique). In all these toothbrushing methods, no one is superior of the other in terms of the effectiveness on plaque removal. However, choice on which tooth brushing method is to be used will depend on the intraoral soft and hard tissue status as well as the dexterity of the individual.

The tooth brushing method mostly used in many populations is the horizontal (scrub-brush) technique, for it is the simplest. The technique mainly utilizes vigorous horizontal brushing strokes, though at times also incorporates the vertical, circular and even vibratory strokes, whereby the toothbrush is applied 90 degrees angle to the tooth surface (Wilkins

1976, Echeverria et al. 2003). The lingual/palatal and occlusal surfaces are brushed with the mouth open while buccal/labial surfaces are cleaned with the mouth closed. The vigorous scrubbing enhances gingival recession and when the dentifrice used has enough large abrasive particles, these results to cervical tooth abrasive lesions with or without tooth sensitivity. In such instances, a softer toothbrush, a vertical tooth brushing method using dentifrices of appropriate size and hardness of abrasive materials is recommended (Rateitschak et al. 1989).

Some of the brushing methods are the Bass and Charters methods. The Bass method of brushing is widely accepted and thus commonly recommended for its ease of use and patients are able to adopt it easily, and for this reason, the method will be described in detail. Toothbrush bristles applied obliquely at a 45 degree angle with the bristles toward the gingival sulcus (Figure 4.9). The brush is moved using short back-and-forth motions while at the same time exerting a gentle vibratory pressure without dislodging the tips of the bristles from the gingival sulcus (Perry and Beemsterboer 2007). This method need to complete several strokes in the same position before lifting up the tooth brush to be applied or adapted to adjacent three or four teeth. The same back- and-forth motions with vibrations is repeated in this new area, and thereafter, continue all round the arch for the upper and lower teeth as well as for the buccal and palatal surfaces. On the lingual surfaces of the anterior mandibular teeth and the palatal surfaces of the maxillary anterior teeth, the toothbrush should be turned vertically i.e. to brush with the heel of the tooth brush. The occlusal surfaces of three to four teeth are brushed with several short, back-and-forth strokes while the bristles are firmly pressed into the pits and fissures.

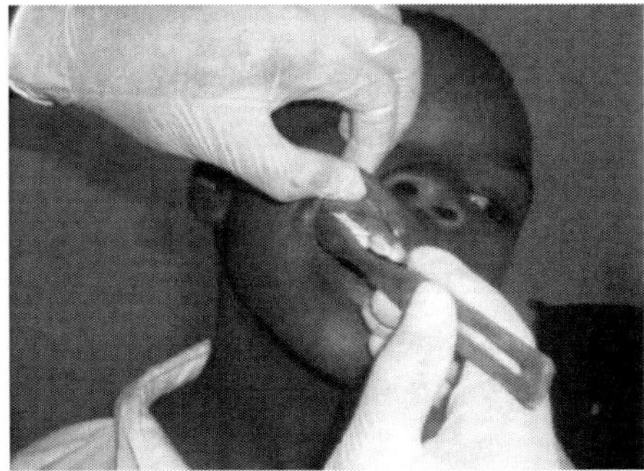

Figure 4.9. Bass technique: Bristle brushes applied in a 45° to the tooth surface bristles directed towards the gingival sulcus (Courtesy of E.G. Mumghamba).

The "modified" Bass technique incoperates the "roll strokes" in that after having applied the vibratory motions, the roll strokes are exerted to lift the debris from the gingival sulcus by rotating the brush towards the occlussal direction. However, it is recommended that the two techniques i.e. the "vibratory" and the "rolling' strokes should be performed separately.

The Charters Method of brushing is also recommended in cases where there are open interdental areas with receded interdental papilla. The purpose is to loosen debris and plaque on the area as well as massaging and stimulation of the blood circulation in the marginal and interdental gingiva. Bristles are applied obliquely at a 45 degree angle towards the occlussal or incisal surfaces. Brush moved back-and-forth with rotatory motion. However the method is diificult to accomplish on the lingual surfaces, brush ends do not engage the gingival sulcus to remove subgingival plaque accumulation, and requires high digital dexterity and therefore not preferred by most patients.

4.6.1.3.2. Tooth Cleaning Devices

Tooth cleaning devices includes the plastic toothbrush (manual or electric), local chewing sticks (meswak, miswak), toothpicks, and dental floss.

4.6.1.3.3. Use of Toothbrushes

The size of a toothbrush bristle should be 0.007 inch. Therefore when the Interdental papilla is absent then an interdental brush is recommended and it is 95% effective. However, for plastic tooth brushes (Figure 4.10), the recommended type should have soft bristles with doom shaped tips to prevent trauma to the soft and hard oral structures during tooth brushing practice. The power to drive the toothbrush may manual or electrical, the former are commonly available type in shops in developing countries while the latter are not readily available due to limited purchasing power of the people.

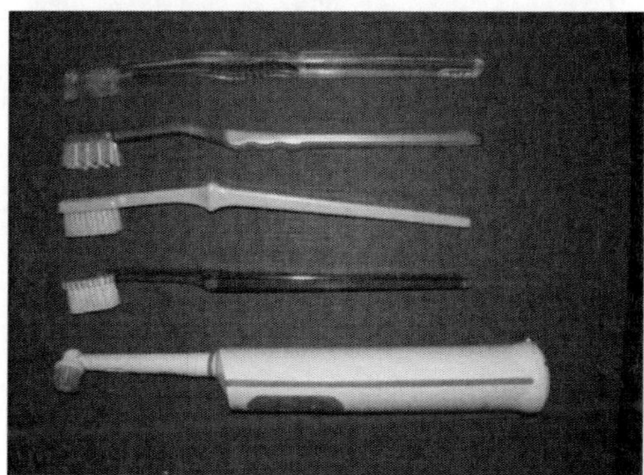

Figure 4.10. Plastic toothbrushes – different types: manual and electric (Courtesy of E.G. Mumghamba).

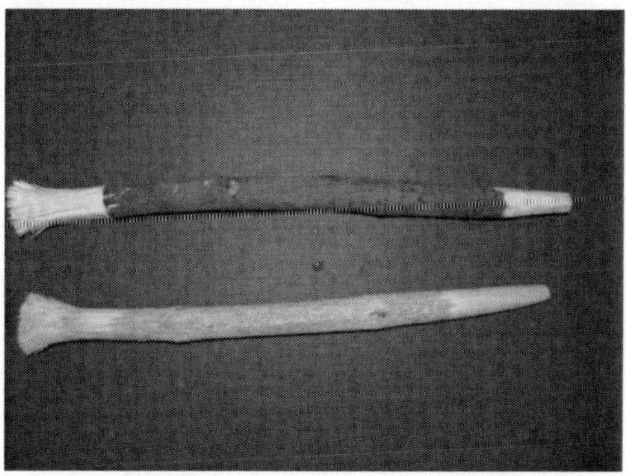

Figure 4.11. Chewing sticks – different types (Courtesy of E.G. Mumghamba).

4.6.1.3.4. Use of Chewing Sticks

Based on the purchasing power of the individual, plastic toothbrush or the "chewing stick" can be used as both of them are almost equally effective when used carefully (WHO

2000, Wu et al. 2001, van Palenstein et al. 1992). Chewing sticks (Figure 4.11) are still very much being used in Africa, Middle East and Asia because they are simple, readily available, and affordable (Wu et al. 2001, Bukar et al. 2004, Varenne et al. 2006). When using chewing stick the practical way to clean the teeth is to apply a technique that involves grasping of the chewing stick is a "modified palm grasp with the thumb-up while the tail of the mswaki is put between the ring and small finger (Figure 4.12). This is a little bit different from the grasp used for normal plastic toothbrush or electrical tooth brush (Figure 4.13). The difference in grasping is accounted by the fact that the chewing stick fibers/bristle for cleaning are at the end of the tip or actually run parallel to the handle while the plastic manual or electric toothbrush the bristles run at right angles to the handle.

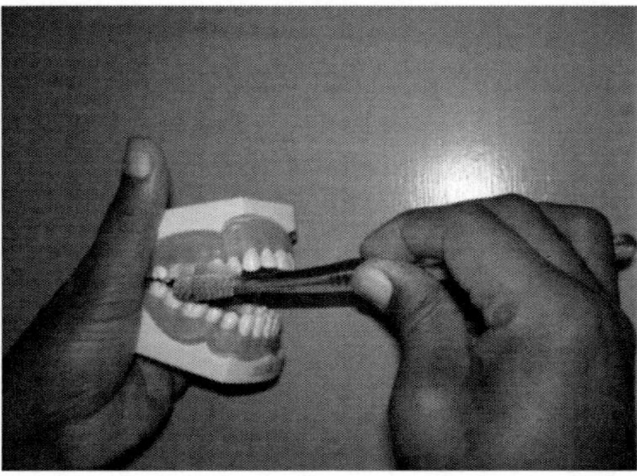

Figure 4.12. Proper toothbrushing – well adapted manual plastic toothbrush (Courtesy of E.G. Mumghamba).

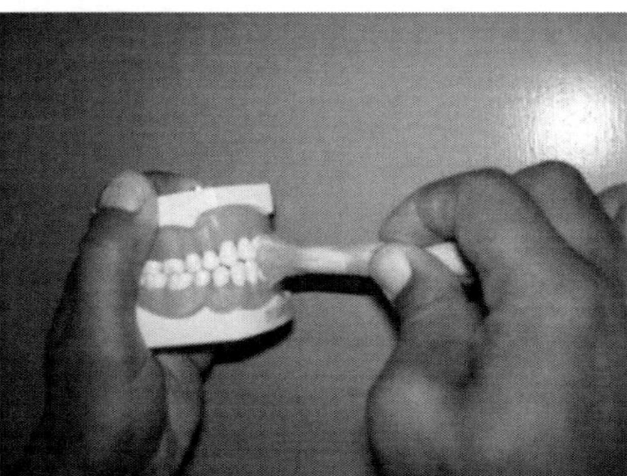

Figure 4.13. Proper tooth cleaning using chewing sticks (Courtesy of E.G. Mumghamba).

4.6.1.3.5. Use of Dental Floss and or Tooth Picks

Flossing is 80% effective in removing interdental plaque in the presence of an interdental papilla. Dental floss penetrates 1.5mm subgingivally (Renvert et al. 1990). In the absence of an interdental papilla, brushing or flossing is only 55% effective. Cleaning of the interdental or approximal spaces using a dental floss (dental thread) (Figure 14) and or tooth picks/sticks (Figure 15) is necessary to remove food impacts and plaque biofilm that contribute to the occurrence of interproximal dental caries as well as interdental gingival and periodontal lesions. At times when people engage on use of tooth picks particularly to remove meat impacts between the teeth, the readily available tooth picks are those that are cylindrical shaped rather the triangular ones. Obviously, then the cleaning of interdental space which is triangular shaped becomes less effective when a cylindrical tooth pick is appliead instead of the triangular tooth pick. Although interdental cleaning is a time consuming practice, it is very common in developed countries but in developing countries and in particular among the SDP it is negligible. The reason for this unpopularity is thought to be ignorance and poverty. The patient's oral home care has to be monitored on a regular basis. Monitoring techniques include, staining plaque with plaque disclosing agents or any of the food colouring material at all appointments and use of an objective plaque index.

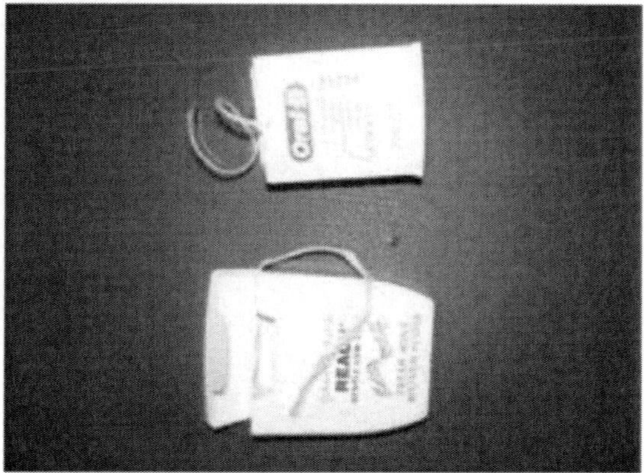

Figure 4.14. Dental floss – Different types. A: Oral B – Ultra floss. B: Reach (Johnson and Johnson).

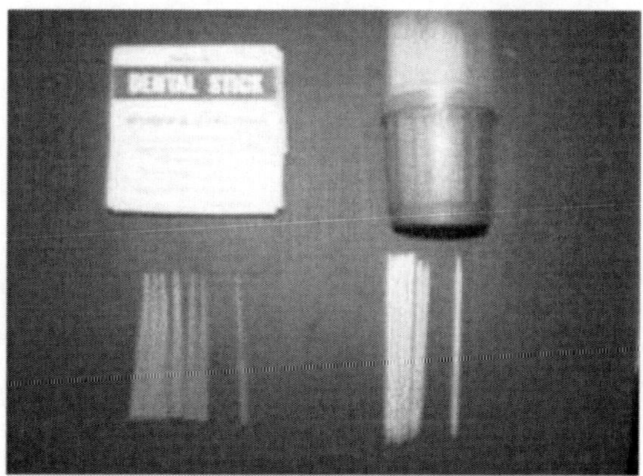

Figure 4.15. Tooth picks – Diffeent types. A: Recommended triangular shaped toothpicks. B: Cylindrical tooth picks – not recommended.

4.6.1.4. Tooth Cleaning Adjuncts

Adjuncts to tooth cleaning are toothpastes which may be fluoridated or non-fluoridated. Fluoridated tooth pastes among other things helps to control dental caries. The cleaning activity of toothpaste is dependent on the incorporation of abrasive particles. It is recommended that abrasive particles should be of ideal size, shape and hardness so that it may not lead to excessive wear of the hard tooth substance which is also rich in fluoride. In SDP where purchase power is extremely low, people use other traditional alternatives such as ashes, charcoal, and sand which may be detrimental to the hard tooth substance.

4.6.1.5. Tongue Cleaning

Tongue cleaning is an important aspect of home oral hygiene procedures. Most people like to have fresh breath. If it happens that the individual is aware of having bad breath, most make efforts either to brush the teeth more and more, use chewing gums and other oral antiseptics to mask the bad breath. A tongue that has not been cleaned for a long time for example for a day (24 hours) will be covered by plaque biofilm which harbors multitudes of oral bacteria whereby some of them contribute to the occurrence of bad breath. A properly cleaned tongue appears pinkish in colour and no whitish deposits (Figure 4.16).

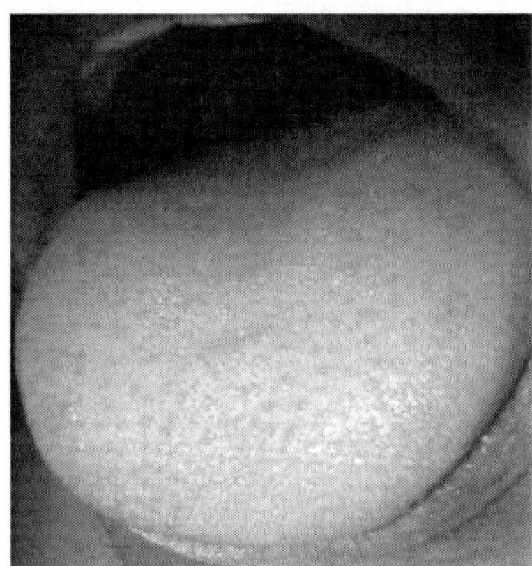

Figure 4.16. Tongue – clean, pink in colour (Courtesy of E.G. Mumghamba).

In a non-cleaned tongue, the plaque biofilm on the tongue makes it appear as whitish or yellow whitish (Figure 4.7). Cleaning of the tongue may be accomplished by brushing it with a normal tooth brush or by a special back-surface of the toothbrush. Also scraping of the tongue surface gently and repeatedly right from the back to the anterior part of the dorsal surface with either a wood spatula or even a spoon would render the tongue clean. Difficulties to clean the tongue may be experienced among individuals who have a "wrenching reflex" or "a feeling like vomiting" particularly when the posterior part of the tongue is touched. A deep breath may help to some extent to control the wrench reflex.

4.6.1.6. Treatment of Plaque Induced Gingivitis

Gingivitis is a reversible disease and the aim of therapy is to reduce the microbial plaque levels at the gingival margin so as to eliminate noxious substances secreted by the microorganisms and allow the tissues to heal. Some patients may have calcified deposits which also have to be removed. Patients with chronic gingivitis, but without significant calculus, alterations in gingival morphology, or systemic diseases that affect oral health, may respond to a therapeutic regimen consisting of improved personal plaque control alone (Axelsson and Lindhe 1981). This should be followed by supportive periodontal care.

Appropriate supportive periodontal maintenance that includes personal and professional care is important even in cases of chronic gingivitis. However, in the underprivileged, compliance with a maintenance regimen that is too frequent may be a problem especially if the patient has long distances to travel to the clinic. In such circumstances, some topical antibacterial agents may assist the patient but that is only if they can afford it. Alternatively, warm salt water rinses would be beneficial in assisting the patient to maintain plaque control in the event that they are unable to purchase a topical antibacterial agent. Chewing sticks have antibacterial properties and can be used if the correct procedure is taught and adopted.

In a 15 year longitudinal study involving 375 patients on a maintenance programme of oral hygiene instructions and supportive periodontal treatment every 2 months for 2 years then every 3 months for the next 4 years was carried out with the control group being seen annually only. After 6 years, the test group was doing so well (mean attachment gain of 0.2 mm) compared to the control (mean attachment loss of 1.2 mm) that the control group was discontinued. The authors concluded that professional and personal plaque control was effective in preventing recurrence of diseases (Axelsson et al. 1991).

In a situation where gingivitis still remains after the removal of plaque and other contributing local factors, evaluation of the underlying systemic factors should be done. If such conditions like diabetes, pregnancy, puberty and blood dyscrasias are present, then once the systemic problem is resolved or controlled, the gingival inflammation will subside after plaque removal.

Treatment procedures for the control of chronic gingivitis include:-

a) Patient education with the aim of getting them to understand the disease process and the extent of their disease.
b) Training in personal oral hygiene.
c) Counselling on control of risk factors like smoking, medical status and stress.
d) Removal of supragingival plaque and calculus and accessible sub-gingival deposits which will involve periodontal scaling.
e) Correction of plaque retentive factors such as caries, ill fitting partial dentures, faulty orthodontic therapy and poor restorations may also be necessary.
f) Following active treatment, the patient should be place on a supportive maintenance programme.

4.6.1.7. Treatment of Chronic Periodontitis

The clinical features include oedema, gingival bleeding on probing, and/or suppuration, loss of clinical attachment, furcation involvement of the molar teeth and periodontal probing depths. Radiographic evidence of bone loss and increased tooth mobility may be present. The mild form is characterized by periodontal destruction of no more than 1 to 2mm clinical attachment loss, the moderate form by 2 to 4mm of clinical attachment loss and the severe form by more than 5mm clinical attachment loss (Smith et al. 1985). The aetiological factors associated with periodontitis are plaque microorganisms, supra- and sub-gingival calculus and plaque retentive factors (Figure 4.17a and 4.17b).

In chronic periodontitis, the goals of treatment include:
a) The reduction or elimination of microorganisms
b) Removal of local retentive factors
c) Control or elimination of contributing risk factors like smoking and diabetes.

d) Arresting the progression of the disease
e) Preserving the dentition
f) Restoring and maintaining a state of health, comfort and function
g) Prevention of recurrence
h) Regeneration of lost tissue – in the underprivileged this may not be possible due to the expense involved in using bone grafts and guided tissue regeneration membranes.

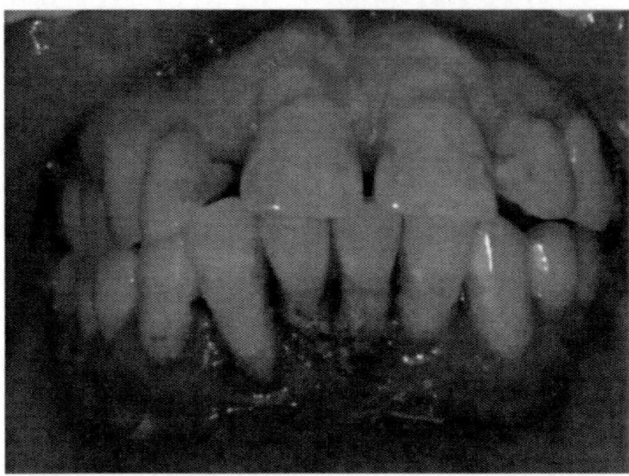

Figure 4.17a. Before treatment (Courtesy of E.G. Mumghamba).

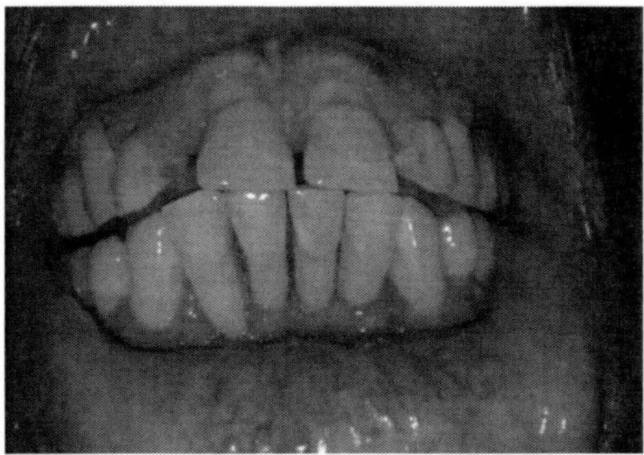

Figure 4.17b. After treatment (Courtesy of E.G. Mumghamba).

Management of chronic periodontitis will first require a comprehensive examination followed by diagnosis of the condition which should include the extent and severity, prognosis and a treatment plan.

In developing a treatment plan, it is important to consider the following risk factors:

a) History of previous Periodontal diseases
b) Systemic health especially the presence of diabetes
c) Smoking
d) Age
e) Stress
f) Nutrition
g) HIV infection
h) Substance abuse
i) Medications

j)   Compliance by the patient
k)   Therapeutic preferences of the patient
l)   Patient's personal plaque control
m) Patient's ability to meet their financial commitments
n)   Clinician's ability to remove sub-gingival deposits
o)   Restorative and prosthetic requirements
p)   The extent and severity of the disease

All these factors mentioned may affect treatment outcome. It is therefore important to eliminate, alter or control these factors. Consultation with the patient's physician is indicated in the case where the patient has systemic illness or is on medication.

4.6.1.8. Treatment Procedures
The treatment procedures include:

a)   Patient education and instruction on plaque control.
b)   Supra-and sub- gingival scaling and root planning.
c)   Antimicrobial agents like mouthwashes or adjunctive systemic antibiotics may be used. Locally delivery antibiotics may be too expensive for the underprivileged but where possible they could be used.
d)   Elimination of local contributing factors like caries, poor restorations and ill fitting dentures and faulty orthodontic treatment.
e)   Splinting of mobile teeth in advance periodontitis.
f)   Restorations of open contacts which have resulted in food impaction.
g)   Correction of occlusal trauma.
h)   Periodontal surgery where indicated.

Where the desired outcome is achieved, then the patient is placed on a supportive maintenance regime which involves regular visits for monitoring the periodontal tissues, the level of plaque control and removal of any accumulated deposits.

In advance disease characterized by bleeding on probing, oedema, suppuration, loss of periodontal support of greater than one third of the supporting tissues, loss of clinical attachment in the furcation exceeding class 1, periodontal probing depths greater than 6mm and clinical attachment loss greater than 4mm, all attempts should be made to eliminate, alter or control risk factors in order to improve treatment outcomes. The treatment procedure is the same as mentioned in the case of chronic periodontitis, but in addition in ths case, extraction of hopeless teeth is indicated.

A tooth where extraction should be considered as an option of treatment, is one where there is advance loss of supporting structures with mobility of grade 3 including movement of a vertical component. Additionally, for reasons of health, non-compliance with plaque control or lack of effectiveness in plaque control, by the patient, a clinician may defer extensive treatment and instead offer a compromised treatment plan which may include extractions and provision of replacements using simple plastic acrylic dentures. However, if a denture is put and there is no plaque control, the tissue response may be worsened.

In the underprivileged, where the distances travelled, the cost of treatment and patient preferences, may affect the treatment plan, initial therapy may be the end point where only scaling and root planning are carried out along with patient education and instruction. Extraction of teeth with advance disease is offered rather than complicated management. The severity and extent of disease, age and health of the patient may also compromise the treatment outcome and therefore complex treatment procedures are not included in the treatment plan. There is also a possibility that the patient may not want treatment and would rather wait for symptoms and have extractions as time goes on or wait for exfoliation in advance bone loss.

4.6.1.8.1. Phases of Treatment

a) Non-surgical:

    i.   Eliminate pain/infection, address chief complaint.
    ii.   Laboratory testing in case of any underlying medical condition. Medical consultation with the patient's physician is important if there is a systemic condition.
    iii.   Improve oral hygiene.
    iv.   Remove etiological factors by mechanical means or ultrasonic instrumentation.
    v.   Caries control, endodontic treatment, extractions, orthodontic treatment,
    vi.   Occlusal adjustment if needed.
    vii.   Antimicrobial therapy like chlorhexidine mouthwash or salt water rinses.
    viii.   Systemic antibiotics if indicated.
    ix.   Evaluation of oral hygiene at every visit.
    x.   Evaluation of tissue response to therapy on each visit.
    xi.   Prepare tissues for surgery if indicated, but in most cases not possible for the SDP.

b) Re-evaluation visit, confirm or alter remaining treatment plan.
c) Surgical phase (corrective phase): The prerequisites for periodontal surgery at this stage are considered to be somehow complicated or too demanding in such a manner that they seem not to be feasible for the SDP. However, oral hygiene instruction should be continue to be emphasized. It needs meticulous orall hygiene, but not all of the patients will be able to comply. The teeth with mobility may be treated by scaling and root planning and after insisting on oral hygiene and observe for possible tooth extraction in later days if there is danger of natural exfoliation and aspiration.
d) Remaining dental care:

    –   Prosthetic replacements if required, final occlusal adjustment if needed.

e) Maintenance phase:

    i.   Monitor and reinforce oral hygiene.
    ii.   Monitor the health of the periodontium.
    iii.   Scale and root plane on a regular basis as needed.
    iv.   Re-probe, not necessary every year in non-active disease patient.

v.   Up-date radiographs every 2 yrs or as needed.

4.6.1.8.2. Scaling and Root Planning

This type of treatment is indicated for those individuals that on examination would be found to have pocket depth deeper than 4 mm together with gingival bleeding on the sites involved. This is the process of removing calculus, planing root surfaces, curetting the gingiva and removing diseased tissues lining the periodontal pockets.

Scaling: This is the process of instrumentation used to remove all supragingival uncalcified and calcified deposits and all gross subgingival accretions.

Root planing: The process of instrumentation used to remove microbial flora on root surfaces or lying free in the pocket, all calculus deposits on the crown and root surface. Also root planning is a process of removing endotoxin in infected cementum which is a complex polysaccharide in gram negative bacterial cell wall. Scaling and root planning has been shown to shift the composition of subgingival plaque from one of gram-negative anaerobes to one dominated with gram-positive facultative bacteria compatible with health (Drisko et al. 2000).

Varieties of instruments are available and are classified according to the purpose they serve, for example:

a)   *Periodontal probe:* Used to locate clinically, measure and mark periodontal pocket depths.
b)   *Explorer:* Used to locate calculus deposits on tooth and root surfaces
c)   *Sickle scaler:* Used to remove supra-gingival calculus only due to its bulkness in size and that it has sharp edges.
d)   *Curettes:* these are fine instruments which are either area specific (Gracey curettes) or universal curettes and are used for removal of both fine supra- and sub-gingival calculus on the root surfaces as well as altered cementum. They may also be used to remove diseased soft tissue lining the pocket (gingival curettage).
e)   *Cleansing and polishing instruments:* These are rubber cups, bristle brushes, dental tape and air-powder abrasive systems which polish the tooth surfaces. The air-powder abrasive system is contra-indicated in patients with histories of respiratory illness, haemodialysis patients, hypertensive patients and patients with infectious diseases (Copulos et al. 1993).

It has been shown that ultrasonic instrumentation is as effective as using hand curettes in the removal of calculus deposits (Nyman et al. 1975).

4.6.1.8.3. Periodontal Surgery

In patients with moderate to advance loss of periodontal support, periodontal surgery should be considered in patients who have demonstrated willingness and ability to maintain an acceptable standard of good oral hygiene. Varieties of surgical treatment modalities are available. These include resective, regeneration and gingival augmentation therapy. These surgical procedures may not be feasible in a patient coming from a socially disadvantaged population due to cost implication. However, what remains to be an important strategy is the willingness and ability to maintain a good plaque control in such patients.

4.6.1.8.4. Management of Teeth with Furcation Involvement

Furcation involvement is the spread of disease to the area between the roots of the teeth. When there is furcation involvement, the prognosis of the tooth is compromised because of the anatomy of the area and the difficulty in access for therapy or maintenance by the patient (Glickman 1953).

Aetiology of Furcation Involvement

a) Primary Factor – bacterial plaque
b) Contributing Factors –

    i. Amount of alveolar bone loss
    ii. Pulpal Pathology
    iii. Iatrogenic Factors

Predisposing Factors

a) Furcation Location. The more coronal the location of the furcation entrance, the higher the chances of the disease process exposing the furcation area.
b) Cervical Enamel Projections (there is no connective tissue attachment in these areas) – 17% Maxillary Molars and 29% Mandibular Molars
c) Thickness of Overlying Gingiva and Bone. When the overlying tissues are thin, exposure of the furcation is more frequent.
d) Root Anatomy
e) Enamel Pearls
f) Root concavities and invagiations.

4.6.1.8.5. Classification of Furcation Involvement

The classification of furcation involvement by Bower (1979) is as follows:

Grade1: early stage of furcation involvement. The pocket is supra-bony and primarily affects the soft tissue. An increase in pocket depth but no radiographic changes

Grade 2: there can be one or more of the furcations affected in the same tooth. The furcation lesion is essentially a cul-de-sac with a definite horizontal involvement of the furcation area. Probing into the furcation area will not communicate with other furcations if present.

Grade 3: in grade 3, the bone is not attached to the dome of the furcation. However the furcation area may be filled with soft tissue and may not be visible. Radiographic changes are present with a display of a radiolucent area in the crotch of the tooth.

Grade 4: the Interdental bone is destroyed, and the soft tissues have receeded apically so that the furcation is clinically visible.

The rationale for Furcation Treatment includes:

a) Regeneration of lost attachment apparatus – treatment of choice but not always possible especially in the underprivileged.
b) Access for oral hygiene.
c) Access for root preparation.

d)   Pocket Elimination.
e)   Treatment of non-periodontic conditions like:-

i.   Root caries
ii.   Fractures
iii. Root resorption
iv.   Endodontic complications like perforations and broken instruments.

The treatment of furcationally involved tooth is a complex issue. The furcation area is complex anatomically and difficult or impossible to clean using the routine periodontal methods (O'Leary 1969).

Grade 1: They are usually associated with supra-bony pockets therefore treatment will involve scaling and root planing, curettage and/or odontoplasty where if the facial groove is exposed, it is reshaped to allow easier plaque control and prevent plaque accumulation.

Grade 2: Treatment for lesions staged as grade 2-4 might not be feasible for the SDP.

Shallow horizontal involvement without significant vertical component, will respond to flap procedures with odontoplasty and osteoplasty.

Grade 3 and 4: non-surgical treatment is not effective. Periodontal surgery, root resection or amputation, hemisection or root separation, endodontic therapy and restoration of the tooth may be necessary.

Tunnelling procedure: When the furcation is exposed clinically, flap procedure together with odontoplasty and osteoplasty is indicated to fully expose the furcation area for cleaning. This reduces the dome of the furcation and makes it easier for the patient to keep clean.

4.6.1.8.6. Management of teeth with mobility

All teeth have a slight degree of physiologic mobility of which varies from tooth to tooth and at different times during the day (Hart 1996). It is more in the morning and less in the evening and more obvious in single rooted teeth as compared to multirooted teeth.

Mobility is tested using two pieces of a single-ended periodontal/ examination instruments, for examole the blunt ends of a mouth mirror and an explorer. With the modified pen grasp of one instrument on the right hand and the other on the left hand and with proper fulcrum, the right hand instrument pushes lingually the crown of a tooth at a right angle to the long axis of the tooth and assess the distance the crwon in being displaced, while the left hand is resting, not pushing against the other. Next stroke is the left-hand instrument pushing the crown of the tooth on a buccal direction and likewise assess the displacement while the right-hand i nstrument is resting. The grade of tooth mobility in a bucco-lingual direction is graded as follows (Cameron et al. 2007):-

Grade 0:   Physiologic mobility only
Grade ½: Clinical mobility that is slightly greater than physiologic mobility but less
              than 1 mm buccolingually (also designated as +)
Grade 1:   Slightly pathologic mobility, approximately 1 mm buccolingually
Grade 2:   Moderately pathological mobility, approximately 2 mm buccolingually, but
              no vertical displacement.

Grade 3:   Severe pathologic mobility, greater than 2 mm buccolingually or mesiodistally, combined with a vertical displacement.

The management of tooth mobility will depend on the cause. Where the mobility is a result of loss of supporting structures i.e the periodontal ligaments and alveolar bone, then treatment of the inflammatory condition may reduce the mobility but this depends on the extent and severity of the loss of alveolar bone support. Where the mobility is a result of trauma from occlusion, then correction of the problem will resolve the mobility. In cases of mobility during pregnancy, the mobility will resolve postpartum. In pregnancy, mobility occurs in individual with or without periodontal diseases and is due to the physicochemical changes in the tissues. When mobility is due to pathological changes in the jaw like tumours and osteomyelitis, resolution is difficult and treatment may be to extract the mobile teeth along with the removal of the tumour or treatment of the osteomyelitis. In tooth mobility of grade 1 or 2, resolution of the underlying cause of mobility may reduce most of the movement of the tooth but in grade 3, it is difficult to resolve the condition and extraction or splinting may be the only option.

4.6.1.8.7. Splinting of Teeth

Indications:-

a)   Mobility of teeth that is increasing or that impairs patient comfort
b)   Migration of teeth
c)   Prosthetics where multiple abutments are necessary.

Before splinting is considered, periodontal inflammation must be resolved because inflammation can produce mobility in the presence of normal occlusal forces. Additionally, any parafunctional habits or deflective tooth contacts must be sorted out first before splinting is considered as they may cause tooth mobility.

Splinting may be done using a more simple approach for example using orthodontic wires with the recommended diameter.

4.6.1.8.8. Occlusal Therapy

Trauma from occlusion is defined as tissue injury to the supporting structures of the tooth as a result of excessive occlusal forces which are beyond the tissues ability to repair or adapt (Stahl 2005). Trauma from occlusion can be caused by alterations in occlusal forces, reduced capacity of the periodontium to withstand occlusal forces or both. There are two forms of trauma from occlusion:-

a)   *Primary trauma from occlusion-* which is excessive occlusal forces causing injury to a healthy periodontium. This can occur when restorations or prosthetic replacements alter the direction of the occlusal forces.
b)   *Secondary occlusal trauma-* this is when the adaptive capacity of the tissues to withstand occlusal forces is impaired by a compromised periodontium. Previously well tolerated occlusal forces become traumatic.

Trauma form occlusion does not initiate pocket formation because the supra-crestal gingival fibres are not affected and therefore prevent apical migration of the junctional epithelium. Trauma from occlusion that occurs concurrently with inflammatory periodontal diseases may result in increased bone loss and progression of periodontitis due to the widened periodontal ligament space and the hyalinization of periodontal ligament fibres caused by the excessive occlusal forces. In such a case, both the occlusal trauma and the periodontal diseases must be addressed separately with the periodontal inflammation being treated first. Failure to treat either the chronic periodontitis or the occlusal trauma will result in tooth loss eventually. The aim of treatment is to restore health of the periodontium, eliminate or reduce excessive force on the teeth and the patient should be able to masticate in comfort without damage to the periodontal tissues. A comfortable and functional dentition should be the end point of treatment. The following are some of the signs and symptoms of occlusal trauma:-

a) Tooth mobility
b) Tooth migration
c) Tooth pain or discomfort when chewing
d) Tenderness of muscles of mastication
e) Temporomandibular dysfunction
f) Presence of wear facets not commiserate with the patient's age and diet
g) Chipped teeth
h) Fremitus
i) Radiographic changes – widening of the periodontal ligament space

Treatment of trauma form occlusion may include occlusal adjustment, management of parafunctional habits, orthodontic tooth movement, and provision of removable or fixed appliances which provide stabilization for the mobile teeth. Tooth extraction of selected teeth may also help resolve the problem.

4.6.9. Management of Aggressive Periodontitis

Aggressive periodontitis is characterized by rapid loss of attachment and bone in an otherwise healthy individual with the amount of microbial plaque being inconsistent with the disease severity. It tends to have a familial aggregation (International Workshop for a Classification of Periodontal Diseases and Conditions 1999) and may be self arresting in some cases (Page and Schroeder 1982). Aggressive periodontitis describes three diseases formerly classified as "early onset periodontitis": Localized juvenile periodontitis, generalized juvenile periodontitis and rapidly progressive periodontitis. The disease is frequently associated with specific microbiota and neutrophil dysfunction. The *Aggregatibacter* (formerly *Actinobacillus*) *actinomycetemcomitans* (A.a.) species have been implicated in the localized form and A.a. and *Porphyromonas gingivalis* in the generalized form.

The aim of treatment is to:-

a) Eliminate or reduce the associated microorganisms,
b) Remove any other deposits or risk factors like occlusal trauma,

c) Restore function and aesthetics and prevent recurrence.

The disease is self limiting in some individuals but may be difficult to completely control in others. This depends on the microbial flora, systemic factors like the immune defects and possibly genetic predisposition of the individual. The treatment is similar to that of chronic periodontitis but adjunctive systemic antibiotics and topical antimicrobial agents are more commonly used so as to eliminate or reduce the associated causative microorganisms. Microbial identification and antibiotic sensitivity testing is indicated in these cases and may assist in the management. Surgical therapy is indicated only in those teeth that are not severely involved and prognosis is favourable. Unfortunately, a lot of times, patients are seen when the teeth are severely involved and extraction is the only option. This may be due to the rapid progression of the disease or the absence of frank inflammation therefore the disease goes un-noticed for some time. The success of treatment will depend on patient compliance and diligence in adhering to the maintenance schedule.

4.6.10. Management of Acute Periodontal Diseases

Acute periodontal diseases are conditions of rapid onset involving the periodontium and associated structures. They are infections characterized by pain and discomfort and can be classified into:-

4.6.10.1. Management of Gingival Abscess

The gingival abscess is a localized acute inflammatory lesion that may arise from a variety of sources, including microbial plaque infection, trauma, and foreign body impaction (Kareha et al. 1981, Meng 1999). It is painful in nature and the tooth along with adjacent teeth is tender to percussion.

The clinical features include a red shiny localized swelling which may become fluctuant and point in 24-48 hours. The aim of treatment is to establish drainage, relieve pain and restore patient comfort and function. This may be done by discharging the purulent exudate through the pointed orifice or by debridement of the area to remove the irritant. It is important to remove the foreign material, if that is the initial cause, for complete healing. If the lesion does not resolve, it is probably due to the incomplete removal of the causative agent or inaccurate diagnosis. If left alone, the abscess will spontaneously drain in time.

4.6.10.2. Management of Pericoronal Abscess

As with the other abscesses mentioned above, the clinical features are similar except that the abscess is localized to the pericoronal flap/operculum overlying an unerupted tooth or an erupting tooth. The treatment is aimed at creating drainage by debridement of the operculum followed by irrigation with sterile saline. If there is regional swelling, lymphadenopathy or systemic signs, systemic antibiotics may be prescribed. Once the acute phase has been controlled, the partially erupted tooth may be treated by surgical excision of the overlying tissues or removal of the tooth. Removal of the opposing tooth is also a treatment option when third molars are involved so as to relieve pain during mastication while waiting for healing of the swelling before definitive treatment. The treatment in this case may also be extraction expecially if the tooth is not erupting in the correct position.

4.6.10.3. Management of Periodontal Abscess

The periodontal abscess is a localized purulent infection of the tissues adjacent to the periodontal pocket (Figure 4.18). The signs and symptoms are mild to severe discomfort, localized red swelling, a periodontal pocket, mobility of the tooth which is elevated in the socket, tenderness to percussion or biting in the involved tooth, exudate from the pocket and in some cases lymphadenopathy, fever and malaise.

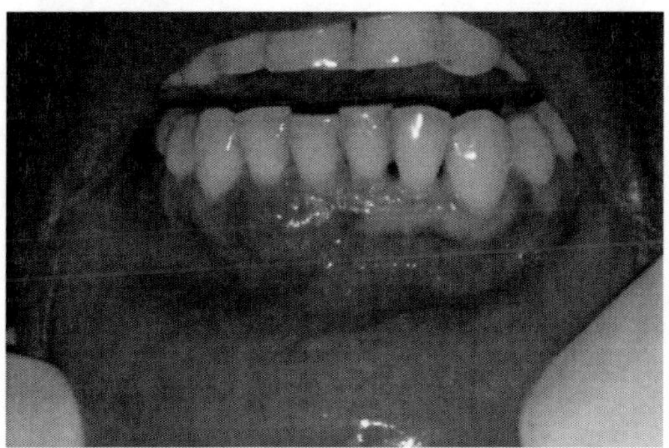

Figure 4.18. Periodontal abscess labial to tooth no. 42 (Courtesy of E.G. Mumghamba).

The treatment options include drainage through the pocket by scaling and root planning or periodontal surgery may be indicated where access to the root surface for debridement is needed (Melnick and Takei 2006). Where there is lymphadenopathy, fever or malaise, cellulitis, a deep inaccessible pocket and in immunocompromised patients, systemic antibiotics are given. Antibiotic of choice is amoxicillin 1.0 gram loading dose followed by 500 mgs three times a day for 3-5 days, or clindamycin for patients that are allergic to penicillin. Tooth removal is also a treatment option especially when the disease is advance and the abscess has spread to involve adjacent tissues.

4.6.11. Management of Necrotizing Periodontal Diseases

Necrotizing ulcerative gingivitis (NUG) is an infection of the marginal gingiva and the Interdental papillae. When the infection extends to involve the attachment apparatus, it is then known as necrotizing ulcerative periodontitis (NUP). The main causative microorganisms associated with the lesions are the *Spirochetes, Prevotella intermedia, Fusobacterium* species, *Treponema* and *Selenomonas* species (Wade et al. 1966). The clinical signs and symptoms include necrosis and ulcerations of the interdental papillae, painful bright red marginal gingivae which bleed easily and a characteristic fetor oris.

The aim of treatment is to alleviate the discomfort and restore function. This can be achieved by gentle irrigation and debridement of the necrotic areas with hydrogen peroxide mouth rinse. Hydrogen peroxide (3%) is used because the associated microorganisms are anaerobes.

This is followed by instructions on oral hygiene to the patient, pain control, and in the presence of systemic involvement, antibiotic therapy (Amir 1997). Once the acute phase is controlled, completion of the debridement process is done with scaling and root planing. Healing may occur with changes in the gingival morphology known as "reverse architecture" due to the punched out lesions of the interdental papillae. In the event of changes in the gingival morphology, gingivoplasty is indicated so as to restore aesthetics.

4.6.12. Management of Herpetic Gingivostomatitis

This is an acute viral infection by herpes simplex type 1 of the gingiva and the oral mucosa. It is a painful inflammatory condition with vesiculation and ulceration of the oral mucous membranes and the gingiva with accompanying lymphadenopathy, fever and malaise. Secondary manifestation includes herpes labialis (Figure 4.19 (a-b) as well as herpes genitalis, ocular herpes and herpetic encephalitis.

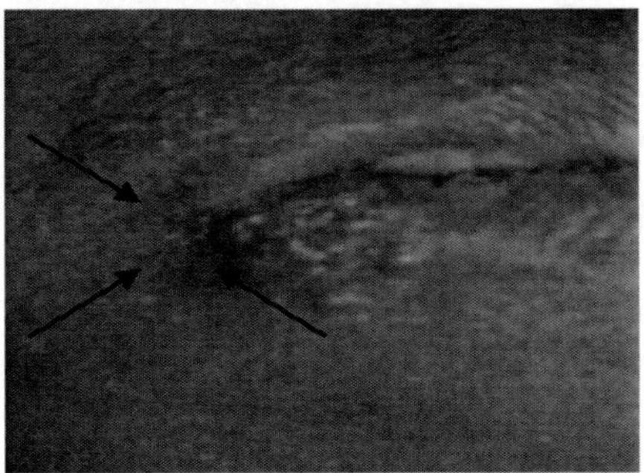

Figure 4.19a. Herpes labialis on lower right side of the lip in a female patient (Courtesy of E.G. Mumghamba).

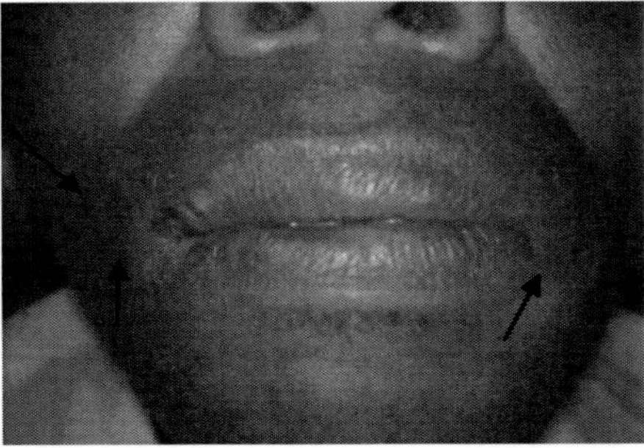

Figure 4.19b. Herpes labialis on both angles (left and right) of the mouth in a male patient (Courtesy of E.G. Mumghamba).

The infection typically occurs in children but can also occur in adults. The aim of treatment is to relieve pain, facilitate maintenance of proper nutrition, hydration and basic oral hygiene. The disease is self limiting but patient comfort may be restored through the use of topical anaesthetic mouth rinse. Treatment is mainly supportive and palliative. It is recommended to use bland (non-spicy) diet, fluid therapy to treat dehydration, analgesics to alleviate pain, and atraumatic professional plaque removal to limit super-infection (e.g. 0.12% or 0.2% Chlorhexidine (Hibitane or Corsodyl")), emollient (softening irritated skin/internal surface/oral mucosa (e.g. orabase, demulcent) and antibiotics in severe conditions with bacterial super-infection.

Recently an anti-viral medication was introduced and it has improved the standard of care that can be offered to patients. Acyclovir is an anti-viral medication which reduces symptoms like fever, decreases development of new lesions and reduces the discomfort experienced during eating. It has been shown that acyclovir 15 mg/kg five times daily for 7 days, when given within three days of onset, will reduce oral lesions presentations to about 4 days only compared to those on palliative care where the oral lesions can take up to 10 days to clear (Wennstrom 1996).

4.6.13. Management of Combined Periodontal and Endodontic Lesions

The combined lesion results from the development and extension of an endodontic lesion into an existing periodontal lesion (Harrington 1979). Differentiation should be made in cases of purely endodontic lesions where the tooth will be non-vital compared to the case of periodontal lesion alone where the pulp status will be vital. In combined perio-endo lesion the tooth involvd would be non-vital. This like the other abscesses is a localized area of infection. The infection may arise primarily from the pulpal tissue and drain through the periodontal pocket and the alveolar bone to the oral cavity or alternatively, the lesion may also be primarily from a periodontal pocket involving the pulpal tissues through the accessory canals or the apex of a tooth. The secondary pulpal infection from the apex of the tooth is known as retrograde pulpitis. The lesion may also arise from a fractured tooth where there is communication between the pulpal and periodontal tissues. The aim of treatment is to eliminate the infection both in the pulp and the periodontium. In periodontal and endodontic lesions, the management begins with treating the endodontic lesion followed by periodontal lesion (Abbot 1998, Gunnar and Gunnar 2006). The pulpal tissues are managed by endodontic treatment. In the periodontium, the treatment may be through periodontal therapy of scaling and root planning and /or surgical therapy to gain access to the root surface. Plaque control is essential. Removal of the tooth is also a treatment option to be considered especially when the lesion is advance or the tooth fractured. Given the fact that both conditions i.e. endodontic and periodontal therapy would mostly need more than one visit to a dentist, compliance of socially disadvantaged patient might be compromised if not impossible and therefore tooth extraction should be considered as the treatment of choice in such cases.

4.6.14. Periodontal Plastic and Aesthetic Conditions

These are conditions where there is an abnormal relationship between the gingival margin and the mucogingival junction. The areas with specific problems are the attached gingiva, shallow vestibules and a frenum interfering with the marginal gingiva.

The examination to detect these defects should be problem focused and include:-

a) A medical history
b) A dental history
c) Relevant findings from probing and visual examination of the periodontium and the intraoral soft tissues

d)   Assessment to identify deficiencies in keratinized gingiva, abnormal frenal attachment and recession
e)   Aetiological factors that may interfere with treatment

Therapy: The goals of periodontal plastic and aesthetic surgery are to maintain the dentition in good function and aesthetics and to reduce the risk of progressive recession (Langer and Langer 1993). This may be accomplished by the following procedures:-

a)   Control of inflammation by plaque control and scaling and root planning.
b)   Root coverage by free gingival autografts, pedicle grafts, lateral repositioned flap, free connective tissue graft, sub-epithelial connective tissue graft (Albandar and Rams 2002) and guided tissue regeneration.
c)   Crown lengthening
d)   Extraction site grafts to prevent ridge collapse
e)   Exposure of unerupted teeth
f)   Frenectomy
g)   Vestibular depth alteration

In all these procedures, the blood supply to the surgical area is the most significant requirement. Without an adequate blood supply, the treatment procedures will fail since the grafts rely on formation of a circulation through anastomosis and angiogenesis from the adjacent gingival tissues.

The desired outcome of treatment should be:-

a)   Healthy periodontium
b)   Correction of the mucogingival condition
c)   Halt the progression of recession
d)   Function and comfort
e)   Satisfactory aesthetics

4.6.15. Management of Gingivitis and Periodontitis Associated with Systemic Conditions

In situations where the periodontal destruction cannot be explained by the local irritants, systemic involvement may be suspected. The following are some of the more common systemic conditions, identified epidemiologically (Rodriguez-Moran and Guerrero-Romero1999), which may alter the response of the periodontium to local irritants or affect treatment outcomes.

a)   Diabetes mellitus
b)   Pregnancy
c)   Leukaemia
d)   Smoking/tobacco use
e)   Osteoporosis/osteopenia

f)   Drug-induced gingival conditions (e.g., phenytoins, calcium channel blockers, immunosuppressants, and long-term systemic steroids

g)   Compromised immune system, either acquired or drug induced

Individuals who are suffering from any of the above conditions or risk factors have to undergo a comprehensive periodontal examination along with laboratory tests to identify the underlying problems. The dental practitioner needs to involve the medical practitioner in the co-management of these patients.

The treatment goal is to achieve periodontal health as well as control of the systemic condition. The involvement of the medical practitioner is important because the periodontal treatment outcome is directly affected by the systemic condition.

4.6.15.1. Management of Periodontal
Conditions among Patients with Diabetes Mellitus

Patients with uncontrolled type 1 or type 2 diabetes are susceptible to periodontal diseases. A meta-analysis that involved cross-sectional studies have shown that there was more periodontal disease in diabetic subjects especially type 2 compared with non-diabetic subjects (Chávarry et al. 2009). In addition, there are studies that have suggested a bidirectional relationship between periodontal disease and glycaemic control with each disease having a potential impact on the other (Mirza et al. 2010, Santacroce et al. 2010, Santos et al. 2010). In patients with uncontrolled diabetes and poor periodontal health, multiple abscesses may be seen. Periodontal infection may worsen glycemic control and should be managed aggressively. Treatment of these individuals will involve control of the underlying systemic condition with the help of the patient's physician as well as treatment of the periodontal condition. The patient should be encouraged to maintain a good level of glycemic control by taking the appropriate medication and controlling the diet as well as maintaining good oral hygiene.

Periodontal therapy has limited success in the presence of poorly controlled or undiagnosed diabetes. Literature shows that most well-controlled diabetic patients can maintain periodontal health and will respond favourably to periodontal therapy (Trevonen and Karjalainen 1997, Westfelt et al. 1996, Offenbacher et al. 1996). Adjunctive systemic antibiotic therapy during the periodontal treatment should be considered especially when multiple abscesses are present or the diabetes is poorly controlled (Grossi 2001, Simpson et al. 2010).

During treatment, it is advisable to minimize stressful long procedures as this will affect the glycemic control. The patient should be advised to also maintain an appropriate diet on the day of periodontal therapy to avoid diabetic complications.

Periodontal treatment among diabetic patients has been reported to improve glycemic control in many patients with both diabetes and periodontal diseases (Teeuw et al. 2010, Mealey and Rose 2008).

4.6.15.2. Management of Periodontal
Conditions among Patients with Pregnancy

The hormonal fluctuations experienced during pregnancy, puberty, and menopause and during the menstrual cycle may alter the patient's response to plaque. There is an exaggerated response to the presence of bacterial plaque.

Hormonal changes during pregnancy can aggravate existing gingivitis. This pregnancy induced gingivitis will get progressively worse until the eight month then resolve a few months after delivery but only if plaque is well controlled and in the absence of plaque retentive factors like calculus. Periodontal diseases have been associated with adverse pregnancy outcome such as preterm birth as well as low birth weight infants (Khader and Ta'ani 2005, Clothier et al. 2007). Consequately, most of the ongoing studies are trying to address issue of treating periodontal disease for the purpose of preventing adverse pregnancy outcomes. However, meta-analysis studies shows results that are more inclined to the view that periodontal treatment does not decrease the incidence of adverse pregnany outcome (Uppal et al. 2010, Polyzos et al. 2010, Macones et al. 2010).

Treatment should include the cause related therapy of oral hygiene instructions, scaling, root planing and prophylaxis with the removal of any plaque retentive factors but periodontal surgery should be postponed to after parturition. Use of systemic antibiotics should be limited and only used if absolutely necessary. Penicillin is the antibiotics of choice in pregnancy.

Hormone-influenced gingivitis appears in some adolescents, and is occasionally a side effect of oral contraceptives in the females. A recent study showed that current users of oral contraceptives had poorer periodontal health (Johnson and Slach 2001). Treatment will include the normal causal related periodontal therapy.

4.6.15.3. Management of Periodontal Conditions among Female Patients on Menopause

The oestrogen deficiency seen after menopause causes a reduction in bone density which can lead to osteoporosis and this condition has been associated with periodontal diseases. Treatment will involve the inclusion of a physician to manage the osteoporosis. Biphosphonates have been used to manage osteoporosis and this also helps in the management of the periodontal condition.

4.6.15.4. Management of Periodontal Conditions among Patients with Leukaemia

Haemorrhagic gingival enlargement with or without necrosis is a common early finding in acute leukaemia. Management of these individuals will have to be done in close cooperation with the patient's physician. Periodontal therapy should be ideally carried out before chemotherapy. These individuals require aggressive periodontal treatment under systemic antibiotic cover with extraction of any hopeless teeth and any teeth which may not have a good prognosis or are potentially infectious in the future.

4.6.15.5. Management of Periodontal Conditions among Smokers

Smoking is associated with poor periodontal health due to the effect of nicotine on the micro-vasculature, the immune system and the response to bacterial plaque. Smokers have been shown by many studies to have more periodontal diseases than non-smokers (Zee 2009, Bergström 2004). Treatment considerations in smokers will include smoking cessation where possible, regular periodontal therapy and when surgical therapy is required, the patient should be fully informed on the risk of delayed wound healing if they do not stop smoking (Hilgers and Kinane 2004, Johnson and Guthmiller 2007, Laxman and Annaji 2008).

4.6.15.6. Management of Drug-Induced Gingival Conditions

The drugs include phenytoins, calcium channel blockers, immunosuppressants, and long-term systemic steroids. These drugs may be associated with gingival enlargement. Treatment should include consultation with the patient's physician and if possible where there is enlargement, the prescription of an alternative drug regimen. Plaque control must be optimum and the patient informed on the recurrence of enlargement if plaque control is inadequate or if the drug modification is not possible.

Surgical therapy to restore aesthetics may be considered in patients with optimum plaque control and in those where a change in the drug regimen is possible. If the change in the drugs taken by the patients is not possible then the patient has to be made aware of the high chances of recurrence. In cases where it is possible to change the drug causing the enlargement and the patient maintains good plaque control, the lesion may subside without surgical intervention.

4.6.15.7. Management of Periodontal Patients with Acquired- or Drug Induced Compromised Immune System

Individuals with a compromised immune system may suffer from more severe forms of periodontal diseases.

a)   Patients with HIV/AIDS
b)   Patients who have received organ transplants and are on immunosuppresants
c)   Patients undergoing cancer therapy
d)   Patients with certain autoimmune diseases

Treatment of these patients must be done in consultation with their physician so as not to compromise their condition. Periodontal therapy should probably be limited to the control of inflammation and maintenance of good plaque control. The extraction of teeth found to have a poor prognosis rather than extensive complicated surgical procedures.

Periodontal therapy should be given to patients who are candidates for the following therapies before they undergo the treatment so as to minimize risk from periodontal infections:

a)   Cancer therapy
b)   Cardiovascular surgery
c)   Joint-replacement surgery
d)   Organ transplantation

4.6.16. Antibiotics in the Management of Gingival/Periodontal Diseases

Generally, antibiotics are not recommended for periodontal therapy since most forms of periodontal diseases will respond reasonably well to conventional mechanical therapy. Additionally, Periodontal diseases is associated with several putative microorganisms rather than one or two species and most of these pathogens will vary in their sensitivity to antibiotics making it difficult to recommend one particular regimen of antibiotic therapy (Haffajee et al. 2003). There is some evidence that use of systemic antibiotic in chronic periodontitis will result in improvement in clinical attachment loss (Olsvik 1995). This line of treatment is still however, not justified because of the resultant antibiotic resistance strains that may develop in time (Slots and Rams 1991). However, there are situations when antibiotic therapy is useful:-

a) Patients with recurrent or refractory disease. These patients will benefit from antibiotic therapy because the recurrent disease may be due to persistent pathogenic species within the periodontal pocket or a compromised host response (Schenkein H and Van Dyke 1994).
b) Patients with acute infections like periodontal /gingival abscesses with accompanying systemic involvement.
c) Patients suffering from necrotizing ulcerative gingivitis/periodontitis. Metronidazole may be useful due to the spirochaetes and obligate anaerobes involved in this condition.
d) Patients with aggressive types of periodontitis (Slots and Ting 2002).
e) Patients with underlying medical conditions like diabetes mellitus may benefit from systemic antibiotics as an adjunct to mechanical therapy.
f) Patients undergoing periodontal surgery may need antibiotic therapy as an adjunct treatment.

The systemic antibiotics should only be given if there is a need for further treatment after a thorough mechanical root debridement followed by surgical access (if needed). The antibiotics prescribed should be based on microbiological testing, the medical status and current medication the patient may be taking. The common antibiotics (and dosage) that are in use for periodontal infections include:-

a) Metronidazole 500 mg/t.i.d./8 days
b) Clindamycin 300 mg/t.i.d./8 days
c) Doxycycline or minocycline 100-200 mg/q.d./21 days
d) Ciprofloxacin 500 mg/b.i.d./8 days
e) Azithromycin 500 mg/q.d./4-7 days
f) Metronidazole + amoxicillin 250 mg/t.i.d./8 days of each drug
g) Metronidazole + ciprofloxacin 500 mg/b.i.d./8 days of each drug

Several studies are available in literature on the use of systemic antibiotics in the treatment of periodontal diseases and for further reading, a review by Slots and Ting, 2002 may be of value in deciding whether or not to use them or which regimen to use. In the underprivileged, use of antibiotics should be limited because of the extra expense involved which may not be necessary.

Therefore careful evaluation and patient selection is important. Topical locally delivered antibiotics are available as an adjunct to periodontal therapy but these drugs are expensive and may not be easily available in the developing countries. Additional uses of antibiotics include root surface conditioning, use with graft materials and use with guided tissue regeneration techniques.

4.6.17. Antiseptics in the Management of Gingival/Periodontal Diseases

This involves the use of antimicrobial mouth rinses in the control of plaque accumulation. Since plaque accumulation has been associated with tissue destruction in gingivitis/periodontitis, it is imperative to keep the levels to a minimum. The inadequacy of mechanical plaque control by many people has been shown in several epidemiological studies where plaque is always recorded in more than 50% of the subjects examined. (Morris et al. 2001). The use of antimicrobial mouth rinses as an adjunct to mechanical plaque control has been studied over the years and the efficacy of several products supported by clinical trials.

4.6.17.1. Mouth Rinses

Essential oils and chlorhexidine have been extensively studied and shown to be effective in plaque inhibition and also in inhibiting the development of gingivitis. They are used as adjuncts and not substitute for plaque control. These rinses penetrate 0.2-1.2mm into the sulcus. This is due to the surface tension and out flowing of the gingival crevicular fluid. Therefore they are mainly used in patients who require extra help. Review and meta-analysis reports shows that formulations containing chlorhexidine, mouthrinses containing essential oils, cetylpyridinium chloride, hexetidine, delmopinol, and dentifrices with amine fluoride/stannous fluoride, triclosan/copolymer dentifrices have been shown to have clinical antiplaque and antigingivitis effects (Baehni and Takeuchi 2003, Gunsolley 2006, Teles and Teles 2009). Also prolonged use of hydrogen peroxide above 1% and less or equal to 3% have been found to reduce plaque and gingivitis as well as enhancing wound healing after periodontal surgery (Marshall et al. 1995). However, the long term incorporation of mouth rinses in the oral health regimen of the underprivileged may not be affordable. Wherever appropriate, their use may be limited to short periods during and after periodontal intsrumentation and periodontal surgery. However, for SDP that are known to be poor, an option to use these antiseptics mostly become impracticle. Therefore most of these populations have been using warm saline gargle and therefore desrve special attention.

4.6.17.2. Warm Saline Gargle

Warm saline gargle is a common mouth wash in some populations and especially socially disadvantaged communities in developing countries where it has been used to treat bleeding gums, gingival inflammation, post extraction cases, post surgical periodontal cases, and apthous ulcers (Malik 2009, Math and Balasubramaniam 2009, Sawair 2010). Warm saline rinse can be used as an alternative to anti-inflammatory drug due to its osmolality and can also be microbicidal. The warm saline rinse solution is made locally at home by adding a pinch of table salt to a cup or glass of warm water and the recommended amount for rinsing is 100-150 mls at least three to four times a day.

4.6.18. Vitamins in the Management of Gingival/Periodontal Diseases

There are no nutritional deficiencics that by themselves can cause gingivitis or periodontitis (Stahl 2005). However, a poor diet deficient in vitamin C and B can contribute to changes in the condition of the periodontium and thus exaggerate the effects of plaque induced inflammation. Vitamin C helps maintain the integrity of the connective tissue and deficiency will result in reduced ability of the periodontium to regenerate and repair itself, increased permeability of the oral mucosa and interference with bone formation leading to poor wound healing, loss of periodontal bone and increased susceptibility to infections. Vitamin B complex group deficiencies can cause oral changes such as gingivitis, glossitis, glossodynia, angular cheilitis and inflammation of the oral mucosa. The gingivitis is due to the deficiencies' modifying effect. There are no studies which demonstrate a relationship between vitamin D or E and periodontal diseases (Stahl 2005). In the management of gingivitis/periodontitis, it is important to also ensure the patients are consuming a health balanced diet to avoid any deficiencies which may accentuate the effects of plaque on the periodontium.

4.6.19. Restorative and Orthodontic Considerations in Periodontal Management

In periodontal treatment, the following procedures may be necessary in order to restore function and aesthetics. These include but are not limited to crown lengthening procedures, tooth exposure, orthodontic tooth eruption, ridge augmentation, gingival augmentation, frenectomy, fiberotomy and extraction and replacement of teeth by partial dentures or implants.

Crown lengthening is a procedure that is done to provide adequate tooth structure for placement of restoration margins coronal to or at the gingival margin. This is so as to avoid the damaging effect to the periodontium of placing restorations subgingivally. Restorations that are placed subgingivally without due consideration of the biological width will lead to destruction of the periodontium.

When teeth are submerged, surgical tooth exposure will restore aesthetics. Orthodontic forced eruption may be necessary in situations where adequate tooth structure is required for restorations. Ridge augmentation, gingival augmentation, frenectomy and fiberotomy are all surgical procedures used to improve aesthetics where the anatomy of the gingival complex has been compromised.

In the underprivileged, some of the above mentioned procedures may be expensive in terms of finances, time and even availability of a periodontist to do the work. The management in such situation may include extraction of the offending tooth/teeth followed by plastic removable partial dentures.

4.6.20. Supportive Periodontal (Maintenance) Therapy

Following active periodontal therapy, it is very important that maintenance of the patient is done on a regular basis to prevent recurrence of the disease (Tan 2009).

This follow up visits should include:-

a)   Update of the medical and dental histories
b)   Evaluation of the current status of the periodontal tissues and the teeth
c)   Assessment of the oral hygiene status

Depending on the findings, the following may be necessary:-

a) Treatment of any new carious lesions, repair of any defective restorations especially those that may be plaque retentive
b) Re-enforcement of plaque control measures and re-treatment of recurrent disease if any. Treatment of any new lesions.
c) Local delivery or systemic chemotherapeutic agents may be used in the case of recurrent disease and when the patient is able to afford the treatment.
d) Establish a suitable interval for periodontal maintenance for each individual patient. The determination of the interval for periodontal maintenance will depend on the findings at the follow up visits. If new lesions are found or the plaque control is inadequate, then the interval is shortened.

The patient should also be informed of problem areas or new areas of disease so that they can pay special attention to these areas. They should also be advised on the need for additional treatment and any other oral changes.

References

Abid A (2004). Oral health in Tunisia. *Int. Dent. J.* 54(6 Suppl 1):389-94.

Abbott P (1998). Endodontic management of combined endodontic-periodontal lesions. *J N Z Soc Periodontol.*;83:15-28.

Albandar JM, Muranga MB, Rams TE (2002). The prevalence of aggressive periodontitis in school attendees in Uganda. *Journal of Clinical Periodontology* 29: 823-831.

Albandar JM, Rams TE (2002). Global epidemiology of periodontal diseases: an overview. *Periodontol.* 2000; 29:7–10.

Albander JM (2002). Global risk factors and risk indicators for periodontal diseases. *Periodontology* 2000. Vol 29, 177-206

Alfaro DP, Ahluwalia KP (2010). Oral care needs, barriers and challenges among community dwelling elderly in New York State and northern Manhattan. *N Y State Dent J.*;76(5):38-41.

Amir J, Harel L, Smetana Z, Varsano I (1997): Treatment of herpes simplex gingivostomatitis with acyclovir in children: a randomized double blind placebo-controlled study, *BMJ*, 314:1800-1803.

Arendorf TM, Bredekamp B, Cloete CA, Joshipura K (2001). Seasonal variation of acute necrotising ulcerative gingivitis in South Africans. *Oral Dis.*;7(3):150-154.

Armitage GC (1999). Development of a classification system for periodontal diseases and conditions. *Annals of Periodontology* 4:1-6.

Armitage GC (2002). Classifying periodontal diseases - a long- standing dilemma. *Periodontology* 2000; 30: 9-23.

Armitage GC, Robertson PB (2009). The biology, prevention, diagnosis and treatment of periodontal diseases: scientific advances in the United States. *Journal of American Dental association*;140 Suppl 1:36S-43S.

Axelsson P and Lindhe J (1981). The significance of maintenance care in the treatment of Periodontal diseases, *J. Clin. Periodontal.*; 8: 281-294.

Axelsson P, Lindhe J and Nystrom B (1991). On prevention of dental caries and Periodontal diseases: Results of a 15 year longitudinal study on adults, *J. Clin. Periodontol* 18; 182-189.

Baehni PC, Takeuchi Y (2003). Anti-plaque agents in the prevention of biofilm-associated oral diseases. *Oral Dis.*; 9 Suppl 1:23-29.

Baelum V, Fejerskov O, Karring T (1986). Oral hygiene, gingivitis and periodontal breakdown in adult Tanzaninans. *J. Periodontal. Res.*;21:221-232.

Baelum V, Fejerskov O, Manji F (1988). Periodontal diseases in adult Kenyans. *J. Clin. Periodontol*; 15: 445–452.

Baer PN (1971). The case of periodontosis as a clinical entity. *Journal of periodontology* 42: 516-520.

Behbehani JM, Scheutz F (2004). Oral health in Kuwait. *Int. Dent. J.;* 54: 401-408.

Bergström J (2004). Tobacco smoking and chronic destructive periodontal diseases. *Odontology;* 92(1):1-8.

Borrell LN, Beck JD, Heiss G (2006). Socioeconomic disadvantage and periodontal diseases: the Dental Atherosclerosis Risk in Communities study. *Am. J. Public Health;* 96(2):332-339.

Bower RC (1979): Furcation morphology relative to periodontal treatment: furcation root surface anatomy, *J. Periodontol.* 50:366-374.

Bower (RC 1979): Furcation morphology relative to periodontal treatment: furcation entrance architecture, *J. Periodontol.* 50:23-27.

Brennan DS, Roberts-Thomson KF, Spencer AJ (2007). Oral health of Indigenous adult public dental patients in Australia. *Aust. Dent. J.;* 52(4): 322-328.

Brindle R, Wilkinson D, Harrison A, Connolly C, Cleaton-Jones P (2000). Oral health in Hlabisa, KwaZulu/Natal--a rural school and community based survey. *Int. Dent. J..*;50(1):13-20.

Bukar A, Danfillo IS, Adeleke OA, Ogunbodede EO (2004). Traditional oral health practices among Kanuri women of Borno State, Nigeria. *Odontostomatol. Trop.*;27(107):25-31.

Burt BA, Ismail AI, Morrison EC, Beltran ED (1990). Risk factors for tooth loss over a 28-year period. *J. Dent. Res.*; 69: 1126–1130.

Cameron CA, Evans GD, Perry DA (2007). Clinical assessment. In Perry DA and Beemsterboer PL. Plaque and disease control for the periodontal patient. In: Peryy DA, Beemsterboer PL (eds). Saunders/ Elevier/ Evolve; *Periodontology for dental hygienist* *Chpt.* 8, pp. 161-200.

Clarke M, Locker D, Murray H, Payne B (1996). The oral health of disadvantaged adolescents in North York, Ontario. *Can J. Public Health*;87(4):261-263.

Clothier B, Stringer M, Jeffcoat MK (2007). Periodontal disease and pregnancy outcomes: exposure, risk and intervention. *Best Pract. Res. Clin. Obstet. Gynaecol.*;21(3):451-466.

Cobb CM, Carrara A, El-Annan E, Youngblood LA, Becker BE, Becker W, Oxford GE, Williams KB (2003). Periodontal referral patterns, 1980 versus 2000: A preliminary study. *J. Periodontol.*;74:1470-1474.

Cobb CM (1996). Non-surgical pocket therapy: mechanical. *Ann. Periodontol.*;1:443–490.

Copulos TA, Low SB, Walker CB, Trebilcock YY and Heifti AF (1993). Comparative analysis between a modified ultrasonic tip and hand instruments on clinical parameters of periodontal diseases. *J. Periodontol.*, 64: 694-700.

Cutress TW, Powell RN, Ball ME (1982). Differing profiles of periodontal diseases in two similar South Pacific island populations. *Community Dent Oral Epidemiol*; 10: 193–203.

Dolan TA, Atchison KA (1993). Implications of access, utilization and need for oral health care by the non-institutionalized and institutionalized elderly on the dental delivery system. *J. Dent. Educ.*; 57(12): 876-887.

Drisko CL, Cochran DL, Blieden T, Bouwsma OJ, Cohen RE, Damoulis P, Fine JB, Greenstein G, Hinrichs J, Somerman MJ, Iacono V, Genco RJ (2000): Position paper: Sonic and ultrasonic scalers in periodontics. Research, Science and Therapy committee of the American Academy of Periodontology. *J. Periodontol.* 71(11);1792-1801

Dye BA, Vargas CM (2002). The use of a modified CPITN approach to estimate periodontal treatment needs among adults aged 20-79 years by socio-demographic characteristics in the United States, 1988-94. *Community Dent Health.*;19(4):215-223.

Echeverria JJ, Sanz M, Rylander H (2003). Mechanical supragingival plaque control. In: Lindhe J, Karring T and Lang NP, editors. Clinical periodontology and implant dentistry. Oxford: Blackwell Munksgaard, chpt. 21, pp.449-463.

Elamin AM, Skaug N, Ali RW, Bakken V, Albandar JM (2010). Ethnic disparities in the prevalence of periodontitis among high school students in Sudan. *J. Periodontol.*;81(6):891-896.

Enwonwu CO, Falkler WA Jr, Idigbe EO, Savage KO (1999). Noma (cancrum oris): questions and answers. *Oral Dis.* 5(2):144-149.

Esan TA, Olusile AO, Ojo MA, Udoye CI, Oziegbe EO, Olasoji HO (2010). Tooth loss among Nigerians treated in teaching hospitals: a national pilot study. *J. Contemp. Dent. Pract.* 14;11(5):17-24.

Finlayson TL, Gansky SA, Shain SG, Weintraub JA (2010). Dental utilization among Hispanic adults in agricultural worker families in California's Central Valley. *J. Public Health Dent.* 70(4):292-299.

Flemming TF (1999). Periodontitis. *Annals of Periodontology* 4:32-38.

Folayan MO (2004). The epidemiology, etiology, and pathophysiology of acute necrotizing ulcerative gingivitis associated with malnutrition. *J. Contemp. Dent. Pract.* 15;5(3):28-41.

Garcha V, Shetiya SH, Kakodkar P (2010). Barriers to oral health care amongst different social classes in India. *Community Dent Health*;27(3):158-162.

Glickman I (1953): Clinical Periodontology, Philadelphia, Saunders.

Grossi SG (2001). Treatment of periodontal disease and control of diabetes: an assessment of the evidence and need for future research. *Ann. Periodontol.* 6(1): 138-145.

Gunnar Bergenholtz, Gunnar Hasselgren (2006). Endodontics and periodontics. In: Lindhe J, Karring T and Lang NP, editors. Clinical periodontology and implant dentistry. Oxford: Blackwell Munksgaard;. Chpt. 14, pp 318-351.

Gunsolley J (2006). Meta-analysis of six month studies evaluating anti-plaque, anti-gingivitis agents. *JADAJ Am. Dent. Assoc.*, Vol 137, No 12, 1649-1657.

Haffajee AD, Socransky SS, Gunsolley JC (2003). Systemic anti-infective periodontal therapy. A systematic review. *Ann. Periodontol.* 8:115-181.

Harrington GW (1979). The perio-endo question: Differential diagnosis. *Dent. Clin. North Am.* 23:673-690.

Hart TC (1996): Genetic risk factors for early-onset periodontitis, *J. Periodontol.,* 67;355-366.

Hilgers KK, Kinane DF (2004). Smoking, Periodontal diseases and the role of the dental profession. *Int. J. Dent. Hyg.* 2(2):56-63.

Holmstrup P (1988). Non-plaque induced gingival lesions, Ann. Periodontol. 4: 20, 1999 *J. Clin. Periodontol.* 15;445-452.

Idigbe EO, Enwonwu CO, Falkler WA, Ibrahim MM, Onwujekwe D, Afolabi BM, Savage KO, Meeks VI (1999). Living conditions of children at risk for noma: Nigerian experience. *Oral Dis*; 5(2):156-162.

Johnson GK, Guthmiller JM (2007). The impact of cigarette smoking on periodontal disease and treatment. *Periodontol* 2000; 44:178-194.

Johnson GK, Slach NA (2001). Impact of tobacco use on periodontal status. *J. Dent. Educ.*; 65:313-21.

Kaimenyi JT (1999). Demography and seasonal variation of acute necrotising gingivitis in Nairobi, Kenya. *Int. Dent. J.*;49(6):347-351.

Kareha MJ, Rosenberg ES, DeHaven H (1981). Therapeutic considerations in the management of a periodontal abscess with an infrabony defect, *J. Clin. Periodontol* 8;375-386.

Khader YS, Ta'ani Q (2005). Periodontal diseases and the risk of preterm birth and low birth weight: a meta-analysis. *J. Periodontol.* 76(2):161-5.

Kikwilu EN, Masalu JR, Kahabuka FK, Senkoro AR (2008). Prevalence of oral pain and barriers to use of emergency oral care facilities among adult Tanzanians. *BMC Oral Health*;8:28.

Kruger E, Jacobs A (2010). Tennant M. Sustaining oral health services in remote and indigenous communities: a review of 10 years experience in Western Australia. *Int. Dent. J.*.;60(2):129-134.

Laher MH (1990). A comparison between dental caries, gingival health and dental service usage in Bangladeshi and white Caucasian children aged 7, 9, 11, 13 and 15 years residing in an inner city area of London, UK. *Community Dent Health.*;7(2):157-163.

Lalloo R, Myburgh NG, Smith MJ, Solanki GC (2004). Access to health care in South Africa-the influence of race and class. S *Afr. Med. J.*; 94(8): 639-642.

1999 International International Workshop for a Classification of Periodontal Diseases and Conditions (1999): Consensus report: aggressive periodontitis, *Ann. Periodontol.,* 4:53-74.

Langer L, and Langer B (1993). The sub-epithelial connective tissue graft for treatment of gingival recession. *Dent. Clin. North Am.,* 37:243-264.

Laxman VK, Annaji S (2008). Tobacco use and its effects on the periodontium and periodontal therapy. *J. Contemp. Dent. Pract.*;9(7):97-107.

Lembariti BS, van't Hof MA, Pilot T, van Palenstein-Helderman WH (1997). Clinical parameters associated with periodontitis in untreated persons. *East Afr. Med. J.*;74(7):427-30.

Lindhe J, Ranney R, Lamster I, Charles A, Chung C-P, Flemming T, Kinane D, Listgarten M, Loe H, Schoor R, Seymour G and Somerman M (1999) Consensus report: Chronic Periodontitis. *Ann. Periodontol.* 4:38-45.

Lindhe J, Socransky S, Wennström J (1986). Design of clinical trials of traditional therapies of periodontitis. *J. Clin. Periodontol.*;13(5): 488-499.

Liu XN, Shinada K, Chen XC, Zhang BX, Yaegaki K, Kawaguchi Y (2006). Oral malodor-related parameters in the Chinese general population. *Journal of Clinical Periodontology*; 33: 31-36.

Locker D, Jokovic A. (1997). Three-year changes in self-perceived oral health status in an older Canadian population. *J Dent Res.*;76(6):1292-7.

Loe H, Theilade E, Jensen S (1965). Experimental gingivitis in man. *J. Periodontol. Res* 36:177-187.

Luhanga C, Ntabaye M (2001). Geriatric oral health issues in Africa: Tanzanian perspective. *Int. Dent. J.*;51(3 Suppl):219-227.

Löe H, Anerud A, Boysen H, Morrison E (1986). Natural history of periodontal diseases in man. Rapid, moderate and no loss of attachment in Sri Lankan laborers 14 to 46 years of age. *Journal of Clinical Periodontology*;13:431-445.

Löe H, Theilade E, Jensen SB (1965). Experimental gingivitis in man. *Journal of Periodontology*; 36: 177-187.

Macones GA, Parry S, Nelson DB, Strauss JF, Ludmir J, Cohen AW, Stamilio DM, Appleby D, Clothier B, Sammel MD, Jeffcoat M (2010). Treatment of localized periodontal disease in pregnancy does not reduce the occurrence of preterm birth: results from the Periodontal Infections and Prematurity Study (PIPS). *Am. J. Obstet Gynecol.*;202(2):147.e1-8.

Malik R (2009). Warm saline rinses. *Br. Dent. J.;* 12; 207(11):520.

Mamai-Homata E, Polychronopoulou A, Topitsoglou V, Oulis C, Athanassouli T (2010). Periodontal diseases in Greek adults between 1985 and 2005--risk indicators. Int. Dent. J.;60(4):293-299.

Manson JD, Lehner T (1974). Clinical features of juvenile periodontitid (periodontosis). *Journal of periodontology* 45: 636-640.

Marshall MV, Cancro LP, Fischman SL (1995). Hydrogen peroxide: a review of its use in dentistry. *J. Periodontol.*; 66(9):786-796.

Math M V, Balasubramaniam P (2009). Water swishing. *Br. Dent. J.*; 207: 304.

Mealey BL, Klokkevold PR (2006). Periodontal medicine: Impact of periodontal infection on systemic health. In: Carranza's clinical periodontology, 10th ed. Newman MC, Takei HH, Klokkevold PR, Carranza FA (eds). St. Louis: Saunders, Elsevier, 312-329.

Mealey BL, Rose LF (2008). Diabetes mellitus and inflammatory periodontal diseases. *Compend. Contin. Educ. Dent.*;29(7);402-413.

Melnick PR and Takei HH (2006). Treatment of periodontal abscess. In: Carranza's clinical periodontology, 10th ed. Newman MC, Takei HH, Klokkevold PR, Carranza FA (eds). St. Louis: Saunders, Elsevier. Chpt. 48, pp. 714-721.

Meng HX (1999): Periodontal abscess, Ann. Periodontol., 4;79-83.

Milgrom P, Reisine S (2000). Oral health in the United States: the post-fluoride generation. *Annu. Rev. Public Health.*;21:403-436.

Mirza BA, Syed A, Izhar F, Ali Khan A (2010). Bidirectional relationship between diabetes and periodontal disease: review of evidence. *J. Pak. Med. Assoc.*; 60(9):766-768.

Miyazaki H, Sakao S, Katoh Y, Takehara T (1995). Correlation between volatile sulphur compounds and certain oral health measurements in the general population. *Journal of Periodontology*; 66: 679-684.

Mombelli A (2003). Periodontitis as an infectious disease: specific features and their implications. *Oral Dis.*;9 Suppl 1:6-10.

Morris AJ, Steele J, White DA (2001). The oral cleanliness and periodontal health of UK adults in 1998. *Br. Dent. J.*;191(4):186–192.

Mumghamba EG, Fabian FM (2005). Tooth loss among habitual chewing-stick and plastic toothbrush users in the adult population of Mtwara, rural Tanzania. *Int. J. Dent Hyg.*;3(2):64-69.

Mumghamba EG, Honkala S, Honkala E, Manji KP (2009). Gingival recession, oral hygiene and associated factors among Tanzanian women. *East Afr. Med. J.*, 86:125-132.

Mumghamba EGS (2009). Periodontal diseases in Tanzania. A PhD-Thesis Summary, University of Turku, Turku, Finland, Annales D-847, (https://oa.doria.fi/handle/10024/44888).

Mumghamba EGS, Markkanen HA, Honkala E (1995). Risk factors for Periodontal diseases in Ilala, Tanzania. *Journal of Clinical Periodontology*;5:347-354.

Ndiaye FC, Bourgeois D, Leclercq MH, Berthe O (1999). Noma: public health problem in Senegal and epidemilogical surveillance. *Oral Dis.*;5(2):163-166.

Novak KF, Novak MJ (2006a). Aggressive Periodntitis In: Carranza's clinical periodontology, 10th ed. Newman MC, Takei HH, Klokkevold PR, Carranza FA (eds). St. Louis: Saunders, Elsevier, pp.506–512.

Novak KF, Novak MJ (2006b). Chronic Periodntitis In: Carranza's clinical periodontology, 10th ed. Newman MC, Takei HH, Klokkevold PR, Carranza FA (eds). St. Louis: Saunders, Elsevier, pp.494–499.

Nunn J, Freeman R, Anderson E, Carneiro LC, Carneiro MS, Formicola A, Frezel R, Kayitenkore J, Luhanga C, Molina G, Morio I, Nartey NO, Ngom PI, de Lima Navarro MF, Segura A, Oliver S, Thompson S, Wandera M, Yazdanie N (2008). Inequalities in access to education and healthcare. *Eur. J. Dent. Educ.*; 12 Suppl 1:30-39.

O'Leary TJ (1969): Tooth mobility, *Dent Clin North Am*; 3:567-579.

Offenbacher S, Katz V, Fertick G, Collins J, Maynor G, McKaig R (1996). Periodontal infection as a possible risk factor for preterm low birth weight. *J. Periodontol.*; 67:1103-1113.

Offenbacher S (1996). Periodontal diseases: Pathogenesis. *Ann. Periodontol.* 1: 821-878.

Oginni FO (2005). Tooth loss in a sub-urban Nigerian population: causes and pattern of mortality revisited. *Int. Dent. J.;* 55(1):17-23.

Okullo I, Astrøm AN, Haugejorden O (2004). Social inequalities in oral health and in use of oral health care services among adolescents in Uganda. *Int. J. Paediatr* Dent;14(5):326-335.

Page RC, Martin J, Krall EA, Mancl L, Garcia R (2003). Longitudinal validatioof a risk calculator for periodontal diseases. *J. Clin. Periodontol*;30(9):819–827.

Page RC, Schroeder HE (1982). Periodontitis in man and other animals: a comparative review, Basel, S Karger.

Page RC (1998). Periodontal diseases: A new paradigm. *J. Dental Educ.*;62(10):812-820.

Page RC (1999). Milestones in periodontal research and the remaining critical issues. *J. Periodontol. Res.* 34:331-339.

Pattison AM, Pattison GL (2006). Scaling and root planning. In: Carranza's clinical periodontology, 10th ed. Newman MC, Takei HH, Klokkevold PR, Carranza FA (eds). St. Louis: Saunders, Elsevier, chpt.51, pp. 749-797.

Perry and Beemsterboer (2007). Plaque and disease control for the periodontal patient. In: Peryy DA, Beemsterboer PL (eds). Saunders/ Elevier/ Evolve; Periodontology for dental hygienist Chpt. 11, pp. 235-258.

Petersen PE (2004). Challenges to improvement of oral health in the 21st century--the approach of the WHO Global Oral Health Programme. *Int. Dent. J.;* 54(6 Suppl 1): 329-343.

Petersen PE, Bourgeois D, Ogawa H, Estupinan-Day S, Ndiaye C (2005). The global burden of oral diseases and risks to oral health. *Bull World Health Organ*; 83(9):661-669.

Polyzos NP, Polyzos IP, Zavos A, Valachis A, Mauri D, Papanikolaou EG, Tzioras S, Weber D, Messinis IE (2010). Obstetric outcomes after treatment of periodontal disease during pregnancy:systematic review and meta-analysis. *BMJ;* 29;341:c7017. doi: 10.1136/bmj.c7017.

Position Paper of the American Academy of Periodontology (1996). Epidemiology of periodontal diseases. *J. Periodontol.*; 67: 935–945.

Quirynen M and van Steenberghe D (2006). Oral malodor. In: Newman MG, Takei HH, Klokkevold PR, Carranza FA, editors. Carranza's Clinical Periodontology Philadelphia, Saunders, chpt. 19; pp. 330-342.

Rateitschak KH, Rateitschak EM, Wolf HF, Hassell TM (1989). Color atlas of dental medicine 1. Periodontology, 2nd revised and expanded edition. Home care by the patient pp.115-129, 148-160.

Renvert S, Wikstrom M, Dahlen G, Slots J, Egelberg J (1990): Effect of root debridement on the elimination of Actinobacillus actinomycetemcomitans and Bacteroides gingivalis from periodontal pockets, *J. Clin. Periodontol*; 17:345-350.

Richards W, Ameen J, Coll AM, Higgs G (2005). Reasons for tooth extraction in four general dental practices in South Wales. *Br. Dent. J.;* 12;198(5):275-278.

Rodriguez-Moran M, Guerrero-Romero F (1999). Increased levels of C-reactive protein in noncontrolled type II diabetic subjects. *J. Diabetes Complications*; 13: 211–215.

Santacroce L, Carlaio RG, Bottalico L (2010). Does it make sense that diabetes is reciprocally associated with periodontal disease? *Endocr. Metab. Immune Disord. Drug Targets*.1;10(1):57-70.

Santos Tunes R, Foss-Freitas MC, Nogueira-Filho Gda R (2010). Impact of periodontitis on the diabetes-related inflammatory status. *J. Can. Dent. Assoc.*;76:a35.

Sanz M, Roldan S, Herrera D (2001). Fundamentals of breath malodour. *J. Contemp. Dent. Pract*; 4: 1-17.

Sawair FA (2010). Recurrent aphthous stomatitis: do we know what patients are using to treat the ulcers? *J. Altern Complement Med.*;16(6): 651-655.

Sayegh A, Hilow H, Bedi R (2004). Pattern of tooth loss in recipients of free dental treatment at the University Hospital of Amman, Jordan. *J Oral Rehabil.*;31(2):124-30.

Schenkein HA, Van Dyke TE (1994). Early-onset periodontitis: Systemic aspects of etiology and pathogenesis. *Periodontol.* 2000;6:7-25.

Simon C, Tesfaye F, Berhane Y (2003). Assessment of the oral health status of school children in Addis Ababa *Ethiop. Med. J.*;41(3):245-56.

Simon EN, Matee MI, Scheutz F (2008). Oral health status of handicapped primary school pupils in Dar es Salaam, Tanzania. *East Afr. Med. J.*; 85(3): 113-117.

Simpson TC, Needleman I, Wild SH, Moles DR, Mills EJ (2010). Treatment of periodontal disease for glycaemic control in people with diabetes. *Cochrane Database Syst Rev.* 2;(5):CD004714.

Slade GD, Spencer AJ, Gorkic E, Andrews G (1993). Oral health status and treatment needs of non-institutionalized persons aged 60+ in Adelaide, South Australia. *Aust. Dent. J.;*38(5):373-380.

Slots J, Bragd L, Wikström M, Dáhlen G (1986). The occurrence of Actinobacillus actinomycetemcomitans, Bacteroides gingivalis and Bacteroides intermedius in destructive periodontal diseases in adults. *J. Clin. Periodontol;* 13: 570–577.

Slots J, Möenbo D, Langebaek J, Frandsen A (1978). Microbiota of gingivitis in man. *Scand J. Dent. Res.;*86(3):174-181.

Slots J, Rams TE (1991). New views on periodontal microbiota in special patient categories. *J. Clin. Periodontol;* 18:411-420.

Slots J, Ting M (2002). Systemic antibiotics in the treatment of periodontal diseases. *Periodontol* 2000; 28:106-176.

Smith BA, Collier CM, Caffesse RG (1985). In vitro effectiveness of dental floss in plaque removal, *J. Clin. Periodontol.;*13: 211-216.

Socransky SS, Haffajee AD (2003). Microbiology of periodontal diseases. In: Clinical periodontology and implant dentistry. Lindhe J, Lang NP and Karring T (eds). Oxford: Blackwell Munksgaard, pp. 106–149.

Socransky SS, Haffajee AD (1997). The nature of periodontal diseases. *Ann. Periodontol.;* 2(1):3-10.

Soder B, Johannson B, So¨der P (2000). The relationship between foetor ex ore, oral hygiene and periodontal diseases. *Swedish Dental Journal;* 24: 73–82.

Sofola OO, Shaba OP, Jeboda SO (2003). Oral hygiene and periodontal treatment needs of urban school children compared with that of rural school children in Lagos State. Nigeria. *Odontostomatol Trop.;*26(101):25-29.

Somkotra T, Detsomboonrat P (2009). Is there equity in oral healthcare utilization: experience after achieving universal coverage. *Community Dent. Oral Epidemiol.;*37(1):85-96.

Song SK, Shon ZH, Kim YK, Kim CH, Yoo SY, Park SH (2009). Characteristics of malodor pollutants and aromatic VOCs around an urban valley in Korea. *Environ Monit Assess.;*157:259-275.

Spalj S, Plancak D, Bozic D, Kasaj A, Willershausen B, Jelusic D (2008). Periodontal conditions and oral hygiene in rural population of post-war Vukovar region, Croatia in correlation to stress. *Eur. J. Med. Res.;*13(3):100-6.

Stahl SS (2005). Repair or regeneration following periodontal surgery, *J. Clin. Periodontol.;* ,6; 389-389.

Syrjälä AM, Ylöstalo P, Knuuttila M (2010). Periodontal condition of the elderly in Finland. *Acta Odontol. Scand.;*68(5):278-283.

Taiwo JO (1996). Effect of social class on the prevalence and severity of necrotising ulcerative gingivitis in Nigerian children. *Afr. J. Med. Sci.;*25(4):357-360.

Taiwo JO (1995). Severity of necrotizing ulcerative gingivitis in Nigerian children. *Periodontal Clin. Investig.;*17(2):24-27.

Tan AE (2009). Periodontal maintenance. *Aust. Dent. J ;* 54 Suppl 1:S110-117.

Tanwir F, Altamash M, Gustafsson A (2006). Perception of oral health among adults in Karachi. *Oral Health Prev Dent.;*4(2):83-89.

Teeuw WJ, Gerdes VE, Loos BG (2010). Effect of periodontal treatment on glycemic control of diabetic patients: a systematic review and meta-analysis. *Diabetes Care.*;33(2):421-427.

Teles RP, Teles FR (2009). Antimicrobial agents used in the control of periodontal biofilms: effective adjuncts to mechanical plaque control? *Braz. Oral Res.*;23 Suppl 1:39-48.

Timmerman MF, Van der Weijden GA, Abbas F, Arief EM, Armand S, Winkel EG, Van Winkelhoff AJ, Van der Velden U (2000). Untreated periodontal disease in Indonesian adolescents. Longitudinal clinical data and prospective clinical and microbiological risk assessment. *J. Clin. Periodontol.*;27(12):932-942.

Timmerman MF, van der Weijden GA (2006). Risk factors for periodontitis. *Int. J. Dent Hyg*;4(1):2–7

Trevonen T, Karjalainen K (1997). Periodontal diseases related to diabetic status: a pilot study of the response to periodontal therapy in type 1 diabetes, *J. Clin. Periodotol*, 24: 505-510

Uppal A, Uppal S, Pinto A, Dutta M, Shrivatsa S, Dandolu V, Mupparapu M (2010). The effectiveness of periodontal disease treatment during pregnancy in reducing the risk of experiencing preterm birth and low birth weight: a meta-analysis. *J. Am. Dent Assoc.*;141 (12):1423-34.

van Palenstein Helderman WH, Munck L, Mushendwa S, Mrema FG (1992). Cleaning effectiveness of chewing sticks among Tanzanian schoolchildren. *J. Clin. Periodontol.*; 19:460–463.

van der Velden U, Abbas F, Armand S, de Graaff J, Timmerman MF, van der Weijden GA, van Winkelhoff AJ, Winkel EG (1993). The effect of sibling relationship on the periodontal condition. *J. Clin. Periodontol.*; 20(9): 683-690.

Varenne B, Petersen PE, Ouattara S (2006). Oral health behaviour of children and adults in urban and rural areas of Burkina Faso, Africa. *Int. Dent. J.*;56(2):61-70.

Wade Ab, Blake G Mirza K (1966). Effectiveness of metronidazole in trating the acute pahse of ulcerative gingivitis, *Dent Pract.*; 16: 440.

Wagaiyu EG, Wagaiyu CK (1992). Prevalence of juvenile periodontitis in national youth service trainees. *East Afr. Med. J.*; 69(1):31-33.

Wells PL, Caplan DJ, Strauss RP, Bell D, George M (2010). An oral health survey of the Lumbee tribe in southeastern North Carolina. *J Dent Hyg.*; 84(3):137-144.

Wennstrom JL (1996). Mucogingival therapy, *Ann. Periodontol.*; 1(1):671-701.

Westfelt E, Rylander H, Blohme G, Jonasson P, Lindhe J (1996). The effect of periodontal therapy in diabetics: results after 5 years, *J. Clin. Periodontol* 23(2):92-100.

WHO (1978). Epidemiology, etiology and prevention of periodontal diseases. Report of WHO Scientific Group, Technical Report Series 621. Geneva.

WHO (1987). Oral health surveys. Basic methods, 3rd ed. Geneva.

WHO (2000). Consensus statement on oral hygiene. *Int. Dent. J.;* 50(3):129-139.

Wilkins EM (1976). Clinical practice of the dental hygienist, 4th Ed. Lea and Febiger, Philadelphia Chpt. 22, pp. 307-328.

Wing S, Horton RA, Marshall SW, Thu K, Tajik M, Schinasi L, Schiffman SS (2008). Air pollution and odor in communities near industrial swine operations. *Environ. Health Perspect.*;116:1362-1368.

Wu DC, Darout IA, Skaug N (2001). Chewing sticks: timeless natural toothbrushes for oral cleaning. *J. Periodont. Res.*; 36:275-284.

Yaegaki K, Coil JM (2000). Examination, classification, and treatment of halitosis; clinical perspectives. *Journal of Canadian Dental Association*; 66: 257–261.

Zee KY (2009). Smoking and periodontal disease. *Aust. Dent. J.;*54 Suppl 1:S44-50.

In: Oral Health Care for Socially Disadvantaged Communities   ISBN: 978-1-62948-287-3
Editors: F.K. Kahabuka, E.N. Kikwilu and I. Anderson © 2013 Nova Science Publishers, Inc.

Chapter V

Surgical Conditions of the Oral and Maxillofacial Region

***Boniphace M. Kalyanyama, Sira S. Owibingire
and Elison N. Simon***
Department of Oral Surgery and Oral Pathology –
Muhimbili University of Health and Allied Sciences

5.1. Introduction

Surgical conditions that occur in the oral and maxillofacial region include trauma, infections, tumour and tumour-like lesions, congenital anomalies and developmental disorders. Others are oral mucosal lesions, neuralgias, temporomandibular joint and autoimmune disorders. These conditions occur in both socially disadvantaged and advantaged individuals but the occurrence, severity and prognosis of such conditions are likely to differ between these two groups with the disadvantaged suffering the most. The conditions that are commonly encountered in authors' daily practice are covered here with the aim of documenting the epidemiology, aetiology, clinical features and management of the common surgical conditions that occur in the oral and maxillofacial region in socially disadvantaged communities.

5.2. Traumatic Injuries in the Oro-Facial Region

5.2.1. Type of Injuries

The oro-facial region is susceptible to injuries from different traumatic afflictions. Trauma to this region may result in injuries to soft tissues or hard tissues (fractures of teeth and bones). In most instances there is a combination of both soft and hard tissue injuries. The major cause of maxillofacial injuries in a given society depends on socioeconomic and socio-cultural factors. In the disadvantaged communities in general and in Tanzania in particular the number of patients suffering from maxillofacial injuries has been increasing (Moshy J et al. 1996, Adebayo et al. 2003, Deogratius et al. 2006,). The main causes of maxillofacial injuries have been reported to be road traffic accidents (Abiose 1986, Oji 1999, Adebayo et al. 2003, Schaftenaar et al. 2009) and assaults (Khan 1988, Mwaniki and Guthua 1990, Olasoji et al. 2002). This is possibly because of the considerable overcrowding in the urban areas and a substantial rural to urban drift. In urban areas an increase in road traffic volume that is not matched with an improvement of the infrastructure, increase in social violence and increasing socio-economic problems are among the contributing factors. Other causes are sports and games, gun shot and explosives, occupational (e.g. falls from heights at construction sites) and attacks by animals. There is an overwhelming majority of males among the patients who present with maxillofacial injuries ranging from 69% to 82% (Oji 1999, Adebayo et al. 2003, Schaftenaar et al. 2009).

5.2.2. Immediate Measures

Maxillofacial injuries are often accompanied by life threatening injuries in other areas of the body. For that matter careful initial assessment and preliminary measures are important to the general wellbeing of the patient (Beek and Merkx 1999). Cardiopulmonary stability evidenced by vital signs i.e. blood pressure, respiratory rate and pulse rate should be assessed immediately to ensure satisfactory airway, breathing and circulation. If there are any signs of airway obstruction appropriate measures should be taken to make sure that the patient is breathing fairly well. Haemorrhage should immediately be controlled by pressure dressing, packing, or clamping of bleeding blood vessels. In disadvantaged communities where there may be shortages of materials crepe bandages, ordinary bandages or any available clean pieces of cloth can be used to apply pressure in a profusely bleeding area. If there are signals of impending shock appropriate measures to reverse it should start promptly. Such measures include lying the patient down with the head slightly inclined below the rest of the body and replacement of blood volume. A patient who is conscious should be put in a sitting position with the head leaning forward. A fainting or semiconscious patient should be put in the recovery position to avoid falling back of the tongue. During these initial processes the health personnel may collect preliminary information. Full case clerkship should be done at a later stage.

Assessment of the cervical spine and head injury is very important since these are structures likely to get involved during injuries of oral-facial structures. Care should be taken not to disturb the spine with unnecessary movements until declared safe. If still in doubt of the safety of the cervical spine a neck collar can be placed. In cases where a clear airway cannot be maintained a nasopharyngeal or an oropharyngeal intubation should be done until when the patient is declared out of danger. In severe crush injuries and comminuted fractures of the oral-facial skeleton accompanied by bleeding and obstruction of the upper airway a tracheostomy is necessary.

The time lapse between injury and presentation to hospital in most instances determines the state of the wounds regarding infection. Delay in presenting for health care is influenced by several factors but the major ones include distances to health facilities, time of the day when the injury occurred (e.g. if a patient is injured at night), ignorance, poverty and cultural beliefs (Deogratius et al. 2006, Schaftenaar et al. 2009). Poor patients living far away from health facilities are most often the ones who face the disadvantage of delay in getting the appropriate care and therefore often present with infected wounds. Infection in a wound can originate from the object which caused the injury, dirt from the skin of the patient or from the ground at the site of injury. In soft tissue injuries and compound fractures there is always a possibility of getting tetanus infection. Tetanus toxoid injection for prophylaxis against tetanus should therefore be given to all trauma patients with open wounds.

5.2.3. Soft Tissue Injuries

Soft tissue wounds encountered in the maxillofacial region fall into the following categories; abrasions, contusions, cut wounds, lacerations, penetrating wounds and avulsions.

Cleanliness of the wound is a very important early measure. Even where a patient cannot, for any reason, attend medical care immediately, the wound should be washed with clean water or antiseptic solution. Wounds of the oral or perioral tissues pose challenges on how to clean them. If the patient can open the mouth, a good rinse with warm saline could suffice. However, the rinsing should not be done vigorously to avert the possibility of restarting bleeding. After carrying out the preliminary life saving and supportive measures a detailed survey of the injuries and patient in general is done followed by a full case clerkship.

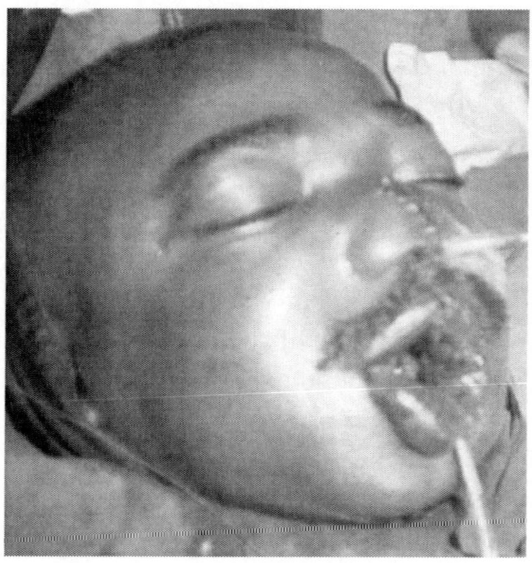

Figure 5.1. A patient with multiple soft tissue and bone injuries in the maxillofacial region (Courtesy of E.N. Simon).

Open lacerated or incised wounds should be sutured promptly. If a patient is to undergo fracture treatment immediately then suturing of such wounds is done at the same sitting after reduction and fixation of the fracture. Treatment should start with debridement, irrigation with saline or other recommended antiseptic and careful closure, preferably using small sutures to avoid formation of unpleasant facial scars. Major wounds may require suturing under general anaesthesia but minor and moderate wounds are normally repaired under local anaesthesia. Analgesics and antibiotics should be prescribed. The type and route of administration will depend on the type and severity of the injury. Patients with big wounds or fractures need strong analgesics like *pethidine* or *morphine* and broad spectrum antibiotics like *ampicillin* or *amoxicillin*. Cases of minor injuries may not require antibiotics. Some avulsed wounds would require reconstructive surgery, which can hardly be done in most health facilities within the reach of the disadvantaged communities. As a result patients with such wounds often remain with unsightly defects in the maxillofacial region that are psychologically depressing.

Explosives, gun shots, animal and human bite wounds commonly present with varying degrees of lost tissue portions. Further, such wounds have the disadvantage of either contamination by the attacker's microbes or presence of substantial amounts of devitalized tissue, both of which pose great challenges in management. This may dictate resorting to delayed primary or secondary suturing. Patients with such wounds may require several operations in the process of restoring aesthetics and function.

5.2.4. Fractures

Studies show that among civilians different bones of the maxillofacial region exhibit differences in the occurrence of fractures (Abiose 1986, Khan 1988, Allan and Daly 1990, Mwaniki and Guthua 1990, Beek and Merkx 1999, Oji 1999, Olasoji et al 2002, Adebayo et al. 2003, Adeyemo et al 2005, Schaftenaar et al. 2009). The nasal bones are the most frequently fractured bones of the face. In many of these fractures there is little displacement and frequently the patient never seeks treatment. The mandible is the second most frequently fractured bone of the face and the tenth most frequently fractured bone in the whole body.

The zygomatic bone is the third most frequently fractured osseous structure of the face. Unless there is marked deformity, interference with mastication, diplopia or numbness in the cheek, many fractures of the zygoma pass unrecognized and therefore untreated. The maxilla is the fourth most frequently fractured bone of the facial skeleton. Fractures of the zygomatic arch are fifth in order of frequency. The depressed segments of the arch frequently limit mouth opening by obstructing the forward and downward movement of the coronoid process. In the absence of such limitation, fractures of the zygomatic arch are frequently overlooked unless there is a notable local depression in the area overlying the fracture.

Fractures of the maxillofacial region are sometimes associated with head injuries. In every case of fracture of the mandible or maxilla the possibility of an associated fracture of the skull should be ruled out before embarking on treatment.

Fractures of the jaw bones may be single, multiple, simple, compound, comminuted or complex. Complex fractures of the middle third of the face, the upper jaw, and associated structures generally involve the nasal, lacrimal and orbital wall bones. The floor or lateral walls of the cranial cavity may also get involved. Accompanying complications include respiratory obstruction, disturbance of vision, obstruction of the nasolacrimal ducts and possibly neurologic complications. Only in very rare situations the frontal and temporal bones accompany midfacial bone fractures.

Before definitive treatment can be instituted, application of a bandage supporting the mandible against the head to limit movements and further displacement of the fragments is strongly advocated. This has several advantages; it stabilizes the fractured bone fragments, limits movements, controls hemorrhage, reduces pain substantially and minimizes the possibility of invasion by microbes. In most instances fractures of the alveolar bone and favourable mandibular fractures can be managed by closed reduction and mandibulomaxillary fixation using either ivy loops or arch bars. Despite the fact that there are many obvious advantages of open reduction and internal fixation (Schwimmer and Greenberg 1980), this may not be the most commonly accessible method of treatment in the disadvantaged communities. Lack of trained personnel, equipment and materials, and the relatively high cost leave closed reduction using maxillomandibular or craniomaxillary fixation as the only options of maxillofacial fracture treatment for this group (Nair and Paul 1986, Ugboko et al. 1998, Schimdt et al. 2000, Motamedi 2003, Deogratius et al 2006).

Complications of treatment of fractures in the maxillofacial region are mainly infection that may lead to osteomyelitis, others are delayed union, malunion and non-union. All of these may have short and long term effects on the patient. To prevent this it is necessary to educate the community on the importance of reporting to hospital immediately after injury and to comply with the instructions given after treatment. Furthermore, it is most important to raise public awareness on the necessity of taking precautions that lead to a reduction in the occurrence of maxillofacial injuries.

5.3. Infections of the Oral and Maxillofacial Region

5.3.1. Origin

The most commonly occurring infections in the oro-facial region are odontogenic in origin. They are almost always caused by mixtures of some of the microorganisms which make up the oral flora. These are primarily aerobic and anaerobic gram-positive cocci and gram-negative cocci and rods. However, if a patient has been on antibiotic therapy most organisms may be killed but a single highly resistant strain (usually *staphylococcus spp*) may survive and produce severe infection. Non-odontogenic predispositions to infection in this region include trauma to soft or hard tissues, iatrogenic and infection from the maxillary sinus.

The commonest source of odontogenic infections is dental caries followed by periodontal diseases (Dymock et al. 1996, Lindhe 1997, Siqueiar et al. 2001). Bacteria from the oral cavity advance through the carious lesions to enter the periapical tissues from where they may migrate to the medullary or cancellous bone of the jaws. In the medulla of either mandible or maxilla the infection may follow the line of least resistance as it spreads. More commonly the infection spreads through the cancellous bone until it reaches the cortical plate. Through the cortex the infection enters the soft tissues. The ensuing soft tissue infection may develop into cellulitis that is soft, doughy and tender to touch. Further developments depend on the anatomy of the region i.e. the delineating muscles and fascia, the immune status of the patient and virulence of the invading microbes (Adekeye and Adekeye 1982, Fermin and Newman 1996, Miller and Dodson 1998, Simon and Matee 1999, Whitesides et al. 2000).

Therefore, the fate of such infection is either resolution without pus formation or local pus formation and/or spread into other soft tissues and blood stream. Other serious complications include osteomyelitis of the jaws, necrotizing fasciitis and carvenous sinus thrombosis. Most odontogenic infections are mild to moderate. Delay in taking action, as is the case in most of the disadvantaged communities, allows the infection to run into serious and often fatal condition. Infection is one among conditions with high mortality in oral surgical patients even in advanced maxillofacial centres in the developing world.

Ignorance and poverty among the people living in remote rural settings expose them to dental caries and periodontal diseases. Lack of health facilities and dental services in these settings deny them the opportunity to get the necessary emergency dental care. Timely extraction of an offending tooth or restorations could prevent suffering from severe pain and occurrence of infection.

5.3.2. Clinical Features and General Management

Thorough history and physical examination of the patient with infection are important in determining the management. When a patient presents with a typical odontogenic infection the most likely picture will be a small swelling in the vestibule (vestibular or dental alveolar abscess). When infection is localized in the periapical region the patient will complain of excruciating throbbing pain and teeth in the region feeling longer than others and extremely tender on slight touch. A periapical x-ray will reveal widened or loss of lamina dura and rarefaction in the spongiosa of the periapical region. The basic principle should be to determine whether the infection is limited to a cellulitis or it has gone to the stage of pus formation (abscess). Other general symptoms of orofacialinfection include trismus, raise in temperature (above 39^0C), general body malaise, headache and loss of appetite. Cellulitis should be treated by aggressive use of antibiotics. Due to the mixed nature of infection of odontogenic origin broad spectrum antibiotics are preferable. When pus collection is present the primary aim should be to perform surgical drainage which may also include removal of the offending tooth.

Extraction of the offending tooth shall not only remove the cause but also provide drainage of pus and prevent propagation of infection. Surgical treatment will range from opening of the pulp chamber and extirpation of the necrotic tooth pulp to wide incision of soft tissue in case of severe orofacial and neck infections. Incision and drainage of pus from any of the fascial spaces may be necessary when manipulation of the tooth alone does not suffice. This will reduce tissue tension, improve blood supply and increase host defenses to the area. Pain killers and antibiotics should be prescribed even after the surgical intervention. Analgesics with anti-inflammatory and antipyretic effects such as *aspirin* or *diclofenac* are preferable. Broad spectrum antibiotics like *ampicillin, amoxicillin* or *erythromycin* are commonly used. Because of the acute nature of odontogenic infection empirical prescriptions are usually used while awaiting the results of culture and sensitivity. In most cases, after removal of the offending tooth infection is easily managed. Only in few cases will the results of culture and sensitivity be necessary. However, since the trend of events cannot accurately be pre determined, where possible it is advisable to take pus for culture and sensitivity in all cases of infection of the head and neck region. In patients with trismus that cannot allow any manipulations on the tooth, antibiotics should be given in order to bring about rapid resolution of the infection and facilitate mouth opening.

5.3.3. Ludwig's Angina

This is one of the most serious fascial space infections of odontogenic origin. It is an acute, rapid, diffuse, indurated bilateral cellulitis of the floor of the mouth and neck. The tissues of the oral cavity are distorted and they force the enlarged tongue upward against the palate and backward into the oral pharynx embarrassing respiration. The pharynx and larynx may also become inflamed thus further restricting respiration and making speech more difficult. Majority of deaths from this condition result from respiration restriction rather than sepsis (Figure 5.2).

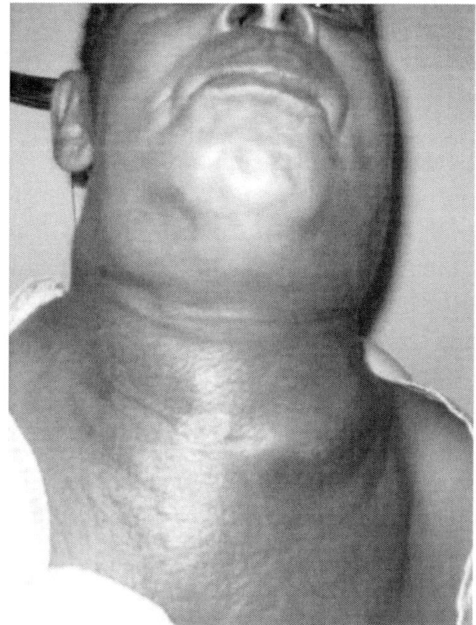

Figure 5.2. Severe odontogenic infection that has spread to involve the neck and chest (Courtesy of E.N. Simon).

Most commonly Ludwig's angina is a result of an odontogenic infection, caused by haemolytic and non-hemolytic *streptococci, staphylococci, pnemococci, Escherichia coli, and Vicent's* organisms (Sandor et al. 1998, Deroux 2001, Bratton et al. 2002).

Patients with Ludwig's angina usually have severe trismus, drooling of saliva, difficulty with swallowing and sometimes breathing. The infection must be aggressively treated with incision and drainage, detoxification and aggressive antibiotic therapy preferably using combinations of *ceftriaxone, gentamycin* and *metronidazole*. The airway must be maintained and emergency tracheostomy should be done in cases of severe airway embarrassment.

5.3.4. Acute Necrotizing Fasciitis

Acute necrotizing fasciitis is a severe form of infection in the cervical facial region that if not well managed may result in patient's death. This condition is characterized by necrosis of the investing fascia and fat (Simon and Matee 1999, Whitesides et al. 2000). The muscles and skin are usually spared. Cervical-facial necrotizing fasciitis, like elsewhere in the body, commonlyaffects patients with debilitating conditions like diabetes mellitus or severe malnutrition. However, any condition in the body that results in lowered body resistance is a predisposition to the occurrence of necrotizing fasciitis. Treatment involves intensive antibiotic therapy and serial debridement until all the necrotic tissue is cleared and new granulation tissue starts forming. In conditions resulting in massive loss of skin, grafting after clearing the infection is necessary in order to avoid unsightly scars and contractures.

5.3.5. Osteomyelitis

Osteomyelitis is an infection of the bone that develops in the bone marrow extending into the cancellous portion then spreads through the cortex and eventually into the periosteum (Shafer et al 1983, Van der Waal 1991). It starts as an acute form (acute osteomyelitis) which if not adequately treated with antibiotics progresses into a chronic form (chronic osteomyelitis). The infection occurs more commonly in the mandible than in the maxilla primarily because the mandible gets its main blood supply from one artery, the inferior alveolar artery. Besides the dominant single main blood supply a dense overlying cortical bone prevents penetration of blood vessels that could have given it additional source of blood supply. On the other hand the maxilla is more porous and has an adequate and richer blood supply derived from several arteries. Osteomyelitis of the jaws can occur as a result of direct extension or haematogenous dissemination of infection from neighbouring bones, sinuses, sockets and soft tissues.

Osteomyelitis of the jaws is a common finding in the developing world mainly because of delay of treatment of odontogenic infections. Improper or inadequate use of antibiotics in the management of odontogenic infections is among the reasons behind occurrence of cases of osteomyelitis.

Osteomyelitis may present as a localized type confined to a small area, or a diffuse type where destruction spreads throughout large areas of bone. Patients with acute osteomyelitis present with deep, severe pain and tenderness, swelling, and on occasion, fever and malaise. Teeth in the affected region are usually very tender and slightly mobile. Chronic stage of osteomyelitis presents with loose teeth, pus discharge from mucosal or cutaneous sinuses and sometimes foul smell from the affected region. There may be periods of acute exacerbations from chronic osteomyelitis.

Acute osteomyelitis is best treated by the use of appropriate antibiotics. Broad spectrum antibiotics with the capacity to reach high concentrations in bone like *amoxicillin* or *amoxicillin with clavulanate (augmentin)* are more preferable. However, the predisposing factor to the occurrence of osteomyelitis must be idientified and eliminated. Deeply carious teeth with periapical infection, fractures of the jaw bones, pericoronitis and post-extraction complications like infected sockets are among the common predisposing factors. Extracting the offending tooth or adequate and prompt treatment of fracture of the jaw bones would reduce the chances of occurrence of osteomyelitis of the jaw bones. In addition to aggressive antibiotic therapy chronic osteomyelitis also needs surgery to remove necrotic bone (sequestrectomy).

5.3.6. Fungal Infections

Fungal infections are rare in this region and are often difficult to diagnose in early stages because of their slow propagation rate. Oral candidiasis (oral thrush) is one of the most common fungal infections in the oral and perioral regions in humans. This condition is caused by *Candida albicans* that cause disease in situations when the body resistance is lowered. It presents as a whitish covering on the dorsum of the tongue and the rest of the oral mucosa depending on the severity of the condition. With the advent of the acquired immunodeficiency syndrome (AIDS) oral candidiasis is commonly seen in patients with lowered body resistance due to the condition. In its different forms it is one of HIV/AIDS defining conditions. For accurate diagnosis smears are taken for microscopy but also culture may be done in the laboratory. Treatment is mainly local application of antifungals like *nystatin* or in severe cases the use of systemic preparations. In cases where topical *nystatin* cannot work *fluconazole* tablets can be used (Patton 2001). Nevertheless improving the immunity of the individual is the basic measure in eliminating candidiasis.

Other fungal infections like actinomycosis also occur in the maxillofacial region more commonly in the mandible than in the maxilla. Trauma in form of tooth extraction or fracture of the jawbones is one of the most common predisposing factors. It is an infection of soft tissues but can invade the mandible or maxilla. Actinomycosis is a relatively uncommon infection of the soft tissues of the jaws and neck, usually caused by *Actinomyces israelii*. Also *A. naeslundii* and *A. viscosus* are sometimes involved. The bacteria are usual inhabitants of the oral cavity. Actinomycosis presents as a tumour- like mass but also as multiple healed scars and chronic purulent drainage from sinus tracts around the jaws. The exudates from the sinus tracts contain sulphur granules.

Treatment of actinomycosis is difficult and includes surgical incision and drainage and excision of all sinus tracts. This ensures that adequate amounts of antibiotics reach the infected area. The antibiotic of choice for actinomycosis is *penicillin* followed by *tetracycline*. Doxycycline or minocycline can also be given for a protracted course.

5.3.7. Viral Infections

Viral (herpetic) infections in the oral and perioral region are quite common in situations of lowered body resistance.

The patient wakes up in the morning with crops of blisters on the corners of the mouth or elsewhere in the oral cavity that later ulcerate. These ulcers are painful and may make eating difficult. Some viral conditions like herpes zoster have an increased incidence in patients suffering from conditions that deplete the body immunity like HIV infection or leukaemia. It is a very painful condition that affects an area of a particular nerve distribution (Figure 5.3). Treatment is usually symptomatic aimed at relieving the patient of pain and making him/her function comfortably (Stewart 1997). The ulcers normally heal spontaneously in seven to fourteen days.

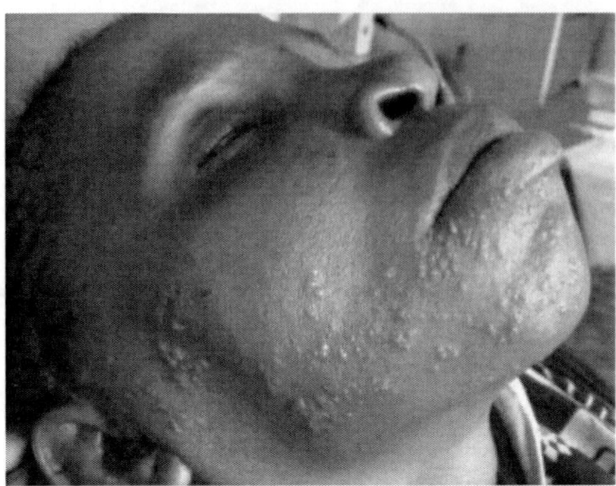

Figure 5.3. A patient suffering from herpes zoster that affected the area of distribution of the trigeminal nerve on the right side (Courtesy of E.N. Simon).

5.4. Tumours of the Oral and Maxillofacial Region

5.4.1. Overview, Clinical Features and Classification

The broadest definition of "benign tumour" encompasses all abnormal tissue masses that are not cancers (Kumar and Cotran 2001). In some cases, certain "benign" tumours later transform into malignancies, which result from additional genetic changes in a subpopulation of the tumour's neoplastic cells. Benign tumours are typically composed of cells which bear a strong resemblance to a normal cell type in their organ of origin. These tumours are encapsulated, not locally invasive; grow slowly and expansively without a tendency of invading surrounding tissues.

Benign tumours could be odontogenic or non-odontogenic in origin. Odontogenic tumours include ameloblastoma, adenomatoid odontogenic tumour, calcifying epithelial odontogenic tumour (CEOT or Pindborg tumour), calcifying odontogenic cyst (Gorlin cyst), odontogenic myxoma, cementoma and odontogenic fibroma (Kramer et al. 1992).

.Non-odontogenic tumours are pigmented cellular nevus, papilloma, keratoacanthoma, fibrous histiocytoma, angiomas (haemangiomas and lymphangioma), neurolemmoma, fibroma, lipoma, leiomyoma, rhabdomyoma, osteoma, chondroma, neurofibroma, central and peripheral giant cell granuloma and fibrous dysplasia. The exact cause of oro-facial benign tumours is not clear; however, some are associated with genetics, environmental and behavioural factors. Trauma and infections have also been implicated as predisposing factors of oral tumours. Benign oro-facial tumours affect almost all ages and their occurrence increases with increasing age of patients with a peak incidence between 29 – 39 years of age (Shafer et al 1983, Kramer et al. 1992, Kumar and Cotran 2001). Tumours (neoplasms) contain a discrete population of cells which proliferate in an independent manner, usually as a result of acquired genetic abnormalities. They are either benign or malignant depending on their properties and behaviour. Occasionally there are entities which may be referred to as "tumours" but are non-neoplastic. These include developmental abnormalities, such as hamartomas and *ectopic rests* (normal tissue in an anatomically abnormal location).

Table 5.1. Differences in behaviour of benign and malignant tumours

Benign tumours	Malignant tumours
Grow slowly and expansively	Grow fast and infiltratively
Do not cause metastases	Cause metastasis far from original place.
Grow to voluminous proportions	Usually larger in size than benign
Do not endanger life unless too big to extent of inhibiting vital functions	Life threatening due to infiltration and spread by metastasis
No microscopically visible difference between tumour cells and tissue of origin	Tumour cells have different microscopic aspect and other biochemical and functional properties than the cells of original tissue.

Benign tumors are very diverse, usually asymptomatic but may cause some specific symptoms depending on their anatomic location, size and tissue type. Features of benign tumours include a painless swelling that gradually increase in size and are usually readily detectable physically and radiologically. On x-ray it is a well circumscribed lesion that does not invade surrounding tissues. Most of the benign tumours are encapsulated with smooth margins. As it increases in size, a benign tumour may compress vital structures for example it may gradually obstruct the airway. Unlike malignancies, benign tumours rarely ulcerate and/or bleed. However, big intra oral tumours are often traumatized by the teeth during mastication resulting in ulceration and infection. These tumours do not compromise the general health of the individual until at very advanced stages. This is one of the characteristics which contribute to the reasons for delay in reporting for health care in majority of the patients from disadvantage communities.

Management

When detected at early stages majority of benign oro-facial tumours are curable with minimal residual effects. Early diagnosis of the disease usually provides a better prognosis and reduces the cost of treatment. Conservative surgical excision of small lesions yield best results and leave behind minimal defects. Curettage with or without cauterization is sometimes used for treatment of locally aggressive tumours, however, if such an approach is chosen there is a big likelihood of recurrence. To prevent recurrence in aggressive benign tumours, like ameloblastoma, a margin of between 1.5 cm and 2 cm of normal tissue is excised or resected together with the tumour. Large benign lesions often require partial resection of the jawbone. This usually leaves the patients with large defects which lead to permanent morbidity and poor quality of life unless reconstruction is done. Reconstruction can be immediate or delayed, and can include use of autologous bone grafts from the anterior or posterior iliac crest or from the rib. Reconstruction of the jaws requires sophisticated equipment. Even if facilities were available, the cost would be rather high to poor people. Immediate reconstruction is preferred because after healing the patient do not necessarily has to undergo another surgery. Majority of the patients tend to be satisfied with the outcome of the first operation and feel cured. As a result they do not see the importance of another operation.

5.4.2. Ameloblastoma

Ameloblastoma is an epithelial tumor arising from odontogenic epithelium. It arises from epithelial rests (of malassez, remnants of dental lamina or enamel organ and the basal layer of the oral epithelium or the Hertwig root sheath). Ameloblastoma is the most common odontogenic tumour accounting for approximately 1% of all oral tumours and cysts in the mandible and maxilla. It usually occurs in individuals aged 20-50 years with a peak in the 3rd and 4th decades; however, the unicystic variant most often occurs in adolescents (Mosadomi A. 1975, Adekeye et al. 1984, Onyango et al 1995, Asamoa et al 1990, Arotiba 1996, Tawfik et al. 2009). This lesion occurs most commonly in the mandible compared to the maxilla (Simon et al. 2005). Less than 10% of ameloblastomas are found in the maxilla. In the mandible they are mostly located in the molar, angle and ramus regions but occasionally occur also in the symphysial region (Figure 5.4). The lesion is distributed equally between males and females.

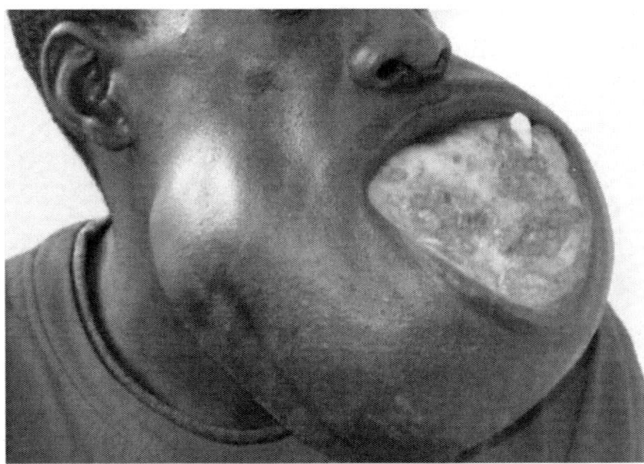

Figure 5.4. A patient presenting with a huge ameloblastoma of the lower jaw (Courtesy of E.N. Simon).

Although ameloblastoma generally is not classified as a malignant lesion (a rare malignant variant exists), it is extremely aggressive and infiltrative (Van der Waal 1991, Kramer et al. 1992). Many have suggested that this lesion should be considered a low-grade or indolent malignancy, similar to basal cell carcinoma. These two lesions have many histologic and behavioral similarities. It generally does not metastasize but is slow growing, persistent, and hard to eradicate. If ameloblastoma is not noticed as an incidental finding on radiographs taken for other purposes, the first symptom is usually a painless bony expansion.

Clinical features:

☐ The tumour is rarely encountered in early childhood. It is usually seen after adolescence although cases of children below 10 years with amelobastoma are occasionally seen. The peak age is the third and fourth decades.

☐ 80% of the lesions occur in the mandible involving mostly the molar, angle and ramus regions while the molar and canine regions are involved in the maxilla.

☐ In the maxilla ameloblastoma may become quite large (filling up the sinus) before it is discovered and nasal obstruction may be the first symptom.

- [ ] It grows slowly, asymptomatically in early stages; and discovered during routine x-ray examination.
- [ ] Clinically it appears as a gradually growing round swelling of the buccal cortical plate; however, ameloblastoma can also cause expansion of lingual cortical plate unlike the odontogenic cysts.

Initially the lesion is bony hard with normal overlying mucosa but as it increases in size, the overlying bone gets thinner and thinner leading to a ping pong like rebounding and later to an egg shell cracking effect.

- [ ] Overlying mucosa is still normal at this stage but later bone is perforated and the tumour may protrude into the oral cavity and the overlying mucosa may ulcerate (Figure 5.5).
- [ ] Teeth undergo progressive loosening and sometimes displacement.
- [ ] Due to mandibular canal involvement, hyposthesia of the lower lip may occasionally be present.

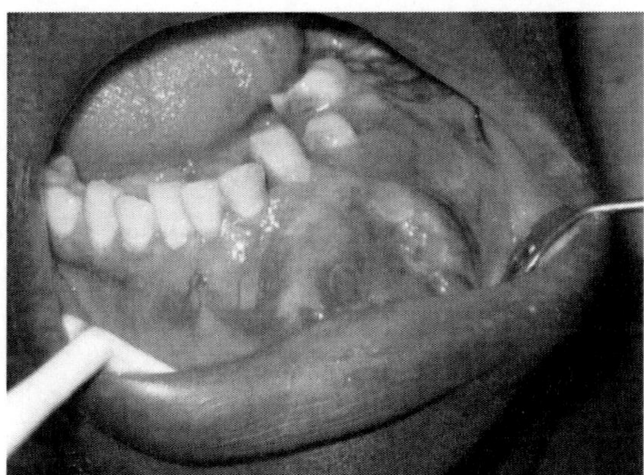

Figure 5.5. Intra oral appearance of ameloblastoma with cortical expansion and tooth displacement (Courtesy of E.N. Simon).

Radiographic findings

- [ ] Ameloblastoma typically appears as an expansile multilocular radiolucency that may be found anywhere in the jaws. It presents with closely trabeculated zones of osseous destruction that gives an appearance of a multilocular cystic cavity.
- [ ] The bone often appears to be replaced by a number of well-defined radiolucent areas that give the lesion a soap bubble or honeycomb configuration (common in ameloblastomas).
- [ ] Teeth are often displaced to the periphery of the tumour and resorption of roots is more frequent in ameloblastomas than in cysts.
- [ ] In most cases radiographic picture shows the unilocular aspect common in cysts.
- [ ] The desmoplastic ameloblastoma may not show complete radiolucency and to a certain extent may present some radiopacity.

Histologic Characteristics

Ameloblastoma does not have a capsule (Van der Waal 1991, Kramer et al. 1992). The neoplastic component is purely epithelial and resembles the cap stage of odontogenesis. The lesion may have a reactive connective tissue component that is not neoplastic. Multiple histologic varieties exist, e.g. the follicular, acanthomatous, granular cell, plexiform, desmoplastic and unicystic ameloblastomas.

To avoid misdiagnosis, which may result in instituting inappropriate treatment, it is necessary that the clinical diagnosis should always be supported by a histological diagnosis.

Treatment

The treatment of choice for ameloblastoma is surgical excision involving wide tumor free margins. The surgical treatment is guided by the local invasiveness of the tumour, the radiological appearance, absence of metastases, absence of invasion of the lower border of the mandible and possible perforation into the oral cavity. The tumour is not radiosensitive. All patients with ameloblastoma, regardless of surgical treatment method or histologic type, must be monitored radiographically throughout their lifetime because if excision is inadequate, recurrence is common.

In most cases it is necessary to perform maxillectomy to remove ameloblastoma of the maxilla because maxillary ameloblastomas are not confined by the strong cortical plate found in the mandible. In addition, the posterior maxilla lies in close relationship to many vital structures. These factors make strong arguments for aggressive and definitive surgical treatment of the maxillary ameloblastoma. In the mandible, complete resection of the affected area of bone including a margin of about 1.5 cm to 2 cm away from the periphery of the tumour are considered the standard. This may be accomplished with block or segmental resection, depending on the relationship of the lesion to the inferior cortical border. Resection of the lesion with dentoalveolar structure preserving the lower border of the mandible (marginal resection) may be done. Reconstruction of the defect with autogenous bone graft from the iliac crest, the rib or the fibula may be performed at the same time or on a later date.

The single exception to this may be the unicystic ameloblastoma. This variant most commonly appears in late adolescence and, as the name suggests, it is characterized by a unilocular radiolucency that is often found in the area of the mandibular third molars. Unlike other types of ameloblastomas, it is believed that this lesion is encapsulated and can be removed by enucleation/curettage procedures alone. These lesions may recur, and recurrences may require more aggressive treatment. Most authors believe that if left untreated, this lesion becomes an ameloblastoma of the classic varieties, leading to the corollary conclusion that these lesions simply represent an early stage in the development of ameloblastoma.

For the rare peripheral (soft tissue) ameloblastoma, a more conservative excision is the standard of care coupled with close clinical follow-up.

5.4.3. Odontogenic Myxoma

An over four years prospective study on odontogenic tumours found odontogenic myxoma (OM) to be the second commonest tumour after ameloblstoma (Simon et al. 2005). Elsewhere, in the African continent OM have been reported to occur with relative frequencies between 1% and 15% among odontogenic tumours(Mosadomi A. 1975, Adekeye et al. 1984,

Onyango et al 1995, Asamoa et al 1990, Arotiba 1996, Tawfik et al. 2009). From China relative frequencies of OM ranging from 1% to 8.4 % were reported (Wu and Chan 1985, Lu et al. 1998, Jing et al. 2007). American and European studies have reported relative frequencies of odontogenic myxoma ranging from 0.5% to 17.7% (Mothes et al. 1991, Daley et al. 1994, Mosqueda-Taylor et al. 1997, Mortellaro et al. 2008). OM essentially occurs intrabony. It has the capacity to cause destruction of both spongiosa and cortex of the jaws which result to tooth displacement and resorption of the roots (Figure 5.6). However, soft tissue OM lesions have been reported to occur on the gingival and periodontal membrane.

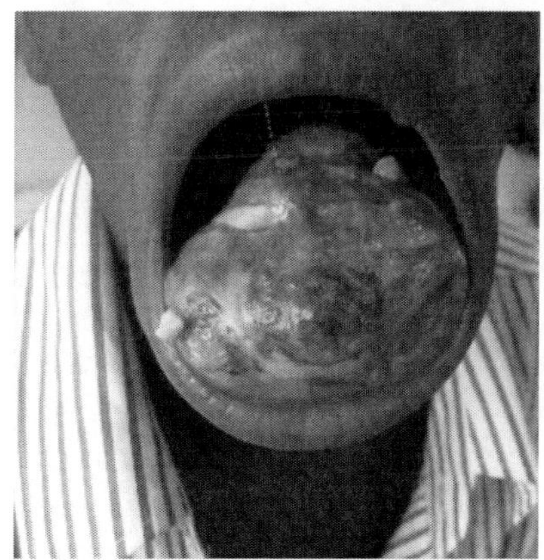

Figure 5.6. Odontogenic myxoma of the mandible (Courtesy of E.N. Simon).

The histological characteristic of OM is generally not pathognomonic and in children, the situation is even more confusing clinically, radiologically and histopathologically because of the concurrent diverse embryologic differentiation of dental tissues. The overlap of the common features of this lesion with several other lesions that also occur in the maxillofacial region is another challenge in reaching to it's correct diagnosis and management (Van der Waal 1991, Kramer et al. 1992). Although to a certain extent improved diagnostic methods and increased population awareness has helped to reduce the complications associated with OM, the most accurate tools like the CT scan, MRI or histopathology services are either not available or are unaffordable to the majority of socially disadvantaged communities such as most Tanzanian patients. As a result patients with OM present to hospitals after considerable delay with big tumours that pose substantial difficulties in management and consequently lead to severe morbidity.

5.4.4. Malignant (Cancer) Lesions

Essentially malignant lesions differ from benign tumours because they are unencapsulated and locally invasive, grow fast, infiltrate surrounding tissues and have a tendency to metastasize to regional lymph nodes in the orofacial region. They include squamous cell carcinoma, verrucous carcinoma, fibrosarcoma, angiosarcoma, chondrosarcoma, osteosarcoma, salivary gland tumours, malignant schwannoma, liposarcoma, leiomyosarcoma, rhabdomyosarcoma, Kaposi's sarcoma and basal cell carcinoma.

Although malignant lesions have been reported in many countries, the frequency of occurrence differs from one country to another. For example, in Canada, oral cancer was reported to account for 2.0% of all cancer cases and in the United Kingdom they accounted for 5.4% of all oral and maxillofacial tumours (Howell et al. 2003, Jones and Franklin 2006). In Indonesia and China malignant tumours were reported to account for 45.3% and 50% respectively of all orofacial tumours (Kuyama et al. 2000, Budhy et al. 2001). In Iran oral cancer accounted for 6% of all oral and perioral tumours (Razavi 2007). In different African countries oral cancer was found to constitute between 18% and 75% of all tumours diagnosed in the orofacial region (Chidzonga 2006, Ajayi et al. 2007, Kamulegeya and Kalyanyama 2008, Parkins et al. 2009, Elarbi et al. 2009).

The advent of the human immunodeficiency virus (HIV) infection and the acquired immunodeficiency syndrome (AIDS) has changed the patterns of occurrence of some disease conditions including malignant lesions. Patients with AIDS have been seen to have an increased risk of getting malignant lesions, higher incidences, widespread clinical dissemination and a more rapidly progressive course of malignant lesions than HIV-negative individuals (Mwakigonja et al. 2008).

The aetiological or predisposing factors of malignant tumours include tobacco in all forms e.g. cigarette or pipe smoking, snuff dipping and tobacco chewing, alcohol consumption, exposure to ultraviolet radiation and x-rays and infection by some viruses (Patel et al. 2008, Idris et al. 1995, Shamaa 2008).

Cancer (squamous cell carcinoma) is mostly diagnosed after 40 years of age and the average age at diagnosis being 60 years. Occasionally cancer is also diagnosed in patients who are younger than 40 years. For decades cancer affected men more than women at the rate of 6 men for every woman. However, currently the ratio has changed to 2 men to 1 woman. This change in the ratio could be primarily due to the changes of lifestyle whereby there has been an increase in the number of women smokers over the last few decades (Ariyoshi et al. 2008, Mumena 2005, Han et al. 2010, et al. 2008). At early stages, these lesions are painless and there are minimal physical changes. The dental surgeon or general practitioner at a primary centre sees or feels precursor tissue changes or the actual cancer in its earliest stages when it is still very small. A cancer lesion may appear as a white or red patch of tissue in the mouth or a small indurated ulcer (Cawson 1996, Regezi 2003, Effiom et al. 2008). Other symptoms include a lump or mass that is either visible or felt on palpation, pain, difficulty in swallowing, speaking or chewing, any warty like mass, persistent hoarseness of voice and any numbness in the orofacial region. In principle for any ulcerative lesion in the oral cavity which does not heal for more than ten days after the suspected cause has been removed should be thoroughly examined by a professional to rule out cancer. In developing countries and in low socioeconomic communities patients report to health facilities late with advanced tumours (Mumena 2005, Ortholan et al. 2009, Otoh 2009).This is the greatest problem in management of cancer in the developing countries. The death rate associated with malignant oro-facial lesions is particularly high because often cancer is discovered late when metastases has taken place (Figure 5.7). The reasons for such delay might possibly include ignorance, socio-economic, strong cultural beliefs and reliance in traditional medicine.

Whether a patient is to be treated by surgery, irradiation and surgery, or irradiation, surgery and chemotherapy is dependent on the stage of the malignant lesion. Majority of malignant lesions go through a pre-malignant state before becoming invasive cancers. Most early stage malignant lesions are curable by surgery. A combination of surgery and radiotherapy or the use of radiotherapy alone in most cases suffices. This usually leaves the patients with minimal disfigurement post therapy depending on the location of the lesion. Advanced stages of disease have poorer prognosis even when combination therapy is used. Once diagnosed the lesion has to be staged according to the TNM system.

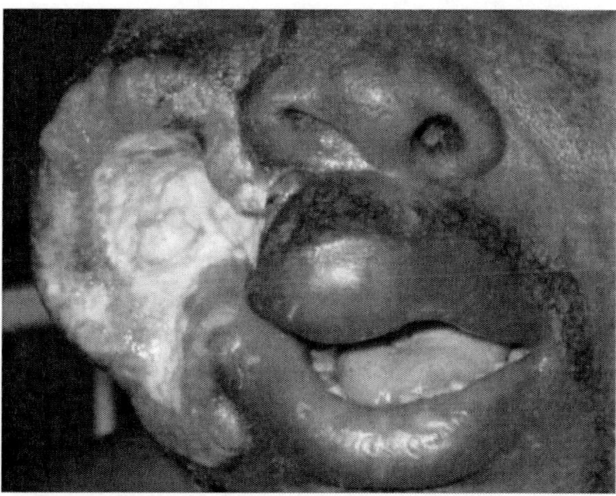

Figure 5.7. A case of late presentation of squamous cell carcinoma of the perioral region (Courtesy of E.N. Simon).

The management plan and prognosis basically depend on the stage of the tumour. Ideally treatment of malignant lesions in the head and neck region as elsewhere in the body is a multidisciplinary approach including oral maxillofacial surgeons, radiation and chemotherapy oncologists, and rehabilitation and restorative specialists. The actual treatment modalities are usually surgery, irradiation and chemotherapy, in most cases used in combination.

In disadvantaged communities, most often patients present with advanced malignant lesions than in developed countries. For such patients two modalities of treatment may be used. When surgery is still possible these lesions are surgically removed along with neck dissection for involved lymph nodes. Such extensive surgery in most cases require reconstruction of which is rarely done in less developed settings. After wound healing the patients are further exposed to radiotherapy or a combination of radiation and chemotherapy. A malignant tumour that is very big with possible metastasis is regarded as inoperable and the patient can only benefit from palliative radiotherapy or a combination of radiotherapy and chemotherapy. In both modalities the patient may require adjunctive therapy to assist in speech, chewing food, problems associated with the lack of normal salivary flow as well as dental or facial prosthesis for the defects created.

Delays in reporting to health facilities make most patients with neoplastic lesions in the disadvantaged communities present with huge tumours that limit reconstruction options. This is mainly attributable to the low level of understanding, socio-economic factors and cultural beliefs of most of the socially disadvantaged communities. As a result after undergoing the mutilating surgeries to remove big malignant tumours these patients end up leading a rather poor quality of life.

5.4.5. Kaposi's Sarcoma

Kaposi's sarcoma (KS) is a proliferation of endothelial cell origin, although dermal/submucosal dendrocytes, macrophages and probably mast cells may have a role in the genesis of these lesions. It is nowadays the second most commonly seen malignant lesion of the oral cavity in adults. Since the advent of HIV/AIDS oral KS is frequently seen in patients with lowered immunity due to HIV. Possible etiologic factors include genetic predisposition, infection (especially HHV8 or KSHV), environmental influences of various geographic regions, and immune dysregulation, such as reduced immune surveillance. Over 80% of the AIDS patients with KS have been found to develop oral lesions, which may be the initial site of involvement or the only site (Vaishnani et al. 2010, Mwakigonja et al.2008).

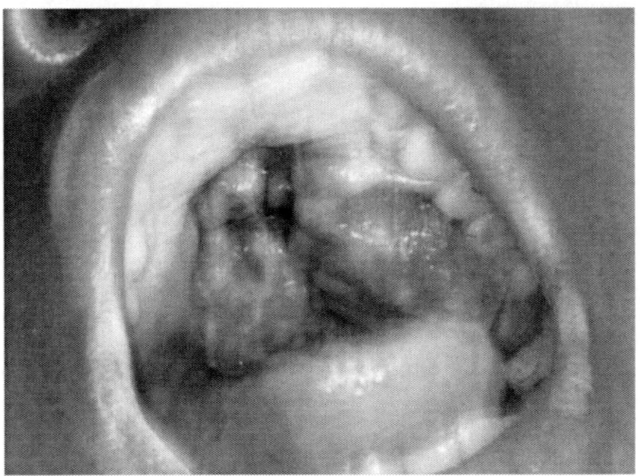

Figure 5.8. Oral Kaposi's sarcoma on the palate (Courtesy of E.N. Simon).

The palate, gingiva and tongue seem to be the most frequently affected sites. Lesions range from a rather trivial appearing, flat lesions to rather ominous, nodular, exophytic, single or multifocal lesions. The colour is usually red to bluish-purple (Figure 5.8). Microscopically, early lesions of KS may compose of hypercellular foci containing bland-appearing spindle cells, ill-defined vascular channels, and extravasated red blood cells. Later, hemosiderin and inflammatory cells may also be seen. The swellings sometimes become very big and extensive such that they interfere with eating or breathing. KS is treated by chemotherapy or a combination of chemotherapy and radiotherapy.

5.4.6. Melanomas

Oral malignant melanoma (OMM) is a rare but dangerous disease accounting for 0.2% to 11% of all malignant melanomas. The palatal region and maxillary gingiva are the most common sites (Ebenezer 2006, Chidzonga et al 2007, Kalyanyama et al.2009). Compared to studies elsewhere, where OMM was reported in generally older patients with a mean age of 56 years, a recent study in Tanzania has reported OMM at a slightly younger mean age of 46 years (Smyth et al. 1993, Hicks and Flaitz 2000, Greenberg and Glic 2003, Chidzonga et al. 2007, Kalyanyama et al.2009).

Although males are reportedly more affected, some studies have found a slight female preponderance (Ebenezer 2006, Chidzonga et al. 2007). Predisposing risk factors include a positive family history, light natural pigmentation, and an acute intermittent exposure to sunlight, especially in childhood. Widespread and unpredictable metastasis to bones, lymph nodes, central nervous system, lungs and liver has been frequently found. Because the disease readily metastasizes it is very important to take note of any suspicious pigmented lesions in the oral cavity that do not have a clear explanation.

In disadvantaged communities, of whom the majority live in rural areas with no dental services, early detection would mainly depend on the non-dental health personnel in rural dispensaries and health centres. There is therefore a great need to educate and raise the awareness of both the general population and the health personnel in these primary centres on the importance of early detection and appropriate referral of patients with oro-facial tumours. Continuing education to health personnel in the primary centres on clinical presentations of different benign and malignant tumours of the oro-facial region would facilitate early detection and appropriate referrals. The role of use of tobacco in its different forms and alcohol consumption in the predisposition to cancer of the oral and peri-oral region should be emphasized. The community at large should be encouraged to undergo voluntary screening for these lesions. At individual level they must be encouraged to report to health personnel suspicious lesions as soon as they see them. It is important therefore to formulate effective education programmes that are targeted to the disadvantaged communities focusing on change of attitudes.

5.5. Congenital Anomalies in the Orofacial Region

The embryological development of the oro-facial region is among the most complex developmental process in the human body. Structures of this region develop from both endoderm and ectoderm. Also some structures are formed from "nest cells" which migrate from remote sites. Occasionally, there occur particular failures of the fusion of several parts and migration of structures including descending of thyroid gland from oral region to the neck. Later in life remnants of these embryological tissues may proliferate and form several pathologies, mainly cysts. Majority of syndromes that have a wide range of malformations often present with one or more defects involving the oro-facial region.

Cleft lip and palate are among the most common congenital anomalies in the orofacial region. Prevalence of cleft lip and palate is about 1 in 600 to 1000 live births and generally affect boys more than girls, with cleft lip being more frequent in boys whereas isolated cleft palate is more common in girls. The clefts are basically due to failure of the migration and complete fusion of lateral and medial nasal swellings and the two maxillary swellings to form structures of the midface. The migration (fusion) should occur systematically in the 5th to 8th weeks of embryological development.There seems to be a hereditary component in the aetiology of the cleft lip and palate due to the familial tendencies seen. Environmental factors which have been implicated for causation of clefts include nutritional deficiencies, radiation, several drugs, hypoxia, and viruses.

Children with cleft lip and palate are likely to suffer problems related to feeding, nasal deformity, ear problems, speech difficulties and malocclusion. All these necessitate management to be started early and to maintain a close follow-up. The goals of management are to permit intelligible speech, to restore oropharyngeal functions including swallowing and to improve orofacial aesthetics in terms of short and long term outcomes.

The corrective surgical interventions should be started early in life. It is recommended that the cleft lip be corrected early basing on the "rule of 10" that is; the baby should be at least 10 weeks of age, weigh 10 pounds (4.55kg) and with haemoglobin of at least 10 g/dl. Since surgical correction of the cleft is an elective procedure, the health of the child should be in an optimal condition before the surgery is done to minimize the risks.

The cleft palate closure (palatorraphy) in children may be more difficult and may be proceeded by cleft lip repair (cheillorraphy) followed by soft palate between 18 and 24 months of age then hard palate later at least before 5 years of age when the child is expected to be enrolled in school. Ideally the team involved in management of cleft lip and cleft palate should include oral and maxillofacial surgeon and/or plastic surgeon, otorhinolaryngologist, an audiologist, paedodontist, orthodontist, paediatrician, speech therapist, psychologist and social worker. The list is long but each of them has a role to play through his/her individual specialized expertise to contribute in the comprehensive management of the patient with cleft lip/palate.

Due to ignorance, in most disadvantaged communities, there is persistence of beliefs which associate congenital anomalies with bad luck and unsacred. For that reason, in the past, children born with uncommon congenital anomalies were left to die by being thrown into heavy forests or were hidden inside houses where they were not seen by the rest of the community. In most of the underprivileged communities children with such congenital malformation are still being hidden or rather locked-in-house.

It is in such disadvantaged communities where up to date you can still find adolescents and young adults with untreated/unrepaired congenital anomalies like cleft lip and palate. When cleft patients report for treatment at a much older age, the deformities often require series of surgical corrections than would have been at a younger age. For example, in a grown up person with cleft lip and palate the dentition is usually grossly affected. Complicated orthodontic treatment is likely to be not only expensive but also likely to be unavailable in such communities. In peripheral health facilities including the district hospitals there are no specialists required to constitute the cleft lip/palate team. This makes the management of facial clefts, especially cleft palate, to be less comprehensive in the underprivileged communities. Treatment of cleft without speech therapy and orthodontic care and sometimes without oral and plastic surgeons services is common in such communities.

It is therefore important to educate the public on cleft lip and palate and encourage parents of children born with such congenital anomalies to take them early to hospital for appropriate care.

5.6. Oral Mucosal and Premalignant Lesions

5.6.1. General Overview

The oral mucosal lesions (OML) are a group of lesions which affect the mucosal lining of the oral cavity. This group of lesions receives less attention compared to other oral diseases/conditions like dental caries, periodontitis, trauma and neoplasms, although they are a common problem in adult population (Pindborg 1977). The types range from white, red, pigmented surface lesions and benign mucosal swellings to ulcerative lesions that can even be malignant. Their presentation may be indolent otherwise normal variants or aberrations on the oral mucosa without any symptoms. This explains why sometimes OML are ignored by individual patients and even overlooked by clinicians. Sometimes these lesions may present as painful, bleeding lesions. Most often this presentation is the reason for attendance at a health facility for care. Unfortunately, oral mucosal lesions especially in socially disadvantaged settings have not received proper attention in the planning of oral health services.

Any symptom and discomfort from the oral mucosal linings may interfere with functions. Painful mucosal ulcers, for instance, may cause difficulty in eating. Also, fear and anxiety from worrying that the ulcer could possibly be cancer make many patients uncomfortable. OML are a significant group of lesions because the oral mucosa sometimes serves as the mirror of the body (systemic) health (Axel 1992). Oral mucosal lesions may signify the presence of unidentified systemic disease e.g. HIV/AIDS and also, there are some OML which are pre-malignant in nature and with time they may transform into oral cancers.

Most studies done on the prevalence of OML among adult populations are from the developed world. Axel's observation on oral mucosal lesions in the 1970's in Sweden is among the oldest documented population studies on OML. In his study the most prevalent mucosal lesion was leukoedema (48.9%). A history of recurrent aphthous ulcer was found in 17.7% while geographical tongue was observed in 8.4% (Axel 1976). The large study samples of Boquot 1986 and Schulman et al. 2004 reported prevalence of 14.8% and 27.9% respectively which are considered average. Among low prevalences of OML documented was in Cambodia whereby the prevalence was 4.9% (Ikeda et al 1991).

The differences in the methodology of studies and differences in the exposure to risk factors of OML may explain the diversity in differences of prevalence of OML worldwide (Kleinman et al. 1991). The WHO guide on the examination and reporting on OML is a useful tool towards standardizing studies on OML. The OML are diverse group of lesions that is summarized in Table 1 below.

5.6.2. Aetiology of Oral Mucosal Lesions

Infective agents such as; bacteria, fungi and viruses cause a significant proportion of oral mucosal lesions. These lesions can present as white lesions like in candidiasis caused by fungal yeasts *(Candida albicans)*, ulcers due to herpes simplex virus or herpes zoster and other oral viruses (Figure 5.9).

The majority of ulcerative lesions are caused by trauma (physical, chemical, radiation) or are due to a malignant process as it is the case for squamous cell carcinoma. There are some few types of OML with multifactorial causes which are non- specific. For example the recurrent aphthous ulcers or stomatitis (RAU/RAS) are caused by several factors like autoimmune reaction, stress, nutritional deficiencies or reaction to certain foodstuffs. Similarly, the vesicullobulous lesions like pemphigus and pemphigoid are caused by autoimmune reaction and appear to have a genetic predisposition. The use of tobacco in form of smoking, snuff and dipping, chewing areca nuts and use of betel quids have been strongly associated with occurrence of various OML. Consumption of strong alcoholic drinks like dry spirits cause certain degree of mucosal damage. The effect of alcohol to the mucosa can also occur indirectly by causing liver cirrhosis hence an imbalance in the synthesis of vitamin A which leads to less protection of mucous membrane making it readily permeable and easily damaged.

Ill-fitting removable dentures can cause constant trauma to the oral mucosa resulting in ulceration. In cases where the care of the denture is inadequate it may be colonized by *candida spp* with resultant stomatitis, focal hyperplasia or angular cheilitis.

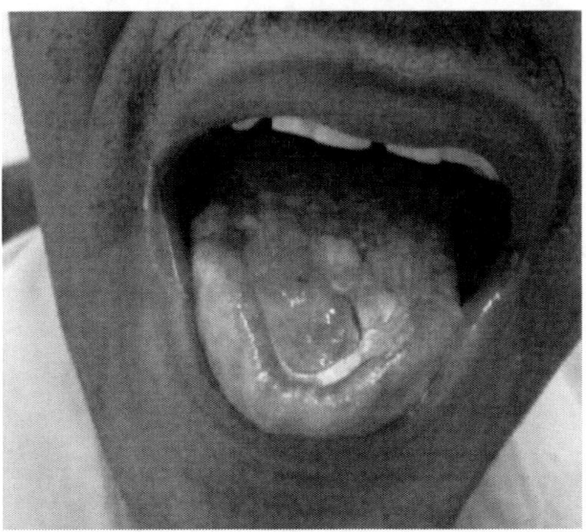

Figure 5.9. A patient with oral candidiasis and angular cheilitis (Courtesy of E.N. Simon).

5.7.3. Management of Oral Mucosal Lesions

Management of oral mucosal lesions depends on the type of lesion. In most lesions which are variants of normal oral mucosa treatment may not be required. They are in a group of white mucosal lesions that include conditions like; linea alba buccalis, leukoedema, keratotic white lesions and geographical tongue (migratory glossitis).

The ulcerative symptomatic OML and malignant ulcers need intervention. Ulcerative lesions in most cases need to be treated by a combination of analgesics, anti-inflammatory drugs and antibiotics to control or prevent infection by oral microbes. Apart from the general supportive therapy ulcers due to infective agents should be treated by specific medications. Where the cause is viral like in recurrent herpetic ulcer or herpes zoster, topical applications and antiviral drugs like acyclovir can be used. For herpes zoster infection systemic acyclovir ought to be considered.

Box 5.1. Summary of Types of Oral Mucosal Lesions

A: *White mucosal lesions:*
Variation in structure and appearance of normal oral mucosa
1. Leukoedema
2. Fordyce granules
3. Linear alba and other areas of normal frictional cornification
4. Non-keratotic white lesions
5. Habitual cheek and lip biting
6. Burns (thermal, due to aspirin, dental medicaments and other causes)
7. Uremic stomatitis
8. Radiation mucositis
9. Conditions caused by specific infectious agents (Koplik spots, Syphilitic mucous patches, Bacterial stomatitis)

Oral Candidiasis
1. Pseudomembraneous (oral thrush)
2. Acute atrophic
3. Chronic atrophic
4. Angular cheilitis
5. Chronic hyperplastic
6. Denture sore-mouth

Keratotic lesions with no increased potential for oral cancer
1. Stomatitis nicotina palatin
2. Traumatic (frictional) keratoses
3. Keratoses associated with dental restorations
4. Focal epithelial hyperplasia

B: *White and red lesions with defined pre-malignancy/ pre-cancerous potential*

1. Leukoplakia
2. Erythroplakia
3. Oral lesions associated with use of tobacco and alcohol
4. Carcinoma in situ
5. Oral submucous fibrosis
6. Actinic (solar) Keratosis,
7. Elastosis, cheilitis
8. Discoid lupus erythromatosus
9. Dyskeratosis congenital
10. Lichen planus

11. Lichenoid reactions

C: *Pigmented Mucosal Lesions:*

Diffuse and bilateral pigmented lesions:

Early onset:
1. Physiologic pigmentation
2. Peutz-Jeghers syndrome

Predominantly adult onset:

With systemic signs and symptoms
1. Addison's disease
2. Heavy metal pigmentation
3. Kaposi's sarcoma
No systemic signs and symptoms
4. Drug induced pigmentation
5. Post-inflammatory pigmentation
6. Smoker's melanosis

Focal pigmented lesions:
Red-blue-purple; Blanching
1. Haemangioma
2. Varix
Red-blue-purple; Non-blanching
3. Thrombus
4. Haematoma
Blue-gray
5. Amalgam tattoo
6. Other foreign body tattoos
7. Blue nevus
Brown-black
8. Melanotic macule
9. Pigmented nevus
10. Melano-acanthoma
11. Melanoma

D: *Ulcerative and vesiculobullous lesions:*
Acute multiple ulcers
1. Herpes virus infections
2. Coxsackievirus infections
3. Varicella zoster infection
4. Acute necrotizing ulcerative gingivitis
5. Erytherma multiforme
6. Allergic stomatitis

Recurring oral ulcers
7. Recurrent aphthous stomatitis

8. Behcet's Disease
9. Recurrent herpes simplex virus infection

Chronic multiple ulcers
10. Pemphigus
11. Bullous pemphigoid
12. Mucous membrane pemphigoid (Cicatricial pemphigoid)
13. Erosive and bullous lichen planus
14. Herpes simplex virus in immunodeficiency
15. Single ulcers
16. Histoplasmosis
17. Blastomycosis
18. Mucormycosis

E: Swellings of oral mucosa
1. Papillary hyperplasia of the palate

2. Squamous cell papilloma and papillomatosis
3. Infectve warts (verruca vulgaris)
4. Condylomata acuminatum
5. Molluscum contagiosum
6. Adenoma of minor salivary gland
7. Others; (e.g. Fibrous polyps, denture induced granulomas, Pyogenic granuloma and pregnancy epulis, Giant cell epulis)

F: Malignant oral mucosal lesions
1. Oral Squamous cell carcinoma
2. Verrucous carcinoma
3. Oral Basal cell carcinoma
4. Oral malignant melanoma

G: Lesions peculiar to tongue mucosa
1. Glossitis
2. The sore, physically normal tongue
3. Georgraphical tongue (benign migratory glossitis)
4. Hairy tongue
5. Median rhomboid glossitis
6. Fissured tongue
7. Lingual varicosities

Adapted and summarized from:

1. WHO: Guide to epidemiology and diagnosis of oral mucosal diseases and conditions. Community Dent Oral Epidemiol 1980;8(1):1-26.
2. Lynch MA, Brightman VJ, Greenberg MS.(eds). Burket's Oral medicine. 9th edition. J. B. Lippincott Co. Philadelphia, 2001.

Some OML need a conservative approach. Lesions which have a well known predisposing/etiological factor should be managed by removal of that factor. For example, trauma from sharp edges of a carious tooth will clear following removal of the traumatizing surface by either tooth extraction or conservation. Similarly, denture stomatitis can clear after abstaining from denture wearing for few days. However, where a denture induced granuloma has occurred then in addition to these measures the granuloma, if significant, should be excised to allow proper fitting of the denture. OML that are associated with tobacco use also do clear following cessation of such use. The risk of oral cancer from smoking decreases significantly following cessation and almost does not exist after 20 years. Pre-malignant lesions must be assessed very carefully. Some may need just a close follow-up if the risk of malignant transformation is low but where the transformation is more likely an aggressive approach will be necessary. A confirmed carcinoma in situ requires excision without delay. Erythroplakia requires a closer follow-up compared to leukoplakia which is homogenous and not changing for a decade. Actinic cheilitis may require observation only. Lesions seen in special groups like albinos need a more aggressive approach. Self examination and reporting in case one sees some suspicious changes on the mucosa is very useful since these lesions may exist for a long time without symptoms. For this to be successful, a community education on OML is necessary, especially to the disadvantaged communities who can not easily get the attention of experts in the field.

References

Abiose B.O. (1986) Maxillofacial skeleton injuries in the Western states of Nigeria. *Br. J. Oral Maxillofac. Surg.* 24: 31-9.

Adebayo E.T., Ajike O.S., Adekeye E.O. (2003) Analysis of the pattern of maxillofacial fractures in Kaduna, Nigeria. *Br. J. Oral Maxillofac. Surg.* 41: 396-400.

Adekeye E.O. and Adekeye J.O. (1982) The pathogenesisis and microbiology of idiopathic cervicofacial abscesses. *J. Oral Maxillofac. Surg.* 40: 100-106.

Adekeye E.O., Avery B.S., Edwards M.B., and William H.K. (1984) Advanced central myxoma of the jaws in Nigeria. Clinical features, treatment and pathogenesis. *Int. J. Oral Surg.* 13:177-186.

Adeyemo W.L., Ladeinde A.L., Ogunlewe M.O., James O. (2005) Trends and characteristics of oral and maxillofacial injuries in Nigeria: a review of the literature. Head and face medicine. 1: 7.

Ajayi O.F., Adeyemo W.L., Ladeinde A.L., Ogunlewe M.O., Effiom O.A., Omitola O.G., Arotiba G.T. (2007) Primary malignant neoplasms of orofacial origin: a retrospective review of 256 cases in a Nigerian tertiary hospital. *Int. J. Oral Maxillofac. Surg.* 36(5):403-8.

Allan B.P., Daly C.G. (1990) Fractures of the mandible, a 35 year retrospective study. *Int. J. Oral Maxillofac. Surg.* 19: 268-71.

Amusa Y.B., Adediran I.A., Akinpelu V.O., Famurewa O.C., Olateju S.O., Adegbehingbe B.O., Komolafe E.O., Faponle A.F., Olasode B.J. (2005) Burkitt's lymphoma of the head and neck region in a Nigerian tertiary hospital. *West Afr. J. Med.* 24(2):139-42.

Andisheh Tadbir A., Mehrabani D., Heydari S.T. (2008) Primary malignant tumours of orofacial origin in Iran. *J. Craniofac. Surg.* 19(6):1538-41.

Ariyoshi Y., Shimahara M., Omura K., Yamamoto E., Mizuki H., Chiba H., Imai Y., Fujita S., Shinohara M., Seto K. (2008) Epidemiological study of malignant tumours in the oral and maxillofacial region: survey of member institutions of the Japanese Society of Oral and Maxillofacial Surgeons, 2002. *Int. J. Clin. Oncol.* 13(3):220-8.

Arotiba G. (1996) A study of Orofacial tumours in Nigerian Children. *J. Oral Maxillofac. Surg.* 54:34-38.

Asamoa E.A., Anyanlere A.O., Olaitan A.A. (1990) Paediatric tumours of the jaws in Northern Nigeria, Clinical presentation and treatment. *J. Cranio-Maxillofac. Surg.* 18:130-135.

Axell T. (1996) A prevalence study of oral mucosal lesions in an adult Swedish population. *Odontol. Revy* 27(Suppl 36): 1-103.

Axell T. (1992) The oral mucosa as a mirror of general health and disease. *Eur. J. Oral Sc.* 100(1):9-16.

Beek G.J., van, Merkx C.A. (1999) Changes in the pattern of fractures of the maxillofacial skeleton. *Int. J. Oral Maxillofac. Surg* 28: 424-8.

Bouquot J.E. (1986) Common oral lesions found during a mass screening examination. *J. Am. Dent. Assoc.* 112:50-57.

Budhy T.I., Soenarto S.D., Yaacob H.B., Ngeow W.C. (2001) Changing incidence of oral and maxillofacial tumours in East Java, Indonesia, 1987-1992. Part 2: Malignant tumours. *Br. J. Oral Maxillofac. Surg.* 39(6):460-4.

Cawson R.A., Langdon J.D., Eveson J.W. (1996) Surgical pathology of the mouth and jaws, 3rd Ed.

Cawson R.A., Langdon J.D., Everson J.W. (eds) (1996) White, red and pigmented lesions of the oral mucosa. In: Surgical pathology of the mouth and the jaws. 1st edition London, Elsevier. Pg 166-188.

Chidzonga M.M. (2006) Oral malignant neoplasia: a survey of 428 cases in two Zimbabwean hospitals. *Oral Oncol.* 42(2):177-83.

Chidzonga M.M., Mahomva L., Marimo C., Makunike-Mutasa R. (2007) Primary malignant melanoma of the oral mucosa. *J. Oral Maxillofac. Surg.* 65:1117-1120.

Daley T.D., Wysocki G.P., Pringle G.A. (1994) Relative incidence of odontogenic tumours and oral and jaw cysts in a Canadian population. *Oral Surg.* 77:276-280.

Deogratius B.K., Isaac M.M., Farrid S. (2006) Epidemiology and management of maxillofacial fractures treated at Muhimbili National Hospital in Dar es Salaam, Tanzania, 1998-2003. *Int. Dent. J.* 56: 131-4.

Dymock D., Weightman A.J., Scully C., Wade W.G. (1996) Molecular analysis of microflora associated with dentoalveolar abscssess. *J. Clin. Microbiol.* 34:537-547.

Ebenezer J. (2006) Malignant melanoma of the oral cavity. *Indian J. Dent Res.* 17:94.

Effiom O.A., Adeyemo W.L., Omitola O.G., Ajayi O.F., Emmanuel M.M., Gbotolorun OM (2008) Oral squamous cell carcinoma: a clinicopathologic review of 233 cases in Lagos, Nigeria. *J. Oral Maxillofac. Surg.* 66(8):1595-9.

Elarbi M., El-Gehani R., Subhashraj K., Orafi M. (2009) Orofacial tumours in Libyan children and adolescents. A descriptive study of 213 cases. *Int. J. Pediatr. Otorhinolaryngol.* 73(2):237-42.

Fermin C.A., Newman M.G. (1996) Clinical periodontology: Periodontal microbiology. 8th edition. Philadelphia. W.B. Saunders. Pp. 84-102.

Greenberg M.S., Glic K.M. (2003) Burket's oral medicine:10th ed. *BC Decker: Hamilton;* p. 131-2,214-5.

Han S., Chen Y., Ge X., Zhang M., Wang J., Zhao Q., He J., Wang Z. (2010) Epidemiology and cost analysis for patients with oral cancer in a university hospital in China. *BMC Public Health.* 10(1):196.

Hicks M.J., Flaitz C.M. (2000) Oral mucosal melanoma: Epidemiology and pathobiology. *Oral Oncol.* 36:152-69.

Howell R.E., Wright B.A., Dewar R. (2003) Trends in the incidence of oral cancer in Nova Scotia from 1983 to 1997. *Oral. Surg. Oral Med. Oral Pathol. Oral Radiol. Endod.* 95(2):205-12.

Ikeda N., Handa Y., Khim S.P., Durward C., Axell T., Mizuno T., et al. (1995) Prevalence study of oral mucosal lesions in a selected Cambodian population. *Community Dent. Oral Epidemiol.* 23:49-54.

Jing W., Xuan M., Lin Y., Wu L., Liu L., Zheng X., Tang W., Qiao J., Tian W. (2007) Odontogenic tumours: a retrospective study of 1642 cases in a Chinese population. *Int. J. Oral Maxillofac. Surg.* 36(1):20-5. Epub 2006 Dec 6.

Jones A.V., Franklin C.D. (2006) An analysis of oral and maxillofacial pathology found in adults over a 30-year period. *J. Oral Pathol. Med.* 35(7):392-401.

Kalyanyama B.M., Shubi F.M., Simon E.N.M. (2009) Oral malignant melanoma in Tanzanian patients. *African Journal of Oral Health Sciences* 5(4): 2-8.

Kamulegeya A., Kalyanyama B.M. (2008) Oral maxillofacial neoplasms in an East African population a 10 year retrospective study of 1863 cases using histopathological reports. BMC Oral Health. 8:19dci:10.1186/1472-6831-8-19.

Khan A.A. (1988) A retrospective study of injuries to the maxillofacial skeleton in Harare, Zimbabwe. *Br. J. Oral Maxillofac. Surg.* 26: 435-9.

Kleinman D.V., Swango P.A., Niessen L.C. (1991) Epidemiologic studies of oral mucosal conditions - methodologic issues. Community Dent Oral Epidemiol. 19:129-140.

Kramer I.R.H., Pindborg J.J., Shear M. (1992) WHO. Histologic Typing of Odontogenic Tumors. Berlin: Springer-Verlag 7-9.

Kuyama K., Yamamoto H., Morimoto M., Meng N., Liang Z., Kobayashi S. (2000) Comparison of occurrence of oro-maxillo-facial tumour types in different regions of the People's Republic of China. *J. Oral Sci.* 42(2):57-62.

Lindhe J. (1997) Clinical periodontology and implantology: Microbiology of periodontal disease. 4th edition. Copenhagen. Munksgaard; Pp.138-188.

Lu Y., Xuan M., Takata T., Wang C., He Z., Zhou Z., Mock D., Nikai H. (1998) Odontogenic tumours. A demographic study of 759 cases in a Chinese population. *Oral Surg.* 86:707-714.

Lynch M.A., Brightman V.J., Greenberg M.S.(eds) (2001) Burket's Oral medicine. 9th edition. J. B. Lippincott Co. Philadelphia.

Miller E.J., Dodson T.B. (1998) The risk of serious odontogenic infections in HIV-positive patients, a pilot study. *Oral. Surg. Oral. Med. Oral. Pathol. Oral. Radiol. Endod* 86:406-409.

Mosadomi A. (1975) Odontogenic tumours in an African population, *Oral Surg.* 40:502-521.

Mosqueda-Taylor A., Ledesma-Montes C., Caballero-Sandoval S., Portilla-Robertson J., Ruiz-Godoy Rivera L.M., Meneses-Garcia A. (1997) Odontogenic tumours in Mexico: a collaborative retrospective study of 349 cases. *Oral Surg.* 84:672-5.

Mortellaro C., Berrone M., Turatti G., Rimondini L., Brach Del Prever A., Canavese F., Pucci A., Farronato G. (2008) Odontogenic tumors in childhood: a retrospective study of 86 treated cases. Importance of a correct histopathologic diagnosis. *J. Craniofac. Surg.* 19(4):1173-6.

Moshy J., Mosha H.J., Lema P.A. (1996) Prevalence of maxillo-mandibular fractures in mainland Tanzania. *East Afr. Med. J.* 73: 172-5.

Mothes P., Kreusch T., Harms D., Donath K., Schmelzle R. (1991) Die Haufigkeit odontogener Tumoren im Wachstumsalter. *Dtsch. Zahnartztl. Z.* 46(1):18-19.

Mumena C. (2005) Oral squamous cell carcinoma. MUCHS Mdent Oral Surgery and Oral Pathology dissertation.

Mwakigonja A.R., Kaaya E.E., Mgaya E.M. (2008) Malignant lymphomas (ML) and HIV infection in Tanzania. *Journal of Experimental and Clinical Cancer Research*: 27:9 doi:10.1186/1756-9966-27-9.

Mwaniki D.L., Guthua S.W. (1990) Occurrence and characteristics of mandibular fractures in Nairobi, Kenya. *Br. J. Oral Maxillofac. Surg.* 28: 200-2.

Olasoji H.O., Tahir A., Arotiba G.T. (2002) Changing picture of facial fractures in northern Nigeria. *Br. J. Oral Maxillofac. Surg.* 40: 140-3.

Onyango J.F., Awange D.O., Wakiaga J.M. (1995): Oral tumours and tumour-like conditions II. Age, sex and site distribution. *East Afr. Med. J.* 72:568-76.

Otoh E.C., Johnson N.W., Ajike S.O., Mohammed A., Danfillo I.S., Jallo P.H. (2009): Primary head and neck cancers in North-Western Nigeria. *West Afr. J. Med.* 28(4):227-33.

Ortholan C., Lusinchi A., Italiano A., Bensadoun R.J., Auperin A., Poissonnet G., Bozec A., Arriagada R., Temam S. (2009) Oral cavity squamous cell carcinoma in 260 patients aged 80years or more. *Radiother. Oncol.* 93(3):516-23.

Parkins G.E., Armah G.A., Tettey Y. (2009) Orofacial tumours and tumour-like lesions in Ghana: a 6-year prospective study. *Br. J. Oral Maxillofac. Surg.* 47(7):550-4.

Patel B.P., Rawal U.M., Rawal R.M., Shukla S.N., Patel P.S. (2008) Tobacco, antioxidant enzymes, oxidative stress, and genetic susceptibility in oral cancer. *Am J Clin Oncol.* 31(5):454-9.

Idris A.M., Ahmed H.M., Malik M.O. (1995) Toombak dipping and cancer of the oral cavity in the Sudan: a case –control study. *Int. J. Cancer* 63(4):477-80.

Pindborg J.J. (1977): Epidemiology and Public Health Aspect of Diseases of the oral Mucosa. *J. Dent. Res.* 56:C14.

Razavi S.M., Sajadi S. (2007) Epidemiological Study of Oral and Perioral Cancers in *Isfahan Dental Research Journal.* 4(1).

Regezi J.A., Sciubba J.J., Jordan R.C.K. (2003) Oral pathology; clinical pathologic considerations. 4th ed. WB. Saqunders, Philadelphia.

Schwimmer A.M., Greenberg A.M. (1986) Management of mandibular trauma with rigid internal fixation. *Oral Surg.* 62: 630-7.

Shamaa A.A., Zyada M.M., Wagner M., Awad S.S., Osman M.M., Azeem A.A. (2008) The significance of Epstein Barr Virus (EBV) and DNA Topoisomerase II alpha (DNA-Topo II alpha) immunoreactivity in normal oral mucosa, Oral Epithelial Dysplasia (OED) and Oral Squamous Cell Carcinoma (OSCC). *Diagn. Pathol.* 3:45.

Shulman J.D., Miles B., Francisco R. (2004) The prevalence of oral mucosal lesions in U.S adults: Data from the Third National Health and Nutrition Examination Survey, 1988 – 1994. *J. Am. Dent. Assoc.* 135:1279-1286.

Simon E., Matee M.I.N. (1999) Cervico-Facial Necrotising Fascitis occurring with facial paralysis. Case report. *East Afri. Med. J.* 76: 472-474.

Simon E.N.M., Merkx M.A.W., Vuhahula E., Ngassapa D., Stoelinga P.J.W. (2005) A four-year prospective study on epidemiology and clinicopathological presentation of odontogenic tumours. *Oral Surg. Oral Med. Oral Path. Oral Rad. and Endod.* 99(5):598-602.

Siqueiar J.F., Rocas I.N., Souto R., de Uzeda M., Colombo A.P. (2001) Microbiological evaluation of periradicular acute abscesses by DNA-DNA hybridization. *Oral Surg. Oral Med. Oral Pathol. Oral Radiol. Endod.* 92:451-457.

Smyth A.G., Ward-Booth P.R., Avery B.S., To E.W.H. (1993) Malignant melanoma of the oral cavity-an increasing clinical diagnosis? *Br. J. Oral Maxillofac. Surg* 31:230-235.

Tawfik M.A., Zyada M.M. (2009) Odontogenic tumors in Dakahlia, Egypt: analysis of 82 cases. *Oral Surg. Oral Med. Oral Pathol. Oral Radiol. Endod.* Dec 5. [Epub ahead of print.

Ugboko V.I., Odusanya S.A., Fagade O.O. (1998) Maxillofacial fractures in a semi-urban Nigerian teaching hospital. A review of 442 cases. *Int. J. Oral Maxillofac. Surg* 27: 286-9.

Van der Waal I. (1991) Diseases of the jaws: diagnosis and treatment. Munksgaard, Copenhagen p 206.

Vaishnani J.B., Bosamiya S.S., Momin A.M. (2010) Kaposi's sarcoma: a presenting sign of HIV. *Indian J. Dermatol Venereol Leprol*, 76(2):215.

Whitesides L., Cynthia C., Roy Meyers R.A.M. (2000) Cervical necrotizing fasciitis of odontogenic origin. A case report and review of 12 cases. *J. Oral Maxillofac. Surg.* 58:144-151.

WHO: (1980) Guide to epidemiology and diagnosis of oral mucosal diseases and conditions. *Community Dent Oral Epidemiol* 8(1):1-26.

Wu P.C., Chan K.W. (1985) A survey of tumours of the jaws in Hong Kong Chinese. *Br. J. Oral Maxillofac. Surg.* 23:92-10223.

In: Oral Health Care for Socially Disadvantaged Communities   ISBN: 978-1-62948-287-3
Editors: F.K. Kahabuka, E.N. Kikwilu and I. Anderson © 2013 Nova Science Publishers, Inc.

Chapter VI

Oral Health Concerns in Children

Febronia Kokulengya Kahabuka[1] and Daniel Iskander Maro[2]
[1] School of Dentistry, Muhimbili University of
Health and Allied Sciences
[2] Tanzania AIDS Prevention Program,
Muhimbili University of Health and Allied Sciences

6.1. Introduction

The chapter *Oral Health Concerns In Children* describes the health conditions of children. Covered in this chapter are health issues of the oral structures (except orthodontic related) among children from birth to adolescence at around 18 years of age. These oral structures include the teeth, the tongue, the gingiva and the tooth supporting structures. The chapter presents the dental development, various oral health conditions in children and adolescents, their preventive measures and management focusing on socially disadvantaged communities with reference to Tanzania, East Africa.

Upon finishing the chapter the reader will have gained knowledge on dental development, the influence of social disadvantage on children's oral hygiene, periodontal health, dental caries, and practices harmful to children's oral care, dental trauma and dental fluorosis. The reader will have also been exposed to different management modalities of these conditions feasible in socially deprived communities.

6.2. Dental Development

Dental development starts around 4-6 weeks intrauterine. Development of the tooth in particular, starts from the dental lamina; that is an epithelial thickening appearing at the sites of the future dental arches, 6-7 weeks intrauterine. Toothbuds of primary teeth are usually formed at 8-9 weeks intrauterine, while the secondary dentition is initiated at around 20 weeks intrauterine. Toothbuds of secondary dentition namely the central incisors to second premolars are formed five months intrauterine to 10 months postnatal. Formation of the second permanent molars is initiated during the first year of life whereas the third molars are initiated during the fourth to fifth year of life.

The process of dental development also includes eruption of deciduous teeth, exfoliation of deciduous teeth and eruption of permanent teeth as presented below:

6.2.1. Eruption of Deciduous Teeth

Tooth eruption is defined as the movement of the developing tooth from within the alveolar bone, through the gingiva into the oral cavity, until it reaches occlusal contact with the opposing tooth (Liversidge and Molleson 2004).

A complete set of deciduous dentition, also termed as milk or primary teeth, has a total of 20 teeth. It comprises of four incisors, two canines and four molars in each jaw. At birth, the crowns of the 20 deciduous teeth are almost completely formed, (www.ada.org/goto/jada November 2005:1619).

On average, the child's first set of teeth will start to emerge in the oral cavity at the sixth month of age, usually with the mandibular central incisors, and will complete at the age of 30 months with the second molars (www.mchoralhealth.org, www.ada.org/goto/jada November 2005:1619). Some communities in east Africa believe that eruption of maxillary incisors before the mandibular ones is a curse in a family. As an attempt to prevent the curse, when the child reaches the tooth erupting age, mothers would rub children's lower gingiva to facilitate eruption of the mandibular incisors. Tables 6.1 and 6.2, show eruption times according to www.mchoralhealth.org and Kahabuka et al (2009) respectively.

In their study, Kahabuka et al (2009) reported that lower central incisors emerge in the oral cavity at around eight months while the upper incisors emerge at ten months of age, boys being ahead of girls. These are followed by upper lateral incisors, lower lateral incisors upper and lower first molars. Canines are the next teeth emerging at 19 months and finally the second molars at 27 to 29 months of age.

Evidence shows distinct variations in the ages at which individual deciduous teeth emerge as well as in the eruption patterns between different ethnic and racial groups (Baghdady and Ghose 1981, Magnusson 1982, Hitchcock et al. 1984, Ramirez et al. 1994, Al-Jasser and Bello 2003).

**Table 6.1. Eruption time of primary teeth
(Age range) www.mchoralhealth.org**

	Lower jaw	Upper Jaw
Central incisor	6 – 10 months	8 – 12 months
Lateral incisor	10 – 16 months	9 – 13 months
Canine	17 – 23 months	16 – 22 months
First molar	14 – 18 months	13 – 19 months
Second molar	23 – 31 months	25 – 33 months

**Table 6.2. Eruption of primary teeth. Mean age (in months)
and standard deviation (Kahabuka et al, 2009)**

	Boys		Girls	
	Mean	S.D.	Mean	S.D.
Upper Jaw				
Central incisor	10.01	1.67	10.47	1.82
Lateral incisor	11.20	2.25	11.55	2.34
Canine	19.30	3.04	19.18	2.86
First molar	16.08	2.45	15.93	1.91
Second molar	28.89	4.12	29.35	3.55
Lower jaw				
Central incisor	7.88	1.86	8.20	2.25
Lateral incisor	13.23	2.84	13.11	3.20
Canine	19.92	3.33	19.47	3.03
First molar	16.39	2.25	16.12	2.08
Second molar	27.14	3.92	27.07	2.94

6.2.2. Exfoliation of Deciduous Teeth

Tooth exfoliation is a physiological process which involves shedding of deciduous teeth to give room to the succeeding permanent teeth. Generally, exfoliation begins with mandibular central incisors between five to six years of age. This is followed by maxillary central incisors then mandibular and maxillary lateral incisors. The last teeth to exfoliate are the canines and second molars (www.mchoralhealth.org). The age ranges for exfoliation of deciduous teeth is shown in table 6.3. It is concomitantly at this age (5-6 yrs) when eruption of first permanent molars and/ or permanent central incisors occurs. Normally the exfoliation process is asymptomatic. However, rarely shedding of teeth may also be accompanied by mild pain or discomfort.

Table 6.3. Exfoliation time of primary teeth (Age range) www.mchoralhealth.org

	Lower jaw	Upper Jaw
Central incisor	6 – 7 yrs	6 – 7 yrs
Lateral incisor	7 – 8 yrs	7 – 8 yrs
Canine	9 – 12 yrs	10 – 12 yrs
First molar	9 – 11 yrs	9 – 11 yrs
Second molar	10 – 12 yrs	10 – 12 yrs

6.2.3. Eruption of Permanent Teeth

Permanent incisors, canines and premolars (successors) erupt in place of their deciduous counterparts, i.e. deciduous incisors, canines and molars (predecessors) respectively, following their exfoliation. The rule does not apply to permanent molars which erupt posterior to the deciduous set, thus do not have predecessors. The set of permanent teeth comprises of 32 teeth, 16 on each jaw (4 incisors, 2 canines, 4 premolars, and 6 molars).

As for deciduous teeth, eruption of permanent teeth is asymptomatic although sometimes it may present with symptoms especially if the gingival tissue above the erupting tooth becomes inflamed.

Eruption of permanent teeth usually starts with the first permanent molars at the age of 5 to 6 years. These are followed by central incisors, lateral incisors, first premolars, second premolars and canines, second molars and lastly third molars (www.mchoralhealth.org). A summary of eruption ages for permanent teeth is presented in table 6.4.

Table 6.4. Eruption time of permanent teeth
(Age range) www.mchoralhealth.org

	Lower jaw	Upper Jaw
Central incisor	7 – 8 yrs	7 – 8 yrs
Lateral incisor	8 – 9 yrs	8 – 9 yrs
Canine	11 – 12 yrs	11 – 12 yrs
First premolar	10 – 11 yrs	10 – 11 yrs
Second premolar	10 – 12 yrs	10 – 12 yrs
First molar	6 – 7 yrs	6 – 7 yrs
Second molar	12 – 13 yrs	12 – 13 yrs
Third molar	17 – 21 yrs	17 – 21 yrs

Generally permanent teeth erupt earlier in girls than in boys and the mandibular teeth erupt earlier than their maxillary counterparts, (Manji and Mwaniki 1985, Mugonzibwa et al 2002). Evidence shows that permanent teeth tend to emerge earlier among African children than among the Caucasians, (Hassanali and Odhiambo 1981, Manji and Mwaniki 1985, Mugonzibwa et al 2002). At five to six years, children still have deciduous teeth that will shed gradually with age. Consequently, children will have early mixed dentition from the age of five to seven years to late mixed dentition or complete permanent dentition at 12 years of age.

6.2.4. Complications in Tooth Eruption

Numerous complications may occur in association with tooth eruption. These include delayed eruption, tooth malpositions, retained deciduous teeth, impactions, pericoronitis, and other complications related to eruption of third molars.

a)   Delayed eruption

A delay in tooth eruption of up to 12 months is of little or no importance in a child who is otherwise healthy. Tooth delays may result from local factors: obstructing the tooth in path of eruption, insufficient space in the dental arch, ectopic positioning and impaction. In addition retardation or delayed eruption of the permanent teeth may occur if, for whatever reasons, deciduous teeth will exfoliate or be extracted more than 2 years earlier than eruption time of their permanent successors. This is due to formation of dense fibrous tissue on top of alveolar crest probably as a result of long standing masticatory strains. Delays can also result, however rare, from systemic causes.

Management

Management of such situations may require surgical interventions to remove the local factors obstructing the tooth such as odontomes, crown exposure to remove obstructing fibrous tissues, disimpaction or orthodontic interventions such as serial extraction, and other orthodontic corrections.

b)   Retained deciduous teeth

Generally the eruption paths of permanent teeth are directed to the root of the deciduous predecessors. This facilitates root resorption and shedding of the deciduous teeth. In some instances, the permanent incisors erupt outside the path, for example lingual or labial to the deciduous incisors. In such a situation, the roots of deciduous teeth may not resorb. It is not uncommon for the deciduous teeth to be retained while the permanent teeth continue to erupt hence the two sets of incisors are present in unison (Figure 6.1a and 6.1b). If this will happen to a child whose parents are well informed, or in a child living in a country where a practice of routine visits to dentists is observed, the condition is usually noted early and prompt management can be done.

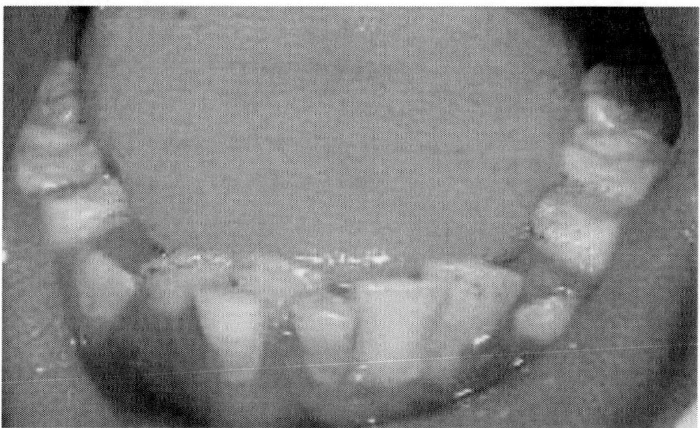

Figure 6.1a. Mandibular anterior crowding in consequence of retained right mandibular central and lateral deciduous incisors. Right central and lateral permanent incisors as well as left lateral permanent incisors are erupted lingually (a courtesy of F. Kahabuka).

Management

Management of overlapping teeth is done by space creation, usually extraction of the retained deciduous tooth/teeth. Given sufficient space, extraction of the retained deciduous tooth will create room for the succeeding permanent tooth and under the help of the tongue movement the permanent tooth will assume the normal alignment. Incase there is lack of enough space for the permanent tooth to erupt, the tooth is likely to emerge outside the arch hence bring about malposition and crowding even if the deciduous tooth sheds in time. This may demand orthodontic intervention to correct the malocclusion.

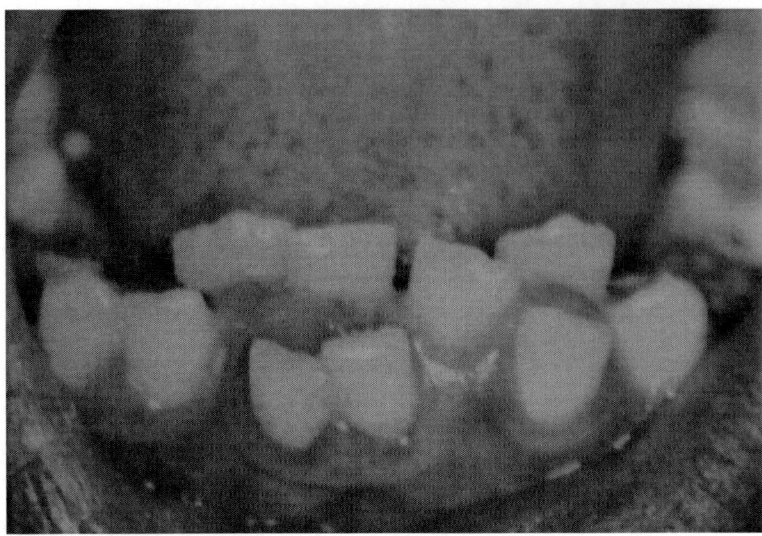

Figure 6.1b. Mandibular anterior crowding due to retained right central and lateral deciduous incisors, left lateral deciduous incisors, with both central and lateral permanent incisors erupted lingually. There is gingivitis around the right central and lateral deciduous incisors (a courtesy of F. Kahabuka).

In a socially disadvantaged setting where the health seeking culture through routine dental check up is not practiced, these conditions are likely to be noted late when the teeth are nearly fully or when fully erupted, causing discomfort to the child due to severe crowding (Figure 6.1). Nonetheless, management of such condition is the same as above but may require longer time intervention due to severity of the condition.

   c)   Impactions

A tooth is said to be impacted, usually with unknown etiology; if it fails to erupt into an exposed position in the oral cavity, thus remains embedded in the bone or surrounding soft tissues. Impacted teeth can usually go unnoticed. Diagnosis of a totally impacted tooth relies on radiographic examination. For an impacted tooth which presents with symptoms, or in case of any risk of developing complications, surgery (disimpaction) is the treatment of choice.

Management

In socially disadvantaged communities where electrical power may be unavailable or unstable and where availability of electrically driven instruments may be scarce, conventional removal of impacted teeth using hammer and chisel can be employed. Use of these instruments renders the procedure long and the patient is likely to get severe headache afterwards. It is therefore important for an operator to learn and master the skill and proper use of these instruments so as to relieve patients of unnecessary strain and pain. Prescription of pain killers is recommended after operative procedures, while prescription of antibiotics should be considered in case of any signs of infection.

6.3. Periodontal Health

Periodontal health simply means the health of the periodontium (periodontal ligament, gingiva, cementum, alveolar and supporting bone). Maintaining periodontal health basically entails practicing proper oral hygiene.

6.3.1. Oral Hygiene

Oral hygiene refers to personal maintenance of cleanliness, or practice conductive to the preservation of the health of teeth and oral structures. Good oral hygiene results in a mouth that looks and smells healthy, (www.ada.org).

Good oral hygiene practice is recommended for all individuals though the methods and means may vary for different age groups. For instance, in newborn babies the responsibility of oral care lies on their parents or caretakers. In these young ones, ideally cleaning should be done by wiping the child's gums with a wet washcloth or a clean gauze pad after each feeding. However, due to poor hygiene conditions that prevail in the populations in the socially disadvantaged communities, such a practice should be recommended with caution.

Tooth cleaning or toothbrushing should be initiated after eruption of the first tooth whereas proper regular toothbrushing should be established when the first primary molars erupt. At about two years of age when nearly all the child's teeth have emerged in the oral cavity, toothbrushing should be done using a small amount of children's toothpaste, until the child is able to spit it out because excessive fluoride may cause fluorosis (www.keepkidshealthy.com). Toothbrushing should be done twice daily: in the morning and at night before bedtime. A soft brush with a small head and big handle is recommended. Instigating good oral hygiene at an early age helps to inculcate positive attitudes among parents and children. Ultimately it aids to prevent gingivitis and periodontitis while the concomitant use of fluoride toothpaste has a benefit in prevention of dental caries (http://kidshealth.org).

Parents should brush their children's teeth up to school age, around six years. At school age children are able to perform their own oral hygiene. Children aged seven years are expected to brush their own teeth, though parents are advised to supervise them from time to time. Tooth cleaning can be done using either manual or eclectic tooth brush. It is important to note that an electric or ultrasonic tooth brush has similar cleaning effect as manual brushing (Costa et al 2010) and may be a motivating tool for disabled children.

In socially disadvantaged communities however, a number of factors may hamper implementation of these otherwise simple and easy recommendations. These factors include large family size, low purchasing power, low education status and prevalent life threatening infectious diseases (Kahabuka 2008). Education status of the family and particularly of the mother has a relationship with the family welfare. An uneducated or lowly educated mother is unlikely to give desired attention to children's oral hygiene. In many societies, even so in East African communities, it is usually the mother who is responsible for taking care of children's hygiene. When the family size is large due to considerable number of children, the mother will be swarming with family chores and consequently unable to give the necessary attention to children's oral hygiene. On the other hand if the family's purchasing power is low, the mother will be occupied with fetching food for the family and put little or no emphasis on issues which are seen to be trivial such as oral hygiene. Additionally, the family will be incapable of including fluoride tooth paste on their regular basic requirement catalog. The general health condition of the family may also influence the amount of effort directed to oral hygiene. If children in the family are often afflicted by infectious (fatal) diseases, the mother will be occupied by the sick children and most likely will not give attention to her young children's oral hygiene.

6.3.2. Gingivitis

Gingivitis is inflammation of the gingivae due to microbial plaque accumulation. It is caused by microbial plaque of polybacterial nature which accumulates on the teeth. Aerobes are the predominant flora with preponderance of the Streptococcus species (Egwari et al 2009). Minimal plaque accumulation and normal functioning defense mechanism result into no symptoms. More pronounced plaque accumulation or defects in the defense reactions result in clinical symptoms.

In children, gingivitis presents with red marginal gingiva, swollen marginal gingiva, distended shiny surface, clinically obvious crevicular exudates and an increased tendency towards gingival bleeding on probing. This is due to inflammation which is, at the time, fortunately limited to the gingiva. The number of children with visible plaque on their teeth surfaces, hence poor oral hygiene, is considerable. Consequently gum bleeding either on brushing or upon probing is a common phenomenon in children.

Prevalence of gingivitis usually varies from country to country and even from one study to another within the same country. A wide range of varying prevalences have been reported worldwide. For example, Cortellazzi et al (2008) reported a low prevalence of 16.6% among 5 year olds while Feldens et al found a prevalence of 77% among 3 to 5 ye-ar olds; both studies done in Brazil. A low prevalence was reported by Cosić et al among 6 and 12 year old children in the Netherlands. Other varying prevalences have been reported by Rebelo et al (2009) among Brazilian children (78.5%), Motohashi et al (2009) among Lao children (25.4%), Shidara et al (2007) among Cambodian children (46.2%), Dhar et al (2007) among Indian children (84.3%) and Mumghamba et al (1995) among Tanzanian children (80 - 94%) and mean sextants with gingivitis as 0.25 among Tanzanian children (Kikwilu and Mandari 2001).

Prevention of Gingivitis

The prevention of gingivitis is through plaque control, mainly by tooth brushing. The practice of tooth brushing is common. More than 90% of the people do it regularly. But the question is; what proportion brush correctly.

Biannual visit to dental clinic is recommended to monitor hygiene and facilitate early detection and management of diseases. However, such a practice is not feasible in socially deprived communities where there are few practicing dental professionals, poor access to dental facilities (Kikwilu et al 2008) and poor awareness about oral health among the communities (Nyandindi et al 1994).

Management of Gingivitis

Management of gingivitis requires proper examination, diagnosis and treatment. Diagnosis of gingivitis is based on clinical symptoms; redness, swelling and bleeding tendencies of the gingiva or through gingival bleeding index (GBI) based on whether or not the marginal gingiva bleeds upon gentle probing. Thorough periodontal probing for examination is not recommended for young children.

Usually, gingival inflammation remains superficial in healthy children. This marginal gingivitis is reversible with plaque control. It heals without any permanent changes in the normal gingival configuration. In severe forms of gingivitis, professional tooth cleaning to ensure removal of subgingival plaque and gentle scaling to remove calculus if present is recommended.

Plaque control may be achieved through mechanical means which include tooth brushing, use of toothpicks and flossing. Therefore education on plaque control and instructions on the use of dental floss are essential.

Tooth Brushing

As stated earlier, it is recommended that tooth brushing should be done twice daily; in the morning and in the evening before retiring to bed. A small (pea sized) amount of fluoride tooth paste is advocated. A plastic as well as a wooden tooth brush can be used. Parents should be encouraged to supervise tooth brushing of their children. For young children, a simple and straight forward method is recommended because of their limited capacity to concentrate for long periods and their dexterity is not yet highly developed. Thus a scrub method is recommended using horizontal movements of a tooth brush along out/inside surfaces of the dental arches. Tooth brushing should be done systematically to cover all tooth surfaces. Bristles should be placed along the gumline at a 45-degree angle, they should contact both the tooth surface and the gumline. Behind the front teeth, the brush should be tilted vertically while for biting surfaces, the brush should be placed against these surfaces (www.adha.org).

Motivation of both parents and children cannot be overemphasized. Parents and children should be instructed on tooth brushing. Dentist should demonstrate to parents and children on proper tooth brushing. Emphasis should be put on the method and frequency of brushing and not on type of tooth brush used.

Additionally, parents should be advised to supervise tooth brushing to make sure that children older than 2 years use only a pea-sized amount of fluoride toothpaste and avoid swallowing it. Parents should teach their children to spit out the remaining toothpaste after brushing. A child should be called upon for follow up visits to monitor the oral hygiene status. *(See tooth brushing methods chapter 4 section 4.6.1.3).*

In the socially disadvantaged communities, the mother who is the main care taker of a child may be over laden with responsibilities and therefore unable to pay enough attention to the child's oral health. The situation may worsen in case of large family size and extended family life which are common in some populations in developing world. Given these circumstances children's oral heath care may be left unchecked, oral hygiene practice may go without parental supervision even before the school age, before the child has developed enough skills and technique for home care.

Poverty, poor infrastructure, lack of awareness, poor oral health knowledge and attitude of parents are additional factors leading to parental failure to proper care and supervision of their children's oral hygiene.

Toothpicks

Gingival tissues in children mostly fill the interproximal spaces. Thus use of toothpicks will result into gingival retraction and exposure of proximal surfaces. For this reason the use of toothpicks in children is recommended only in very specific cases under instructions of a dentist or dental hygienist.

Flossing

A dental floss is a thread mostly made of plastic ribbon or nylon filaments whose main purpose is to remove any food or plaque that gets lodged in interproximal areas. Flossing require wounding the floss around middle fingers and leaving at least 2 inches in between. Using a thumb and index finger the user should direct the floss in between teeth, use a zig zag motion and follow the shape of the teeth. Then move the floss outside thus dislodge debris stuck between teeth and get rid of plaque that sticks to the tooth surface itself. If properly carried out flossing can benefit subjects whose gingival health is less satisfactory. Young children up to the age of six years are unable to floss, parents are therefore responsible to floss their children.

The prohibitively high cost of dental floss makes it inaccessible to majority in socially disadvantaged communities. On the other hand, Berchier et al (2008) in their review article concluded that routine instruction to use floss is not supported by scientific evidence.

Chemical Plaque Control

Chemicals used to control plaque function as inhibitor of plaque formation and/or inhibitor of plaque metabolism. Chlorhexidine 0.2% is the most thoroughly investigated chemical agent. It is available as a mouth rinse, a dental gel or a varnish. Its regular or intermittent long use is justified in high risk patients (Silk et al 2008, Liena Puy and Forner Navarro2008.).

Use of home care products containing chemical antimicrobials has been proved to have additional value in gingivitis reduction than use of brushing or flossing alone. The products can reach difficult to clean areas such as interproximal surfaces and they reduce growth of biofilms on oral soft tissues.

These should be recommended for patients who have difficulties achieving proper biofilm control when using mechanical means alone (Teles RP, Teles FR 2009).

6.3.3. Periodontal Conditions

Periodontal conditions such as calculus, plaque, and increased periodontal pockets, gingival recessions, gingival clefts, and in severe cases spontaneous gum bleeding and even tooth mobility are a result of complication of complex bacterial activities and body reaction to bacteria. Anaerobes such as Porphyromonas, Prevotella, Fusobacterium and Actinobacillus eg *Actinomyces actinomycecomutans* are the predominant species in periodontal diseases, (Egwari et al 2009). The disease conditions develop following long term poor oral hygiene that leads to accumulation of plaque and calculus. Fortunately these are not common among children and adolescents.

Periodontal conditions are among the oral health challenges in developing and socially disadvantaged communities. Apparently substantial proportions of the people in these communities have poor oral health knowledge. They have low awareness of gum disease, tooth decay, and poor knowledge about the causes and prevention of these diseases (Nyandindi et al 1994). Most likely they have not been informed of oral health issues during their childhood and therefore they have not adopted good oral hygiene practices. They are likely to have poor attitude towards tooth brushing and poor tooth brushing techniques. Other important factors for concern in these communities include poor access to oral hygiene facilities such as tooth brushes, dental floss and lack or poor access to dental care services which could serve as a key source for oral health information (Kikwilu et al 2008).

A patient would present with gingivitis, bleeding on gentle probing, gingival recession, gingival clefts, horizontal or vertical bone loss etc. Severe forms of gingivitis may signal presence of a general disorder. Thus severe generalized periodontal disease should be regarded as mandatory need for investigating the child's general health. Early recognition increases the chances of preventing loss of tooth support. As such early treatment is very effective. If left untreated, in a later life, periodontal conditions can lead to loss of teeth following excessive bone loss.

Management

The mainstay of periodontal therapy is the physical disruption of the plaque biofilm and use of adjunctive chemical where required (Tan AE 2009). Scaling and root planning, and instruction to home care are recommended. Tooth brushing twice daily is the recommended regimen supplemented with 0.2 % chlorhexidine mouthwash rinsing, (Addy 2003). However, in socially disadvantaged communities where chlorhexidine may not be easily accessible, alternative mouthwash such as 3% hydrogen peroxide solution which is relatively less expensive and readily accessible can be used. In addition, use of mouth washes in between meals, dental floss and toothpicks may be recommended. In disadvantaged communities dental floss and mouthwashes are expensive for the majority, emphasis should be put on proper tooth brushing using either plastic or wooden tooth brushes. Yearly visits for dental check-ups and care is farfetched because of limited dental personnel and poor accessibility of oral health services, *(see chapter 4 section 4.6 for details of management of periodontal diseases)*.

6.4. Dental Caries

Dental caries is a progressive demineralization and disintegration of the calcified dental tissues that occurs underneath a layer of bacteria on the tooth surface. It is a complex disease with multifactorial etiology. For caries to occur there has to be an interplay of four factors, the susceptible host (tooth), microflora with cariogenic potential (plaque), suitable substrate (dietary carbohydrates) and time, that is; the frequency of consumption of the dietary carbohydrates (Parisotto et al 2010). The dietary carbohydrates that are fermentable by bacterial plaque to produce acids which demineralize the tooth to cause caries are sugars both mono and disaccharides: sucrose, glucose, lactose and maltose. Of these sugars, sucrose is known to be the most cariogenic (Moynihan and Petersen 2004).

6.4.1. Dental Caries in Deciduous Dentition

In deciduous dentition, dental caries commonly affect molar teeth particularly the lower posteriors, (Carvalho et al 1989, Rugarabamu et al 2002, Maro and Kahabuka 2007). These days the most common form of caries found in deciduous dentition is termed early childhood caries (ECC). However, from time to time, rampant caries may be seen. This is the form of caries which affect incisors as well as canines, also called severe early childhood caries (SECC). If the cariogenic challenge is still strong, the decayed teeth will present with active caries which usually appear as opaque, whitish or light brownish. Alternatively, if the caries was mainly due to feeding practices in infancy, at later ages most lesions will be arrested usually appearing brown or black in colour.

6.4.1.1. Early Childhood Caries (ECC)

Early childhood caries (ECC) is defined as the presence of one or more decayed (non cavitated or cavitated lesion), missing (due to caries) or filled tooth surface on any primary tooth in children up to 71 months of age (Drury 1999). Other terms used to describe this condition include baby bottle syndrome, breast milk tooth decay, nursing bottle syndrome, bottle mouth caries, nursing caries, rampant caries, milk bottle syndrome and faciolingual pattern of decay (Ismail and Sohn 1999). ECC can develop soon after the first tooth erupts. Maxillary deciduous incisors are mostly affected and this pattern of caries attack is known as severe early childhood caries or in short SECC (Drury 1999). An example of SECC is shown in Fig 6.2a and 6.2b.

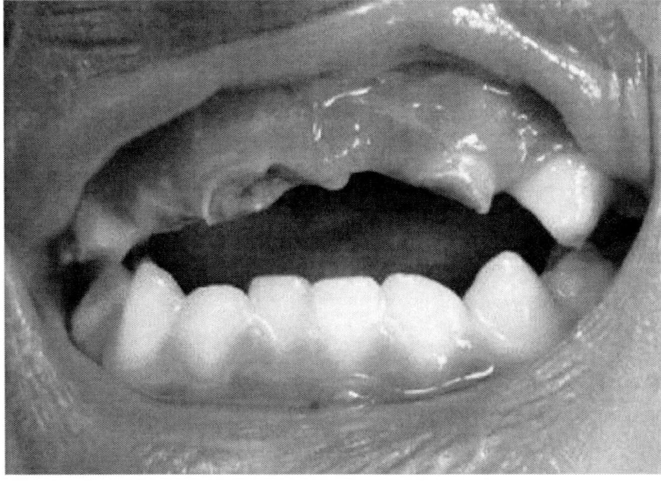

Figure 6.2a. Rampant caries affecting maxillary incisors and molars sparing mandibular incisors. This is because; usually mandibular incisors are protected by the tongue from contacting residual milk during sucking (a courtesy of F. Kahabuka).

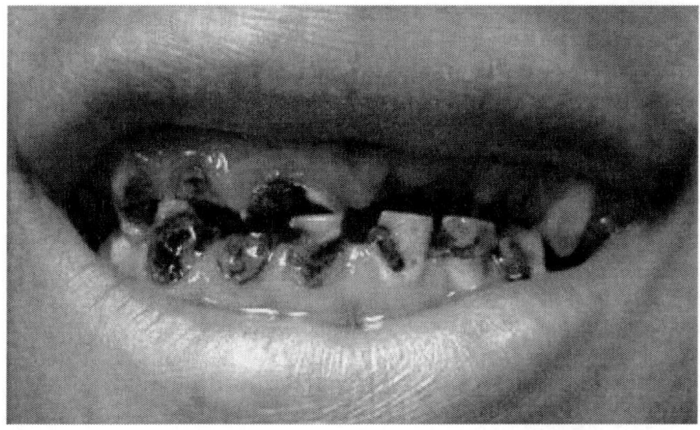

Figure 6.2b. Rampant caries affecting most of the teeth (maxillary and mandibular) (a courtesy of F. Kahabuka).

Numerous risk behaviours are known to be significantly linked to ECC. These include breastfeeding at will after 6 months of age, the habit of sleeping with the breast nipple in the mouth, frequent use of medicinal syrups, extensive bottle feeding and extensive use of sweetened pacifier (Rosenblatt and Zarzar 2004). Extensive and prolonged bottle feeding practice especially, when the bottle is used to induce sleep or if the bottle is used often to provide the child sweet drinks as a comforter, predisposes a child to development of rampant caries. Similarly, a practice of breast feeding at will after six months of age particularly by leaving a nipple in a child's mouth puts a child at risk of developing rampant caries, (Matee et al 1994, Du et al 2000, Van Palensetin- Helderman 2006, Savani and Kahabuka 2008). Certainly all children need to feed on milk for their development; breast milk being superior. Therefore, WHO recommendation of exclusive breast feeding for the first six months of life has to be supported by all medical disciplines.

Accordingly, both human and bovine milk are suitable cariogenic substrates. Once an individual eats a suitable substrate, bacteria metabolize the substrate to produce acids that demineralize the tooth enamel. If the substrate is provided at reasonable intervals of about two hours, the buffering property of the saliva will bring about enamel remineralization. In such a situation therefore, no caries activity will occur. But if the substrate is availed frequently or constantly, demineralization of the enamel continues without an opportunity for remineralization and therefore caries process ensures. The moment the cariogenic challenge becomes stronger than the buffering system as in the case of residual milk left in the child's mouth when the child sleeps with a nipple in the mouth, an aggressive form of ECC called rampant caries occurs. In other words, if the milk is allowed to stay in the oral cavity for a long time, it is fermented to acids by the bacteria present on the biofilm on the teeth. This results in a shift towards demineralization process and thus active caries development. Saliva is known for its protection of teeth due to its buffering capacity. However at night the body reduces the amount of saliva it produces i.e. the salivary flow decreases. The decrease of saliva production in the oral cavity means one is exposed to higher risk of developing caries since the natural protective balance of the buffering effect of saliva is deficient. Thus as the child sleeps with a nipple or with milk in the mouth at night, the residual milk results in a compounded shift to demineralization due to constant sugar exposure coupled by decrease in salivary flow.

Prevalence of Early Childhood Caries (ECC)

The prevalence of ECC has been widely studied, and reports indicate a wide range between different communities. Al Dashti et al (1995) found a prevalence of 18% among preschool children in Kuwait, Khan (1998) a prevalence ranging between 37 to 63% in 3 to 5 years old South African children. Wyne et al. (2001) found a prevalence of 27.3% in Saudi preschool children whereas in Brazil Rozenblatt and Zarzar (2004) reported 28.4% among 12-36 months. In Tanzanian children, the prevalence has been reported by Matee et al. (1994) to be 6.8%, Mosha et al. (1994, 2005) 24% and 25% among 5-6 year old children respectively, Mziray and Kahabuka (2006) 26.4% among children aged 6-36 months, Maro and Kahabuka (2007) 59.1% in 2-6 years, and Savani and Kahabuka (2008) 16.7% among 13-36 months. Among underprivileged Tanzanian children of a similar age group of 2 to 6 years, Maro and Kahabuka (2007) reported a prevalence of 42.5%.

Management of Early Childhood Caries (ECC)

Generally, management of dental caries is focused on prevention and repair. When caries manifest in children below 9 years of age, it becomes a major challenge to dentists not only in terms of the work load but also because the age of the affected children is difficult to handle (Wyne et al 1995).

Likewise, caries poses a challenge to the parents due to its nature, presentation and associated complications at the child's tender age. Even though some parents doubt the importance of treating deciduous teeth, with reasoning that they are ultimately destined to exfoliation.

There are numerous reasons to prevent and treat caries in the primary dentition;

a)   Prevent pain and discomfort
b)   Prevent infection of jaws and germs of permanent teeth
c)   Prevent negative attitudes towards dentistry that may arise following pain due to toothache or during dental treatment
d)   Promote interest in keeping good oral health
e)   Maintain good masticatory function and esthetics
f)   Prevent caries in permanent teeth by introducing them to a sound oral environment
g)   Prevent malocclusions

Among the major challenges faced during caries management in children is management of children's behaviour. Having a confident and relaxed patient in the dental chair is one of the most important prerequisite for successful treatment. This is extra important when managing children considering the anatomy of children's teeth which demands great care from the operators while performing restoration procedures.

In the past, treatment for dental caries was centered at "drill and fill". In recent years, diet counseling and educating parents about undesirable feeding practices has contributed in the success of decreasing rampant caries in high-risk groups of children. Ultimately, optimal long-term results may be achieved by treatment of the underlying caries process.

The Medical Model

The modern approach to caries management is described under the *"medical model."* The medical model is aimed at treating the underlying caries process. The model has 4 steps namely:

1) Gaining control of the bacterial infection
2) Reduction of risk levels
3) Remineralization of teeth
4) Long term follow-up

Gaining Control of the Bacterial Infection

The goal of caries control is to reduce the bacterial burden in the mouth of the child. Interceptive treatment approach is preferred, aiming at arresting the caries activities. Restoration of the lost tooth substances is postponed. Here, the minimally invasive caries control procedure, also called Atraumatic Restorative Treatment (ART), can be done whereby plaque and soft tooth substances are removed using hand instruments and then a thin layer of glass ionomer sealant is applied. The main problem usually encountered is uncooperative behavior of the child.

Reduction of Risk Levels

Step two in the medical model is reduction of the risk levels for patients. First, sugar intake must be reduced. A dietary assessment should be done to identify when sugar consumption needs to be decreased. Fluorides are known for their constructive value in caries protection. Increasing fluoride use at home will also reduce the risk of dental caries.

If the cause of rampant caries was due to breastfeeding at will; advice the mother to cover her breast at night and to avoid leaving the nipple in the child's mouth. The recommended practice is that the mother should wake up and breastfeed the child. If the cause of rampant caries is the use of bottle with milk or sweetened soft drink, advise the mother to use sugar free soft drinks or water when putting the child to sleep.

Remineralization of Teeth

Step three in the medical model of caries management is the reversal of active caries site by remineralization. There are three parts to this step: 1). Fluoride varnish should be applied 3 times in a 10 day period; 2). Fluoride application at home whereas fluoridated dentifrice should be used twice daily. For the very high risk children with dentin caries, application of 1.1% NaF gel by toothbrush is recommended. 3). Xylitol gum (a chewing gum that is not sugar added) is recommended.

Long Term Follow-Up

The last step in the medical model is long term follow-up of patients at home and in the dental clinic. The clinical recall frequency is recommended to be three months for high risk patients and six months for low risk cases. Caries activity and risk should be re-evaluated each time during the dental recall visits.

Limitation of Medical Model in Socially Deprived Communities

In socially disadvantaged communities, application of the medical model may face a number of challenges. For instance, breast feeding at will is recommended as one of the measures to combat malnutrition. On the other hand, dentists will discourage breast feeding at will especially after the child is one year old when children's teeth are erupted and continue to erupt. This may bring controversy as how to combine the messages from two health disciplines i.e. one message encouraging the practice and the other discouraging it. Since malnutrition is of more serious health concern, the dentist ought to join their medical colleagues and advice mothers to breast feed at will but not to leave the nipple in a child's mouth especially at night and more importantly after the child is one year old.

Fluoride application may also be a challenge since it is expensive but in some areas fluoride in drinking water is too high, thus its topical application may not be recommended. Finally, long term follow up may require additional resources which are not available in these communities.

Management Considerations for Caries in Different Age Groups

Due to different challenges encountered in children of different age groups, management of dental caries for children under age groups 0-3 years, 3-6 years and 6-12 years is presented below:

Age Group 0-3 Years

The major problem in children under this age group of 0-3 years, is the uncooperative behaviour. The major goal in the management is to arrest caries. Restoring the lost tooth substance may be postponed. If necessary, light sedation may be used in the clinic or general anaesthesia and deep sedation may be used (a specialist in anaesthesia is required). Generally, interceptive approach is preferred.

Treatment Strategy

Treatment strategy for caries in this age group should involve all options for arresting or decreasing the caries activity. The general technique should include three parts: Information, motivation and instructions.

The general caries arresting and preventive measures e.g dietary advice, oral hygiene instructions and use of fluoride should be adopted and these procedures should be done at subsequent visits.

On the other hand, local technique: professional cleaning, careful removal of debris and soft tissue, and application of fluoride varnish or a thin layer of glass ionomer sealant can be employed.

Teeth with good prognosis should be selected. Incisors and first molars may be extracted. But canines and second molars are more important for normal development of the jaws and the eruption of the permanent dentition. Therefore, as much as possible these teeth should be treated conservatively.

In more serious cases treatment should be done under general anaesthesia. However, this should be radical, that is more extractions and less restorations to minimize the time the child has to be under GA since long periods of time under GA puts a child at risks. In socially disadvantaged communities, the use of general anaesthesia may be limited due to unavailability of resources. Consequently, if several extractions are to be done, a child may have to be brought to the dental clinic several times in order to complete treatment.

Age Group 3-6 Years

The most frequently affected surfaces are occlusal surfaces of second and first molars as well as approximal surfaces of first molars. When restoring caries on occlusal surfaces, atraumatic restorative treatment is preferred. The technique is friendly to children since use of rotary instruments is not required. In addition, the technique is feasible in areas where electrical supply is lacking or unreliable. Stainless steel crowns can be used for primary molars with extensive destruction of the crown. When stainless steel crowns are not available, or may not be done due to various resource limitations, extensively damaged molars may be extracted and a space maintainer prepared if the economic situation allows.

Age Group 6 To 12 Years

Children under this age group have mixed dentition and later permanent dentition. Pits and fissures of the permanent first molars are the most frequent sites for caries. Fissure sealing is thus of major importance. Preventive resin/ glass ionomer restoration used for combinations of restoration and sealing techniques is of great value. Diagnosis and treatment of approximal caries is also essential in this age group.

Prevention of Caries in Deciduous Dentition

Parents of infants and toddlers should be advised to avoid leaving nipples in children's mouth especially at night and to use fluoridated tooth paste. If these measures will be instituted early they will facilitate enamel remineralization and prevent progression of the caries process. Parents of older children should be advised to restrict consumption of sugary snacks and beverages. If caries will occur, parents should be advised to seek dental consultation for early detection and treatment. In areas where children's visit to a dentist twice a year is feasible, it will facilitate early detection and prompt treatment.

Chemical plaque control using chlorhexidine is indicated for patients at high microbiological risk; it is more effective at controlling caries when used in combination with fluorides (Llena Puy and Forner Navarro 2008)

Parental attitudes and practices on dental care and dental hygiene have considerable influence to their children. As it was reported by Parhar, et al 2009 that mothers who brush their teeth with fluoridated tooth pastes are likely to have children who use fluoridated tooth pastes and mothers who take sweets are likely to have children who take sweets. So it is important that both parents as well as their children are given dental education.

Child's First Visit

The child's first visit to a dentist primarily is a two way mutual assessment session. The visit should be utilized to encourage the child to accept the dentist and the dental environment without fear. It should be organized in such a way that it becomes an enjoyable experience for the child. Previously, it was recommended that a child's first visit be at 2 ½ to 3 years old. Currently, the first appointment is recommended at the child's first birthday.

At the first visit examination of infants and toddlers is centred on introduction of a child and their parents to dentistry to provide them with a foundation for the development of positive attitude towards dentistry. Secondly, it is aimed at assessment and oral examination, for early detection of evidence of any dental disease and third, prevention and counselling the parents regarding their role in prevention of their child from developing dental diseases.

In socially disadvantaged communities, visit at the child's first birthday is not feasible due to limited resources as well as lack of oral health awareness among the public.

Complications of Early Loss of Primary Teeth

Early loss of primary teeth especially loss of the second deciduous molars may result into mesial drift of the first permanent molar and/or distal drift of the second premolars. Both drifts lead to crowding and thus aesthetic disturbances. Multiple early losses of deciduous teeth may have functional interference and lowered self esteem, (Figure 6.3a and 6.3b).

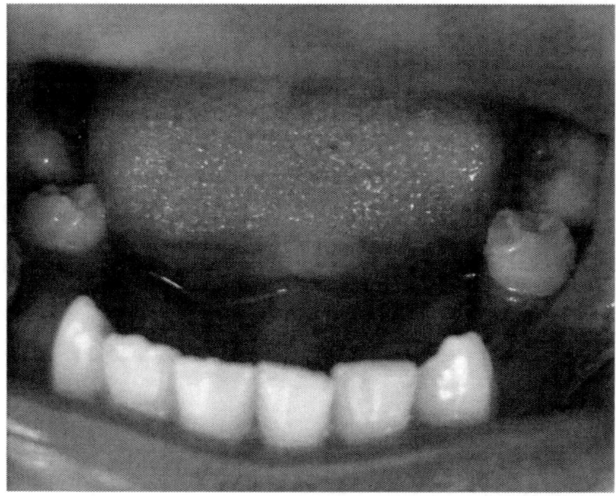

Figure 6.3a. Distal drift and 90° twist of premolars (a courtesy of F. Kahabuka).

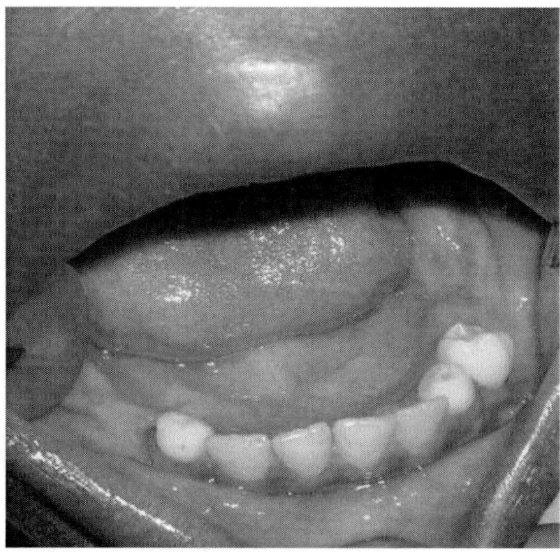

Figure 6.3b. Early loss of deciduous teeth in a child aged 8 years (a courtesy of F. Kahabuka).

6.4.2. Dental Caries in Permanent Dentition

Dental caries in the permanent dentition affect children aged six years and above.

Active lesions are most frequently found in young and newly erupted teeth and in individuals with other signs of caries activity. Usually the active lesions present with pain and discomfort. On the other hand, arrested (inactive) caries, which are usually dark brown or black in colour, are often seen in older teeth in children with no or low caries activity.

Mandibular first molars are the most frequently affected teeth, and pits and fissures of the permanent first molars are the most frequent sites for caries (Maro and Kahabuka 2007). Although in a study conducted among Tanzanian children by Rugarabamu et al (2002), mandibular second molars were found to be the most frequently affected by new caries lesion followed by mandibular first molars. Furthermore, Rugarabamu et al (2002) demonstrated that progression of lesions at a follow-up examination after 1, 2 and 3 years was generally slow in occlusal surface lesions of first molars compared to lesions in second molars.

Dental caries in permanent dentition like in deciduous dentition have multifactorial causation similar to earlier description. At this juncture, the causative factors may be addressed as snacks at home and at school as well as the frequency of consumption of these snacks.

Snacks

Parents and relatives usually give snacks to children as a means to express love and warmth. Parents should be warned that frequent consumption of sugary snacks put children at increased risk of developing dental caries.

Children above six years of age, especially those who go to school, are relatively more independent than the younger ones. They may buy and eat snacks of their choice. Studies show that at many schools, there are places selling snacks to school children (Roder, 1970; American Academy of Paediatrics Committee 2004, Kahabuka 2004). This gives children an opportunity to buy snacks of their choices and hence the risk to developing caries.

Time (Frequency)

The frequency of consumption of sugary foods is related to occurrence of dental caries. Consumption of sugary snacks and drinks more than five times per day significantly increases the risk of developing dental caries.

Management of Caries in Permanent Dentition

The child's history on eating pattern particularly in-between meal snacks should be investigated and recorded. This information is useful in planning dietary information or counseling.

After history taking, examination should be done with a child seated on a dental chair. For young children, it is advisable to start examination by visual inspection, assuming sharp eyes. Later instruments may be used depending on individual child's cooperation. If required one may utilize a blunt probe. Plaque and debris should be removed then the tooth or teeth be dried to visualize the caries lesion. When required, conventional bitewing radiography may be done.

As much as it is possible decayed permanent teeth should be conserved. When situations allow, conventional cavity preparation using minimal intervention technique may be done.

Caries management for children, like in adults, includes both simple and sophisticated restorative treatment. Bearing in mind the limitation in availability of sophisticated materials and tools for dental restorative treatment in the socially disadvantaged communities, one may resort to atraumatic restorative treatment (ART), for more details on ART refer chapter 3 section 3.2.7.2 to 3.2.7.4.

Prevention of Caries in Permanent Dentition

Children should be educated on causes of dental caries and be advised to limit their sugar consumption. They should also be advised to use fluoride tooth paste to gain the advantage of remineralization but also to help inhibit adherence of microbial biofilm on the tooth surfaces (hydroxyapatite) as was reported by Li et al (2009). Parents should be urged to take note of the first permanent molars that erupt at six years of age. Often parents assume these teeth to be part of the deciduous dentition thus they do not give them due attention. Children and parents should be instructed and encouraged on proper oral hygiene and proper diet so as to minimize risks of developing dental caries. Parents should be encouraged to inspect their children's oral cavity in order to detect the disease at early stages and consult a dentist for treatment. Additionally, places selling foods within school premises should be monitored in order to control children's consumption of sweet snacks. If monitoring is not feasible, school authorities may plan to provide school meals as a preventive measure not only of dental caries but also of ensuring attendance and concentration in classes (Kahabuka 2004). Furthermore, primary school teachers may be trained to recognize early dental caries and refer children to dentists for management.

The magnitude of dental caries is relatively low in the developing countries and socially disadvantaged communities in general (World Health Organization 2002). This is mainly due to low frequency of taking sugary food stuffs as a result of limited access to sugary food substances. Besides the relatively low caries prevalence, most caries among these communities go neither noticed nor treated (Mosha et al 2005, Massarente et al 2009). With the adoption of western life style especially in urban areas, the risk for developing caries in these communities is likely to increase due to easy access to sugary food substances and increased frequency of sugar consumption (Kahabuka 2004). Other factors prevalent among socially disadvantaged communities include limited use of fluoridated tooth paste and lack of basic oral health knowledge. In such settings access to fluoridated tooth paste is limited and oral health knowledge and awareness are relatively poor. Many of these communities are unable to adopt water fluoridation as a method for prevention of caries because only a small proportion of the population have access to piped water. Routine yearly visits to dentists are unheard and furthermore access to dental services is very limited especially to those in rural settings (Kikwilu et al 2008).

In established economy communities pits and fissure sealing is advocated as a preventive measure of dental caries in the permanent dentition. But it should be noted that this practice is not cost effective in low caries prevalent communities as it is the case in socially disadvantaged communities.

Complications Which May Result from Untreated Caries

Delay in seeking treatment for dental caries leads to further progression of the disease and therefore may necessitate resorting to complicated treatment measures or even extraction of the affected tooth. Extraction of permanent teeth in children has untoward effects on the dentition. For instance, early loss of first permanent molars is often complicated by mesial drift of the second permanent molars or distal drift of the premolars (fig 6.3a) and consequently may result into malocclusion. Loss of other permanent teeth may result into functional and or aesthetic disturbances. On the other hand, delayed treatment of dental caries may lead to dental abscess.

Dental Abscess

An abscess is a collection of pus in a tissue, organ or confined space, commonly caused by infection with pyogenic bacteria. Generally dental abscess occurs following infection of the pulp from a carious lesion. More often than not, dental abscess among young children is associated with extensive tooth decay which was left untreated. The condition frequently presents with severe pulsating pain which compel the child to avoid chewing on the offending side. In socially disadvantaged communities inadequate oral health knowledge and practices are contributing factors to late seeking of dental consultation thus increasing a possibility for a child to get dental abscess.

Management

The treatment of choice for dental abscesses in primary dentition is extraction of the offending tooth thus establish drainage. Concomitant administration of wide spectrum antibiotics is recommended. For permanent dentition drainage of the abscess followed by root canal treatment (RCT) is recommended.

6.5. Myths and Practices Detrimental to Oral Structures

Myths are traditional stories accepted as a history, serves to explain the world's view of people handled down from old times. A myth is thought to be a lesson in story form which has explanatory resonance for a certain culture. The stories may be imaginary or invented but they become very famous. Myths known to influence children's oral health are; nylon teeth myth and teething myth. Traditional uvulectomy and association of tongue tie with speech problems are some of the detrimental practices (Kahabuka 2008).

6.5.1. Nylon Teeth Myth

With respect to nylon teeth myth, people are made to believe that un-erupted primary canine tooth bud causes amongst other illnesses; diarrhea, vomiting, fever and growth retardation in infants (Mosha 1983, A/Wahab 1987, Mutai et al 2010). It is propagated that worms infest the un-erupted tooth bud, accordingly removal or gouging of the tooth bud is necessary to cure the diseases (Hassanali et al 1995, Halestrap 1971). Sharp and often un-sterile instruments e.g. bicycle spokes or nails are used to penetrate the gingiva and the jaw bone, without using local anesthesia nor employing aseptic techniques, (Baba and Kay 1989). Canine tooth buds are the most vulnerable sites for tooth bud removal because they are prominently seen as shiny elevated spots over the baby's gingiva. The removed tooth buds are not fully mineralized, they appear jelly-like and hence the term "nylon teeth" (A/Wahab 1987). This belief gained momentum in early 1980's in many rural areas in Africa, particularly in the horn of Africa but also in some parts of East Africa (Jones 1992).

Literature show that traditional healers spread the myth through inducing fear and panic among communities that if the "nylon teeth" are not removed the baby will die. Certainly, some children do die of childhood diseases like malaria, gastrointestinal diseases or respiratory tract infections following which, the death is linked with failure or delay to remove the killer "nylon teeth". Thus out of panic some parents subject their new born babies to tooth bud removal as a preventive measure to the killer "nylon tooth" (Pindborg 1969).

The tooth bud may be removed totally or partially. If total removal was achieved the after effect is the absence of deciduous canines. If the bud was partially disturbed, a malformed tooth will erupt.

Furthermore, tooth buds of primary lateral incisors and sometimes permanent canines, lateral incisors or premolars may be accidentally removed.

Other complications of tooth bud removal are hypoplasia of the permanent successors and adjacent primary and permanent teeth, displacement or dilacerations of permanent teeth, midline shift to the extraction side and distal eruption of permanent lateral incisors, leaving their primary predecessors retained. Occasionally, the practice of tooth bud extraction may be complicated by infection following unhygienic practice and extensive bleeding, at times resulting into death (Pindborg 1969, Mosha 1983, Welbury et al 1993, Masiga and Musera 2003). Figures 6.4-6.7 show some consequences of tooth bud gouging performed in association to "Nylon teeth myth".

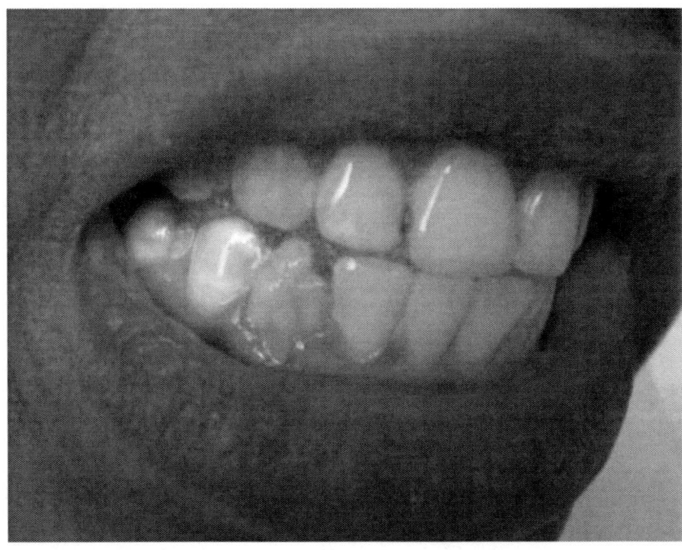

Figure 6.4. Dilacerated right mandibular canine (a courtesy of F. Kahabuka).

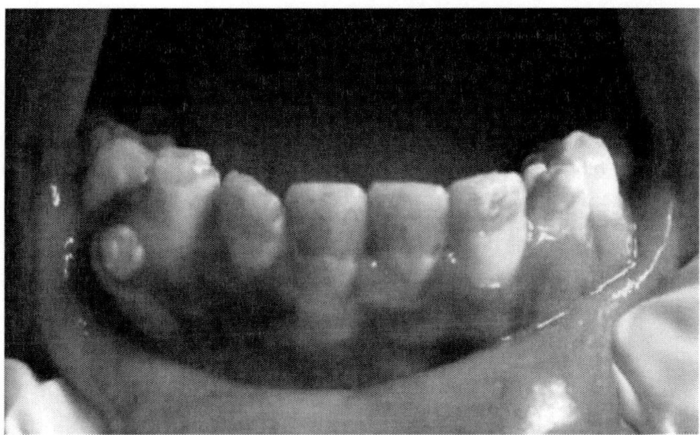

Figure 6.5. Ectopic eruption and dilacerated right mandibular canine. The teeth displays forms of fluorosis (a courtesy of F. Kahabuka).

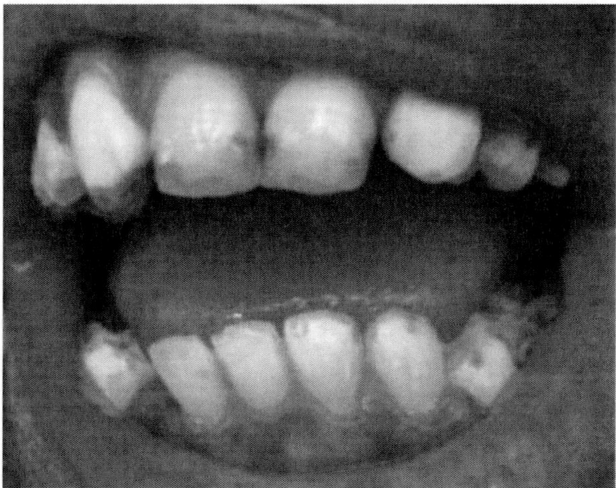

Figure 6.6. Missing maxillary lateral incisors and lower canines, with tilting of mandibular incisors and midline shift to the right (a courtesy of F. Kahabuka).

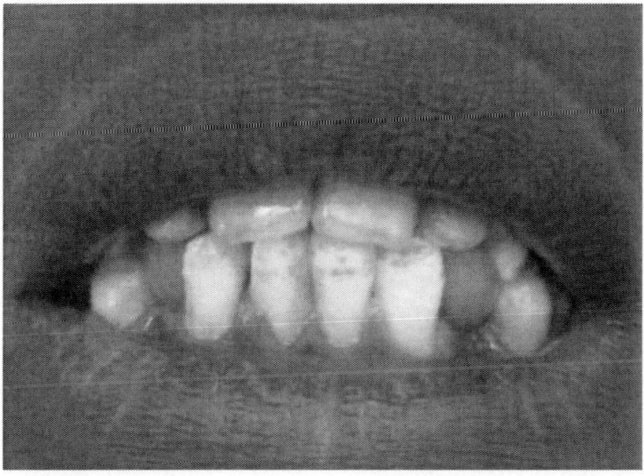

Figure 6.7. Missing left and right mandibular canines as well as fluorosis (a courtesy of F. Kahabuka).

Different reports reveal that tooth buds are gouged in as much as 15% to 59% of the examined children (Baba and Kay 1989, Hiza and Kikwilu 1992, Welbury et al 1993, Holan and Mamber 1994). Some communities have abandoned the practice of grouping primary toothbuds while others still believe on the existence of "nylon teeth" and the myth is associated with possible causes of childhood diseases. The belief is deeply rooted and practised despite sensitisation interventions (Mutai et al 2010). Whenever a new born child has a suspicious finding in the oral cavity, parents are prompted to believe on the existence of "nylon teeth". Some clusters of minority groups are still practicing digging out of the tooth buds. Even when people move from their indigenous countries, they persevere with the nylon teeth belief and the practice of tooth bud removal as was reported among Ethiopian immigrants living in Israel (Holan and Mamber 1994) and Somali immigrants living in Sheffield, the United Kingdom (Rodd and Davidson 2000).

Although the nylon teeth myth is deeply rooted among different cultures, the dental profession does not support the belief. Education and rising public awareness is necessary to eradicate the belief.

6.5.2. Teething Myth

Teething myth refers to a worldwide belief of associating local and systemic symptoms with teething. Common teething symptoms are: gingival swelling (Hesketh et al. 2000), irritation (Cunha et al 2004), redness of the gums (Jones 2002), thumb sucking and gum rubbing (Leung A.K 1989, Oyejide and Aderikonun 1991, Sarrell et al 2005). Some common local and systemic disturbances associated by lay communities with teething include; loss of appetite, crying, increased salivation, drooling, diarrhoea, boils and general irritability (Leung 1989, Jaber et al 1992, Chakrabort et al 1994, Bankole et al 2004, Macknin, et al 2000, McIntyre and McIntyre 2002, Wilson and Mason 2002, Peretz et al 2003, Baykan, et al 2004, Sarrell et al 2005, Kawia and Kahabuka 2009). Other symptoms are fever, runny-nose, conjunctivitis, thumb sucking, gum rubbing and some day-time restlessness (Cunha et al 2004, Oyejide and Aderikonun 1991, Leung 1989, Sarrel et al. 2005, Kawia and Kahabuka 2009). Increased biting, wakefulness, ear rubbing and facial rashes have also been reported to be associated with teething (Baykan et al 2004, Wilson 2002, Macknin et al 2000).

Symptoms associated with teething may be local or systemic. Local teething symptoms are; gingival swelling (Hesketh et al. 2000), irritation (Cunha et al 2004) redness of the gums (Jones 2002), thumb sucking and gum rubbing (Aderinokun and Oyejide 1991, Leung A.K 1989, Sarrell et al 2005). The systemic disturbances include; loss of appetite, crying, increased salivation, drooling, diarhoea, boils and general irritability (Leung 1989, Jaber et al 1992, Chakrabort et al 1994, Peretz et al 2003, Bankole et al 2004). Also reported are; fever, runny-nose, conjunctivitis, and day-time restlessness (Leung 1989, Aderinokun and Oyejide 1991, Cunha et al 2004, Sarrel et al. 2005).

Normally the eruption of deciduous teeth begins when other changes in the infant's immune system, growth and development are also occurring; that is, around six months of age. This is coincidentally, when infants have lost most of their maternally derived antibodies' protection. This predisposes an infant to a variety of infections like respiratory tract infections, urinary tract infections and middle ear infections (Wake et al 1999). This means that teething and occurance of childhood diseases are merely coincidental. The inherent danger in the persistence of teething myths is that, signs and symptoms of some diseases and conditions may be ignored if they are viewed as being merely a part of teething process. Such behaviour could sometimes be detrimental to the child's health (Bankole et al. 2004).

6.5.3. Association of Tongue Tie with Delays or Inability to Speak

Tongue-tie also known as *Ankyloglosia or lingua fraenata* is a congenital condition in which tongue mobility is limited due to abnormality of the lingual frenulum. The lingual frenulum is either too short or placed anteriorly too near to the tip thus limiting the mobility of the tongue (Hong et al 2010). Early in fetal development, the tongue is attached to the floor of the mouth. With cell death and atrophy, the only attachment left for the tongue to the floor of the mouth is the frenulum. Tongue tie is just one reason a baby may be experiencing difficulty breastfeeding, however its impact on breast feeding is poorly understood (Post et al 2010, Forlenza 2010, Hong et al 2010).

A restrictive frenulum may cause any, or all, of the symptoms listed below. First, a heart-shaped tongue tip. The tip of the tongue may be heart shaped or have a "V" shape indentation in the center when the baby sticks out the tongue or cries. But it is possible to have a restrictive frenulum without this classic symptom or to have a tongue that functions adequately, yet has the heart shaped tip.

Secondly, a square or a round tongue tip, that is when extended, the tongue looks square, or round on the tip instead of being pointed. The third possible symptom is difficulty in extending the tongue.

Usually, tapping the tip of the tongue should cause the tongue to come forward, and should be able to cross the gums. If the tongue is tied, the baby has difficulty extending the tongue past the gum line. Fourth symptom is difficulty in moving the tongue from side to side. Nonetheless, it may not be easy to appreciate this symptom in young babies. Lastly, in some instances, the frenulum can be attached very close to the tip of the tongue. In this case, babies have frenulum attached near the front, but the frenulum is very elastic and allows effective breastfeeding without a need for treatment. The known speech problems if mobility of the tongue is reduced include slight, moderate or high deviation of sounds from proper ones (Ostapiuk 2006).

Tongue tie is believed by the lay people to cause delay or inability to speak. Most of the parents whose children are allegedly said to have a tongue tie seek attention of traditional healers for freeing the tongue.

Some parents seek attention of a dentist with a child who is allegedly said to have speech problems due to tongue tie. However, most of such children are found to have normal tongue movements and normal frenulum, although they may have speech problems that are unrelated to the movements of the tongue.

Preventive steps to this problem may include advice to parents to seek experts' opinion if they will notice or suspect a tongue tic problem. Adequate information to the public is also important to avoid early attempts, to go for alternative treatments from traditional healers and other unqualified personnel, which more often result into harm.

6.5.4. Traditional Uvulectomy (TU)

Uvula is one of the three muscles that form the soft palate. It is located at the median plane extending posteriorly to the hard palate. Uvulectomy (*uvula+ Gr.ektome= excision*) is the term used to refer to excision of the uvula. Where as, traditional uvulectomy (TU) is a partial or radical removal of the uvula by traditional practitioners. TU has been reported to be widely practiced in parts of Africa, Tanzania included, and in some Middle Eastern countries (Ijaduola 1981, Ijaduola 1982, Wind J 1984, Ovelami 1993, Mboneko and Fabian 2006, Machumu and Fabian-Taylor 2008). TU is performed among children from one to five years old, majority (68%) at two years. Communities believe that traditional healers have skills and tools required to perform TU (Mboneko and Fabian 2006). Accordingly, studies report a prevalence of TU practice to range from 3.6% to 34% (Mboneko and Fabian 2006, Machumu and Fabian-Taylor 2008).

The reasons given for practicing TU include: cultural or traditional beliefs that children grow well following TU, prevention of death from swollen uvula (Ijaduola 1981, Ijaduola 1982, Wind 1984), prevention of and / or treatment for upper respiratory tract infections (Ovelami 1993, Manni 1984, Prual et al 1994, and Hartley and Rowe-Jones 1994), cough (Machumu and Fabian-Taylor 2008), treatment of recurrent upper respiratory tract infections and chronic diarrhea (Hartley and Rowe-jones 1994).

Some communities believe that an unusually long uvula cause throat infections (Prual et al 994). However, there is no standard measure for the length of the uvula and very rarely medical personnel will recommend and perform uvulectomy for medical reasons due to too long uvulae, (Magardino and Tom 1999). Possibly there is a lot of exaggeration with regard to the length of the uvulae as being the cause of upper respiratory tract infections but also there is lack of knowledge among parents. There are reports on professional uvulectomy which sited sleep apnea, snoring and chronic cough as major reasons for performing the procedure (Margadino and Tom 1999, Najada and Weinberg 2002, Jones and Earis 2005). Nonetheless other findings show that TU has no medical or health benefits (Wind 1984, Manni 1984, Magardino and Tom 1999, and Jones et al 2005).

The practice of TU is associated with a number of complications and secondary infectrion: anemia (mainly secondary to severe bleeding post TU), septicemia, gangrene, airway obstruction, HIV infection (Ijaduola 1981, Wind 1984, and Miles and Ololo 2003, Machumu and Fabian-Taylor 2008), and also increased morbidity and mortality rates among under fives (Ovelami 1993, Asefa et al 1998, and Jones 2005). Other reported complications and infections include severe deformities of the palate, which may lead to problems in speech (rhinolalia operta), tetanus, otitis media, epiglositis, and hepatitis B virus (Ijaduola 1982, and Prual et al 1994) and rejecting foods or difficulties in swallowing (Mboneko and Fabian 2006, Machumu and Fabian-Taylor 2008).

A study done in Tanzania by Wind (1984) showed that many of the children subjected to TU were brought to hospital due to complications resulting from TU and that anemia reached almost epidemic proportions. From the same study it was reported that Tanzanian mothers submitted their children to TU in the belief that by so doing they were increasing the child's well being and prospects of longevity. The study also reported that more than 80% of the children who had tetanus were reported to have undergone TU.

Management of Myths and Practices
It is essential to give education to the general public about the dangers of the above myths and practices. Parents who bring their children to a dentist with allegedly having nylon teeth, speech problems due to tongue tie and/ or complains of long uvula should be given the correct information and be empowered to resist attempts of traditional practices. Treatment of symptoms or rehabilitation of the damages should be done in children who have been subjected to different practices.

6.6. Traumatic Dental Injuries

Traumatic dental injury is any harm to a tooth and /or tooth supporting structures occurring as a result of trauma. Most of these injuries happen as an outcome of children's day to day activities. The majority of dental injuries occur around homes (inside or outside), at schools, on roads, at playgrounds and swimming pools. Dental injuries are common especially in children, affecting both the deciduous and the permanent dentition. Studies conducted in different populations report that 7-50% of the child population has sustained an oro-dental injury by the age of 15 years (Çaliskan and Türkün 1995, Mestrinho et al 1998, Hargreaves et al 1999, Marcenes 1999, Kahabuka et al 2001, Adekovo –Sofowora et al 2005).

The difference in the prevalence is attributed to by type of study; retrospective or prospective, area of study; hospital or community and also age and sex of the study population. Boys are affected twice as much as girls. The most affected teeth are the anteriors with the maxillary central incisors being most frequently involved (Kahabuka et al 2001, Rocha and Cardoso 2001, Shulham and Peterson 2004, Baus et al 2004). In the young age group, a peak of traumatic dental injuries is observed at 2-4 years, while in the older age group, the peak is observed at 8-12 years, (Glendor 1996).

The common causes of dental injury in children are; fall, being struck by an object, sport related accidents, traffic accidents, collision with another child, violence or fight, and child abuse (Marcenes et al 2000, Nicolau et al 2001, Traebert et al 2003; Malikaew et al 2006, Traebert et al 2006). Of these causes, accidental fall during play is the most common cause of dental injuries for children (Adekova-Sofowora et al 2000, Adekova –Sofowora et al 2005, Caidas and Burgos 2001, Rai and Munshi 1998). Motor traffic accidents also give a significant contribution to the magnitude of the problem.

Studies further indicate that increased overjet, insufficient lip closure and being a boy are significant predisposing factors to dental injury (Burden 1995, Petti and Tarsitani 1996, Brin et al 2000, Baus et al 2004, Kahabuka and Mugonzibwa 2009). Lack of proper sports grounds, lack of protective sports gear, less supportive social environments and poor supervision during play, which is a common picture among socially disadvantaged communities, are among the predisposing factors to dental trauma, (Malikaew et al 2003).

Clinical Presentation
The presentation of dental trauma will depend on the nature and degree of injury. The commonest type of injury is the uncomplicated crown fracture. Simple crown fractures present with a loss of a tooth structure, often not accompanied with pain. Large crown fractures and/ or crown root fractures present with pain and aesthetic disturbances.

Complicated crown and crown root fractures are invariably accompanied with severe pain. Injury to the tooth supporting structures and the alveolar bone presents with bleeding, pain and disfigurement depending on the degree of the injury.

A patient who has sustained traumatic injuries may present with swelling, laceration and hemorrhage of oral mucosa and gingiva, abnormalities in occlusion, tooth loss, displaced or loosened teeth, fractured crowns and roots or cracks in the enamel.

Management of Injuries

While knowledge of dentists about dento-alveolar trauma is critical to the prognosis of traumatised teeth especially for those that are avulsed, prompt and appropriate emergency management which in turn depends on lay-people's knowledge and awareness on dental trauma is also important (Hu et al 2006, Al-Jundi SH 2006, Zadik 2007). It has been noted that the most favourable treatment outcome of traumatic dental injuries is observed when patients are attended within twenty four hours after injury. For good prognosis, all patients who sustain dental trauma should seek dental consultation as soon as possible following injury. In other words, the immediate care of traumatized teeth and hence prognosis of dental trauma depends on the actions taken early on ie. actions taken by the lay people. It also depends on knowledge and skills of the dentist who will treat the patient, (Hu et al 2006, Cohenca et al 2006, de França et al 2007).

For proper diagnoses and management, thorough oral examination is important and radiographic examination is mandatory. Treatment options will depend on the presenting condition. These may include arresting bleeding, debridement of the wounds, fixation of loosened teeth, replantation and restoration of fractured teeth as well as tooth extraction.

In socially disadvantaged communities, where oral health knowledge is poor, immediate seeking of dental care services after injury is not common. Similar to dental caries problems, patient who sustain injury seek dental treatment late ranging from one day to seven days (Zerman and Cavalleri 1993, Onetto et al. 1994, Oulis and Berdouses 1996), often after getting complications like pain, swelling, pus discharge etc. On the other hand, skills of the practitioners may be a stumbling block. For instance, in a study by Kahabuka et al (1998) equal proportions of practitioners who were interviewed, about one-third each, reported correct, unnecessary and wrong treatment options Additionally, radiographic services are not available at some health facilities. Practitioners at such facilities make diagnoses and treatment planning purely basing on history and clinical examination findings.

6.6.1. Treatment of Injuries to the Permanent Dentition

Treatment of dental injuries is presented in accordance to American Academy of endodontics 2001, Andreasen and Andreasen (2000, 2007) grouped into injuries to the hard dental tissues and the pulp, and injuries to the periodontal tissues.

6.6.1.1. Injuries to the Hard Dental Tissues and the Pulp

Enamel infraction is an incomplete fracture (crack) of the enamel without loss of tooth substances. The recommended treatment of this injury is observation for pulp symptoms.

Enamel fracture (uncomplicated crown fracture) is a fracture confined to the enamel. The management of enamel fracture is selective grinding of the injured part.

Enamel-dentine fracture (uncomplicated crown fracture) is a fracture involving enamel and dentine, but not exposing the pulp. The aim of treatment for this injury is to seal dentinal tubules from bacterial contamination. Treatment is accomplished either through composite resin build up, or re-attachment of the fractured crown fragment hence restoring aesthetics.

Complicated crown fracture is a fracture involving enamel and dentine, and exposing the pulp. The aim of treatment is to maintain the pulp as healthy as possible. This allows complete root development to take place if the injured teeth have open apices. Pulp capping is done in small exposure (1mm or less) attended within 24 hours from the time of injury. Otherwise pulp amputation is recommended when the exposure of the pulp is big (more than 1mm) or the patient is attended later than 24 hours from the time of injury. This is followed by composite build-up or re-attachment of a fractured fragment.

Uncomplicated crown-root fracture is that fracture involving enamel, dentine and cementum but not exposing the pulp.

Complicated crown-root fracture is a fracture involving enamel, dentine and cementum and exposing the pulp.

For both these fractures the prognosis is usually poor if a conservative approach is chosen. Therefore, extraction is often the best alternative. Later a prosthesis can be prepared.

Root fracture; a fracture involving dentine, cementum and the pulp. Treatment of choice is repositioning of the fractured fragment, followed by immobilization of the involved tooth or teeth for 3 months using a rigid splint. The tooth is observed for any signs of pulp necrosis. If this occurs, the tooth is then treated endodontically.

6.6.1.2. Treatment of Injuries to the Periodontal Tissues

Concussion; an injury to the tooth-supporting structures without abnormal loosening or displacement of the tooth but with marked reaction to percussion.

Subluxation (loosening); an injury to the tooth supporting structures with abnormal loosening but without displacement of the tooth.

Basically, no treatment is required for both concussion and subluxation (loosening). Occlusal relief and soft diet are advocated. Follow-up to monitor pulp changes is essential. Should pulp necrosis occur, root canal treatment is done.

Intrusive luxation (central dislocation); vertical displacement of the tooth into the alveolar bone.

For a tooth with immature root formation, await spontaneous re-eruption. If it does not occur within one to one and a half months, orthodontic extrusion is advocated. Then reposition an intruded tooth and apply a flexible splint for 2-4 weeks. Make radiographs at each follow-up visit to monitor pulp conditions. Should pulp necrosis occur, root canal treatment is done.

In case the tooth has fully developed apices there are two possibilities. First, if part of the crown is visible in the oral cavity; root canal treatment should be done as soon as possible and postpone orthodontic extrusion to a later date. If no part of the crown is visible in the oral cavity; surgically extrude the tooth to its original position, apply a flexible splint for 2-4 weeks then do root canal treatment immediately or just before removing the splint.

Extrusive luxation (peripheral dislocation, partial avulsion); partial vertical displacement of the tooth out of its socket.

Lateral luxation; displacement of the tooth other than axially.

Management of extrusive and lateral luxation will also depend on the status of root maturity to whether the involved tooth has open or closed apex. For a tooth with an open apex; reposition the tooth, apply a flexible splint for 2-4 weeks, and observe the tooth for pulp conditions at follow-up visits. If the involved tooth has a fully developed apex; reposition the tooth, apply a flexible splint for 2-4 weeks and do root canal treatment just before removing the splint.

Avulsion (exarticulation); complete displacement of the tooth out of its socket.

The treatment of avulsion is replantation of the injured tooth and application of a flexible splint for one week. Advise good oral hygiene, supplemented by chlorhexidine mouth-wash. Observe the tooth for pulp condition at follow-up visits. In case pulp necrosis occurs, root canal treatment is done.

Replantation of an avulsed tooth, transported in a recommended medium will yield best results if the tooth is re-planted within four hours after injury (American Association of Endodontics 2001). In other words, successful periodontal healing of the avulsed tooth depends on; storage conditions and on the length of extra-oral period (Petrovic et al 2010).

Recommended transport media for avulsed teeth include Henk's Balanced Salt Solution (HBSS), cow milk, normal saline, child's vestibule/saliva, and water as a last resort, (American Association of Endodontics 2003, Moreira et al 2009).

Patient instruction

Following injuries to the tooth supporting structures, patient(s) should be advised to take soft diet, to brush teeth with a soft tooth brush after each meal, and use *chlorohexidine* (0.1%) or *hydrogen peroxide* (3%) mouthwash twice a day for two weeks.

6.6.2. Treatment of Injuries to the Deciduous Dentition

Superficial enamel fractures of deciduous teeth should be treated by slight grinding of sharp edges.

The recommended treatment for *enamel-dentine fracture* is restoration of a fractured crown whereas in enamel-dentine fracture with pulp exposure, pulpotomy can be performed. If a child is uncooperative, extraction is the treatment of choice.

Almost always, extraction is the treatment of choice for crown root fracture of deciduous teeth.

When a deciduous tooth sustains a *root fracture;* spontanenous healing may occur despite mobility at the fracture line. In case infection occurs: it is recommended to extract the coronal fragment only. The apical part can be left to resorb physiologically.

Unless occlusion dictates otherwise, *a laterally luxated* deciduous incisor can be left untreated. If the laterally luxated deciduous tooth is displaced with the apex forced into the follicle, then extraction is indicated.

Intrusion; under normal circumstances the roots of primary incisors are tilted labially. Most roots of *intruded primary incisors* will be forced through the labial bone plate. In such cases, spontaneous re-eruption should be anticipated. When the root is displaced into the follicle zone, extraction of the involved tooth is inevitable.

Avulsion; replantation of an avulsed deciduous tooth is contraindicated due to chances of pulp necrosis and risk of further injury to the permanent tooth germ by the replantation procedures.

Prevention of dental trauma

The preventive measures against dental trauma to children in socially disadvantaged communities may be reinforced through education to the public at large as well as enforcing the already existing laws so as to achieve prevention as follows;

i.   Use of car seat belts

    a)   Drivers and passengers must use car seat belts
    b)   Drivers of public transport should be educated and motivated to observe traffic rules
    c)   Use of seat belts in public transport should be reinforced.

ii.   Special car seats for young children. Individuals owning private cars should be educated and motivated to use special car seats for their young children.
iii. Integral use of motorcycle helmets by drivers and passengers. Integral use of motorcycle helmets must be emphasized
iv. Mandatory use of oralfacial protectors during some organized sports. In organized sports such as hockey and boxing use of oralfacial protectors must be mandatory
v.   Dental practitioners should undertake careful monitoring of children's occlusal development and undertake timely orthodontic intervention in individuals with large overjet and/or insufficient lip coverage
vi. Education in the prevention of dental injuries to parents, school teachers and sports coaches should be enhanced
vii. For both parents and dental personnel, efforts should be directed in advocating the importance of immediate consultation of dental treatment following injury
viii. Modification of traditional practices for example to avoid climbing up the trees to pick fruits thus minimize instances of falls from trees
ix. Blunt sharp edges e.g. tables and chairs within the homes

6.7. Dental Fluorosis

Dental fluorosis or mottled enamel is a condition where teeth are brown discolored due to excess fluoride incorporated in the tooth structures during mineralization. Teeth are generally composed of hydroxyapatite and carbonated hydroxyapatite; when fluoride is present, fluoroapatite is created. Excessive fluoride can cause white spots, and in severe cases, brown stains or pitting or mottling of enamel. Fluorosis is an irreversible condition which occurs during tooth forming years of a child. The critical period of exposure is between 1 and 4 years old; children above 8 years are not at risk (Alvarez et al 2009).

The condition is mainly found in regions where there is excessive fluoride concentration in drinking water or in food stuff e.g. tenderizers, (Mabelya et al 1997, www.who.int/ water sanitation health/ publications/ fluoride drinking water, 2006). According to Kaseva (2006), excessive fluoride ingestion predominantly comes from drinking water sources. However, prevalence and severity of dental and skeletal fluorosis in northern Tanzania have been reported to be higher than would be expected from ingestion of fluoride through drinking water alone. Studies done in the regions affected by fluorosis in Tanzania have shown that the consumption of food tenderizers, the trona (magadi) is the major source of the observed high prevalence of fluorosis in the affected regions (Mabelya et al 1997, Yoder et al 1998, Awadia et al 1999, Awadia et al 2000). Fluorosis is likely to occur where drinking water has fluoride content of more than 1ppm and in children who have poor intake of calcium.

Like many elements, trace amounts of fluorine which generally occurs in nature as fluoride, is beneficial to human health, but can be toxic if taken in excess. Fluoride is a powerful calcium seeking element. When ingested during tooth formation period, it becomes incorporated in calcified structures of teeth thus damaging the enamel forming cells; the ameloblast, during teeth formation resulting into dental fluorosis or skeletal fluorosis when bones are affected. The enamel is the only hard tissue which permits an early diagnosis of biological effects of even low fluoride doses on the human body (Wenzel et al 1982). Usually dental fluorosis is the first visible sign of over exposure to fluorides during the child's early years of life.

Posterior teeth are mostly affected (Wenzel et al 1982, van Palestein et al 1997). The severity of fluorosis is directly associated with increased concentrations of fluorides (Rischards et al 1989). Fluorosis usually presents with increased porosity of the enamel (Aoba and Fejerskov 2002). In milder forms the porosity is mostly limited to the subsurface enamel. But in more advanced forms, the porosity reaches the surface enamel as well, causing extensive pitting, chipping, fracturing and decay of the particular tooth or teeth. Therefore, the affected teeth usually presents as porous and relatively drier. It is due to these porous surfaces that the tooth picks up dye from food materials and hence the darkish/ brownish discoloration. Due to dryness and porosity, fluorotic teeth would usually fragment easily.

Prevalence of Dental Fluorosis

Fluorosis is prevalent in regions with high concentrations of fluoride available in food or drinks. The prevalence of fluorosis varies widely between different regions of the world. A wide range of prevalence of fluorosis have been reported among Tanzanian populations in different levels of fluoride as 16% in low fluorosis communities and around 97% in high fluorosis communities (van Palestein et al 1997, Mabelya et al 1997, Awadia et al 1999). A number of authors have also reported prevalence of fluorosis in various European populations with different levels of Fluoride in drinking water ranging from 7.1% to 90% (Fordyce et all 2007, Kukleva et al 2007, Momeni et al 2007, Nyvad et al 2009). Recently, Fomon et al (2000) in the United states of America found the prevalence of fluorosis in permanent dentition to be increasing in both communities with and without fluoridated water supply.

Management of Fluorotic Teeth

Fluorotic damage to the enamel is irreversible. Management of dental fluorosis is mainly for esthetic purposes aimed at covering the discoloration as well as repair of enamel fragments with simple restoration or crown capping.

The choice between treatment options depends on the severity of the presenting fluorosis (Akpata 2001).

In mild fluorotic cases tooth whitening procedures by the bleaching or micro-abrasion of the outer layer of enamel may be adequate. Aesthetically offensive discoloration of fluorosed teeth in severe cases where a tooth presents with porous enamel may be managed by more advanced treatment procedures such as composite bonding and porcelain veneering or crowning. The tooth whitening procedures are not recommended for severe fluorosis.

Conservative composite bonding and porcelain veneer caps provide excellent cosmetic results. However, these treatment procedures may be too expensive for general populations (Akpata 2001) especially in socially disadvantaged communities like Tanzania.

Prevention

It is possible to prevent dental fluorosis. To avoid developing fluorosis, expectant mothers and children in their tooth forming ages should avoid ingestion of excessive amount of fluorides. This can be achieved through advocacy and by provision of alternative sources of tenderizers or drinking water to people living in areas whose water sources contain excessive fluoride.

Preventive management of dental fluorosis includes de-fluoridation of drinking water in endemic areas, cautious use of fluoride supplements and supervision of the use of fluoride toothpaste by children aged below 5 years (Akpata 2001).

Furthermore, prevention of fluorosis includes parental involvement such as avoiding use of fluoride toothpaste for children below 2 years unless recommended by a dentist; use only pea sized amount of fluoride toothpaste on a toothbrush during each time they brush for children 2 years and above, always supervise use of fluoride containing dental products for children below 6 years to ensure that they do not swallow the toothpaste.

Further Reading

1) Koch G, Poulsen S. (2003) Pediatric dentistry. A clinical approach. First Edition Blackwell Munksgaard, Copenhagen
2) Andreasen JO, Andreasen FM. Andersson L. (2007) Textbook and color atlas of traumatic injuries to the teeth Fourth Edition. Wiley-Blackwell
3) JO Andreasen, Andreasen FM. (2006) Essentials of traumatic injuries to the teeth: a step-by-step treatment guide. Second edition Blackwell Munksgaard, Copenhagen
4) Pinkham JR, Casamassimo PS, Fields HW, McTigue DJ, Nowak A. (2005) Pediatric Dentistry, Fourth edition. WB Saunders Company.

References

A/Wahab M.M. (1987) Traditional practice as a cause of infant morbidity and mortality in Juba area (Sudan). *Annals of tropical Paediatrics*;7:18-21.

Adekoya-Sofowora C., Bruimah R., Ogunbodede E. (2005) Traumatic Dental Injuries Experience in Suburban Nigerian Adolescents. *The Internet Journal of Dental Science;* Volume 3 Number 1.

Adekoya-Sofowora C. Sote E., Odusanya S., Fagade O. (2000) Traumatic dental injuries of anterior teeth of children in Ile - Ife, Nigeria. *Pediatric Dental Journal*;10:33–39.

Aderinokun G.A., Bankole O.O., Denloye O.O. (2004) Attitudes, beliefs and practices of some Nigerian nurses toward teething in infants. *Odontomastol Tropical*; 07(105):222-226.

Addy M. The use of antiseptics in periodontal therapy. In Linde J., Karring T., Lang N.P. (2003). Clinical periodontology and implant dentistry. Fourth edition. *Black well Munksgaard*; 464-518.

Akpata E.S. (2001). Occurrence and Management of Dental Fluorosis. *Int. Dent. J.*; 51(5):325-333.

Al Dashti A.A., Williams S.A., Cursor M.E. (1995) Breast feeding, bottle feeding and dental caries in Kuwait. A country with low fluoride level in water supply. *Community Dent Health*; 12: 42-47.

Al-Jasser N.M., Bello L.L. (2003). Time of eruption of primary dentition in Saudi Children. *J. Contemp. Dent. Pract.*; 15:65-75.

Al-Jundi S.H. (2006) Knowledge on Jordanian mothers with regards to emergency management of dental trauma. *Dental Traumatol*;22: 291-295.

Alvarez J.A., Rendez K.M.P.C., Marocho S.M.S., Alves F.B.T., Celiberti P., Ciamponi A.L. (2009) Dental fluorosis: exposure, prevention and management. *Med. Oral Patol. Oral. Cir. Bucal.*: 14(2):E 103-107.

American Academy of Paediatrics Committee on School Health. (2004) Soft drinks in schools. *Pediatrics*;113:152-154.

Aoba T., Fejerskov O. (2002) Dental fluorosis: chemistry and biology. *Crit. Rev. Oral Biol Med.*;3:155-170.

Armfield J.M. (2007) Socioeconomic inequalities in child oral health: a comparison of discrete and composite area-based measures. *J. Public Health Dent.*;67:119-125.

Asefa M., Hewison J., Drewett R. (1998) Traditional nutritional and surgical practices and their effects on the growth of infants in south-west Ethiopia. *Pedriatr Perinat Epidemiol*; 12: 182-198.

Awadia A.K., Haugejorden O., Bjorvatn K., Birkeland J.M. (1999) Vegetarianism and dental fluorosis among children in high fluoride area of Tanzania. *Int. J. Paediatr. Dent.*: 9:3-11.

Baba S.P., Kay E.J. (1989) The mythology of the killer deciduous canine tooth in southern Sudan. *Journal of Pedodontics*;14:48-49.

Baghdady V.S., Ghose L.J. (1981) Eruption time of primary teeth in Iraq children. *Community Dent. Oral Epidemiol.* 9:245-246.

Bankole O.O., Denloye O.O., Aderinokun G.A. (2004) Attitudes, beliefs and practices of some Nigerian nurses toward teething in infants. *Odontostomatol Trop.*;27(105):22-26.

Barlow B.S., Kanellis M.J., Slayton R.L. (2002) Tooth eruption symptoms: a survey of parents and health professionals. *ASDC J. Dental Child*;69:148-150.

Baus O., Rohling J., Schwestka-Polly R. (2004) Prevalence of traumatic injuries to the permanent incisors in candidates for orthodontic treatment. *Dental Traumatology*;20:61-66.

Baykan Z., Sahin F., Beyazova U., Ozcakar B. and Baykan A. (2004) Experience of Turkish parents about their infants' teething. *Child Care Health Dev* 30:331-336.

Bentley L.P. (2007) Disparities in children's oral health and access to care. J Calif Dent Assoc. Sep;35(9):618-23. Comment in: *J. Calif. Dent. Assoc.* 2007 Dec;35(12):831.

Berchier C.E., Slot D.E., Haps S., van der Weijden G.A. (2008) The efficacy of dental floss in addition to a toothbrush on plaque and parameters of gingival inflammation: a systematic review. *Int. J. Dent. Hyg*;6:265-279.

Bissar A.R., Oikonomou C., Koch M.J., Schulte A.G. (2007) Dental health, received care, and treatment needs in 11- to 13-year-old children with immigrant background in Heidelberg, Germany. *Int. J. Paediatr. Dent.*;17(5):364-370.

Bradley C. (2003) The dental health of 5-year-old children from disadvantaged schools in the Eastern Regional Health Authority area 2000. *J. Ir. Dent. Assoc.*;49(4):133-138.

Brin I., Ben-Bassat Y., Heling IBrezniak N. (2000) Profile of an orthodontic patient at risk of dental trauma. *Endodontics Dental Traumatology*;16:111-115.

Burden D.J. (1995) An investigation of the association between overjet size, lip coverage, and traumatic injury to maxillary incisors. *European Journal of Orthodontics*;17:513-517.

Caidas A.F. Jr, Burgos M.E. (2001) A retrospective study of traumatic dental injuries in a Brazillian Dental Clinic. *Dent Traumatol*; 17:250-253.

Çaliskan M.K., Türkün M. (1995) Clinical investigation of traumatic injuries of permanent incisors in Izmir, Turkey. *Endod. Dent Traumatol*;11:210-213.

Chakraborty A., Sarkar R. and Dutta B.B. (1994) Localised disturbances associated with primary teeth eruption. *J. Indian Soc. Pedod Prev. Dent.*; 12:25-28.

Cohenca N., Forrest J.L., Rotstein I. (2006) Knowledge of oral health professionals on treatment of avulsed teeth. *Dental Traumatol*; 22: 296-301.

Costa M.R., da Silva V.C., Miqui M.N., Colombo A., Cirelli J.A. (2010) Effects of ultrasonic, electric, and manual toothbrushes on subgingival plaque composition in orthodontically banded molars. *Am. J. Orthod Dentofacial Orthop.*;137 (2):229-235.

Cunha R.F., Pugliesi D.M., Garcia L.D., Murata S.S. (2004) Systemic and local teething disturbances: prevalence in a clinic for infants. *ASDC J. Dental child*;71:24-26.

De França Rí., Trebert J., de Lacerda J.I. (2007) Brazilian dentists' knowledge regarding immediate treatment of traumatic dental injuries. *Dental Traumatol*; 23: 287-290.

De Reu G., Vanobbergen .J, Martens L.C. (2008) The influence of social indices on oral health and oral health behaviour in a group of Flemish socially deprived adolescents. *Community Dent Health*;25(1):33-37.

Dewhurst S.N., Mason C. (2001) Traditional tooth bud gouging in a Ugandan family: a report involving three sisters. *Int. J. Paediatr. Dent.*; 11:29.

Drury T.F., Horowitz A.M., Ismail A.L., Maertens M.P., Raizer G.R., Selwitx R.H. (1999) Diagnosing and reporting early childhood caries. *J. Public Health Dent*; 59: 192-197.

Du M., Bian Z., Gun L., Holt R., Champion J., Bedi R. (2000) Caries patterns and their relationship to infant and socio-economic status in 2-4 year old Chinese children. *Int. Dent. J.;* 50: 385-389.

Egwari L.O., Obisesan B., Nwokoye N.N. (2009) Microbiological status of periodontal diseases in Lagos, Nigeria. *West Indian Med. J.;*58(4):392-397.

Fisher-Owens S.A., Barker J.C., Adams S., Chung L.H., Gansky S.A., Hyde S., Weintraub J.A. (2008) Giving policy some teeth: routes to reducing disparities in oral health. *Health Aff* (Millwood);27(2):404-412.

Fomon S.J., Ekstrand J., Ziegler E.E. (2000) Fluoride intake and prevalence of dental fluorosis: trends in fluoride intake with special attention to infants. *Journal of Pulblic Health Dentistry*; 60:131-139.

Fordyce F.M., Vrana K., Zhovinsky E., Povoroznuk V., Toth G., Hope B.C., Iljinsky U., Baker J. (2007) A health risk assessment for fluoride in Central Europe. *Environment Geochem Health*; 29(2): 83-102.

Forlenza G.P., Paradise Black N.M., McNamara E.G., Sullivan S.E. (2010) Ankyloglossia, exclusive breastfeeding, and failure to thrive. *Pediatrics;*125(6):e1500-1504.

Glendor U., Halling A., Anderson L., Eilert-Peterson E. (1996) Incidence of traumatic tooth injuries in children and adolescents in the country of Vastmanland, Sweden. Swed Dent J;20:15-28.

Halestrap D.J. (1971) Indigenous dental practice in Uganda. *British Dental Journal*;131:463-464.

Hans R., Nicoli A.D., Adavi P.M., Pinc C.M. (2004) Risk factors for dental caries in young children. A systemic review of literature. *Community Dent Health*; 21:71-85.

Hargreaves J.A., Cleaton-Jones P.E., Roberts G.J., Williams S., Matejka J.M. (1999) Trauma to primary teeth of South African pre-school children. *Endod Dent Traumatol;*15:73-76.

Hartley B.E., Rowe-Jones J. (1994) Uvulectomy to prevent throat infects. *J. Laryngol Otol*; 108:65-66.

Hassanali J., Amwayi P., Muriithi A. (1995) Removal of deciduous canine tooth buds in Kenyan rural Maasai. *East African Medical Journal*;72:207-209.

Hassananli J., Odhiambo J.W. (1981) Ages of eruption of permanent teeth in Kenyan African and Asian children. *Ann. Human Biol.*;8:425-434.

Hesketh K.D., Hulland S.A., Lucas J.O., Wake M.A. (2000) Eruption of the primary dentition in human infants. *Pediatr. Dent.* 22:415-421.

Hitchcock N.E., Gilmour A.I., Gracey M., Kailis D.G. (1984) Australian longitudinal study of time and order of eruption of primary teeth. *Community Dent. Oral Epidemiol.* 12:260-263.

Hiza J.F.R., Kikwilu E.N. (1992) Missing primary teeth due to tooth bud extraction in a remote village in Tanzania. *Int. J. Paediatr. Dent.*; 2: 31-34.

Holan G., Mamber E. (1994) Extraction of primary canine tooth buds: prevalence and associated dental abnormalities in a group of Ethiopian Jewish children. *Int. J. Paediatr. Dent.*;4:25-30.

Hong P., Lago D., Seargeant J., Pellman L., Magit A.E., Pransky S.M. (2010) Defining ankyloglossia: A case series of anterior and posterior tongue ties. *Int. J. Pediatr. Otorhinolaryngol.*;74:1003-1006. Epub 2010 Jun 16.

jada.ada.org/cgi (2005) (Accessed February 2011) Tooth Eruption: the primary teeth. *J. Am. Dent. Assoc.*;136:1619.

Hu L.W., Prisco C.R.D., Bombana A.C. (2006) Knowledge of Brazilian general dentists and endodontists about the emergency management of dento-alveolar trauma. *Dental Traumatol*; 22:113-117.

Huntington N.L., Kim I.J., Hughes C.V. (2002) Caries risk factors for Hispanic children affected by early childhood caries. *Pediatr. Dent.*; 24: 536-542.

Ijaduola G.T. (1981). Uvulectomy in Nigeria. *J. Laryng. Otol.;* 95: 1127-1133.

Ijaduola G.T. (1982) Hazards of Traditional Uvulectomy in Nigeria. *East African Medical Journal*; 59: 771-774.

Ismail A.L., Sohn W. (1999) A systematic review of clinical diagnostic criteria of early childhood caries. *J. Public Health Dent*; 59: 171-191.

Jaber L., Chohen I.J, Mor A. (1992) Fever associated with teething. *Arch. Dis. Child.* 67:233-234.

Jones A. (1992) Tooth mutilation in Angola. *British Dental Journal*;173:177-179.

Jones M. (2002) Teething in children and the alleviation of symptoms. *J. Fam. Health Care* 12:12-13.

Kahabuka F.K. (2004) Availability of snacks and drinks within primary school premises in Ilala District, Dar es Salaam. *Tanz. Dent. J.;*10:15-17.

Kahabuka F.K., Fabian F.M., Muze K. Timing and pattern of eruption of deciduous teeth in Tanzanian children (Accepted to *International Journal of Dental Anthropology*, 2009).

Kahabuka F.K., Mugonzibwa E.A. (2009) Risk factors for oral injuries among 8-14 year olds in Dar es Salaam, Tanzania. *Int. J. Paediatr. Dent.*;19:148-154.

Kahabuka F.K., Plasschaert A., van't Hof M.A. (2001) Prevalence of teeth with untreated dental trauma among nursery and primary school pupils in Dar es salaam, Tanzania. *Dental Traumatol*;17: 109-113.

Kahabuka F.K. (2008) Implications of myths, beliefs and practices on children's oral health in developing countries. In R. W. Pierce, R. I. Schwartz "New Perspectives on Knowledge, Attitudes and Practices in Health". Chapter VIII; pp. 187-198 Nova Science Publishers, Hauppauge, N.Y.

Kaimenyi T.J. (1998) Occurrence of midline diastema and frenulum attachments amongst school children in Nairobi, Kenya. *India J. Dent. Res.*;9:67-71.

Kaseva M.E. (2006) Contribution of trona (magadi) into excessive fluorosis--a case study in Maji ya Chai ward, northern Tanzania. *Sci. Total Environ.*;366(1):92-100.

Kawia H.M., Kahabuka F.K. (2009) Symptoms associated with teething in Tanzania Japanese Paediatric *Dental Journal*; 19(1): 9-14.

Khan M.N., Cleaton-Jones P.E. (1998) Dental caries in African preschool children: Social Factors as disease markers. *J. Public Health Dent*; 58: 7-11.

Kikwilu E.N., and Hiza J.F.R. (1997) Tooth bud extraction and rubbing of herbs by traditional healers in Tanzania: prevalence, and sociological and environmental factors influencing the practices. *Int. J. Paediatr. Dent.*;7:19-24.

Kikwilu E.N., Mandari G.J. (2001) Dental caries and periodontal conditions among primary school children in Morogoro municipality, Tanzania. *East Afr. Med. J.*;78:152-156.

Kikwilu E.N., Masalu J.R., Kahabuka F.K., and Senkoro A.R. (2008) Prevalence of oral pain and barriers to use of emergency oral care facilities among adult Tanzanians *BMC Oral Health.*; 8: 28. Published online 2008 September 29. doi: 10.1186/1472-6831-8-28.

Kukleva M.P., Isheva A.V., Kondeva V.K., Dimitrova M.M., Petrova S.G. (2007) Prevalence of dental fluorosis among 4-14year old children from the town of Dimitrovgrad (Bulgaria). *Folia Med.* (Plovdiv).; 49(1-2):25-31.

Lee J., Kiyak H.A. (1992) Oral disease beliefs, behaviors, and health status of Korean-Americans. *J. Public Health Dent.*;52:131-6.

Leung A.K. (1989) Teething. Am Fam Physician 39:131-134.

Lewis H.A., Rudolph M.J., Mistry M., Monyatsi V., Marambana T., Ramela P. (2004) Oral health knowledge and original practices of *African traditional healers in Zonkizizwe and Dube*, SADJ:59:245-246.

Li M.Y., Wang J., Lai G.Y. (2009) Effect of dentifrices containing peptides of streptococcal antigen 1/11 on the adherence of mutans streptococcus. *Arch. Oral Biol.;* 54(11):1068-1073.

Liena Puy C., Forner Navarro L. (2008) Evidence concerning the medical management of caries. *Med. Oral Patol. Oral Cir. Bucal.* 1;13(5):E325-30.

Mabelya L., van Palestein H.W., van't Hof M.A., König K.G. (1997) Dental fluorosis and the use of high fluoride-containing trona tenderize(magadi). *Community Dent. Oral Epidemiol..*; 25(2): 170-176.

Macknin M., Piedmonte M., Jacobs J., Skibinski C. (2000) Symptoms associated with infant teething. *Pediatrics* 105:747-752.

Magnusson T.E. (1982) Emergence of primary teeth and onset of dental stages in Icelandic children. *Community Dent. Oral Epidemiol.* 10:91-97.

Malikaew P., Watt R.G., Sheiham A. (2006) Prevalence and factors associated with traumatic dental injuries (TDI) to anterior teeth of 11-13 year old Thai children. *Community Dent Health*;23(4):222-227.

Manji F., Mwaniki D. (1985) Estimation of median age of eruption of permanent teeth in Kenyan children. *East Afr. Med. J.*;62:252-259.

Manni J.J. (1984) Uvulectomy, a tradition surgical procedure in Tanzania. *Ann. Tropical Medicine Parasitol*; 78: 48-53.

Marcenes W., Al Beiruti N., Tayfour D., Issa S. (1999) Epidemiology of traumatic injuries to the permanent incisors of 9-12 year-old schoolchildren in Damascus, Syria. *Endod Dent. Traumatol*;15:117-123.

Marcenes W., Alessi O.N., Traebert J. (2000) Causes and prevalence of traumatic injuries to the permanent incisors of school children aged 12 years in Jaragua do Sul, Brazil. *Int. Dent. J..*;50(2):87-92.

Maro D., Kahabuka F.K. (2007) Prevalence of early childhood caries among 2-6 years old underprivileged and privileged children in Dar es Salaam *Tanz Dent. J.;*14:53-58.

Masiga M.A., Musera D.K. (2003) Iatrogenic hypodontia following traditional excision of deciduous canine tooth buds:case reports. *African Journal of Oral health Sciences:*4:173-174.

Massarente D.B., Domanesch C., Antunes J.L. (2009) Untreated dental caries in a Brazilian paediatric AIDS patient population. *Oral Health Prev. Dent.*;7(4): 403-410.

Matee M., van't Hof M., Maselle S., Mikx F., van Palenstein Helderman W. (1994) Nursing caries, linear hypoplasia, and nursing and weaning habits in Tanzanian infants. *Community Dent. Oral Epidemiol..*;22(5 Pt 1):289-293.

Matee M.I.N. and van Palenstein Helderman W. (1991) Extraction of nylon teeth and associated abnormalities in Tanzanian children. *Afr. Dent. J.*;5:21-25.

McIntyre G.T., McIntyre, G.M. (2002) Teething troubles? *Brit. Dent. J.* 192:251-255.

Mestrinho H.D., Bezerra A.C.B., Carvalho J.C. (1998) Traumatic dental injuries in Brazilian pre-school children. *Braz. Dent. J.*;9:101-104.

Miles S.H, Ololo H. (2003). Traditional surgeons in sub-Saharan Africa: images from south Sudan. *Int. J. STD AIDS*; 14: 505-508.

Mohamed N., Barnes J. (2008) Characteristics of children under 6 years of age treated for early childhood caries in South Africa. *J. Clin. Pediatr. Dent.*;32:247-252.

Momeni A., Neuhauser A., Renner N., Heinzel –Gutenbrunner M., Abou-Fidah J., Rasch K., Kroplin M., Fejerskov O., Pieper K. (2007) Prevalence of dental fluorosis in German schoolchildren in areas with different preventive programmes. *Caries Res.*; 41: 437-444.

Moreira-Neto J., Gondim J.O., Raddi M.S., Pansani C.A. (2009) Viability of human fibroblasts in coconut water as a storage medium. *Int. Endod J.*;42:827-830.

Mosha H.J., Ngilisho L.A.F., Nkwera H., Scheultz F., Poulsen S. (1994) Oral health status and treatment needs in different age groups in two regions of Tanzania. *Community Dent. Oral Epidemiol.*;22:307-310.

Mosha H.J., Senkoro A.R., Masalu J.R.P., Kahabuka F., Mandari G., Mabelya L., Kalyanyama B. (2005) Oral health status and treatment needs among Tanzanians of different age groups. *Tanz. Dent. J.*;12:18-27.

Mosha H.J. (1983) Dental mutilation and associated abnormalities in Tanzania. *Tropical Dental Journal*;6:215-220.

Moynihan P., Petersen P.E. (2004) Diet, Nutrition and the prevention of dental diseases. *Public Health Nutrition*;7:201-226.

Mugonzibwa E.A., Kuijpers-Jagtman A.M., Laine-Alava M.T., van't Hof M.A. (2002) Emergence of permanent teeth in Tanzanian children. *Community Dent. Oral Epidemiol.*;30:455-462.

Mumghamba E.G., Markkanen H.A., Honkala E. (1995) Risk factors for periodontal diseases in Ilala Tanzania. *J. Clin. Periodontol.*; 22:347-354.

Mutai J., Muniu E., Sawe J., Hassanali J., Kibet P., Wanzala P. (2010) Socio-cultural practices of deciduous canine tooth bud removal among Maasai children. *Int. Dent. J.*;60:94-98.

Mziray H., Kahabuka F.K. (2006) Prevalence and awareness of early childhood caries among attendees of a reproductive and child health clinic at Mnazi Mmoja dispensary, Dar es Salaam. *Tanz. Dent. J.*; 12: 35-41.

Najada A., Weinberg M. (2002) Unusual causes of chronic cough in a four-year old cured by uvulectomy. *Pediatr. Pulmonol.*; 34: 144-146.

Nicolau B., Marcenes W., Sheiham A. (2001) Prevalence, causes and correlates of traumatic dental injuries among 13-year-olds in Brazil. *Dent. Traumatol.*;17:213-217.

Nyandindi U., Palin-Palokas T., Milén A., Robison V., Kombe N. (1994) Oral health knowledge, attitudes, behaviour and skills of children entering school in urban and rural areas in *Tanzania Public Health*;108:35-41.

Nyvad B., Machiulskiene V., Feferskov O., Baelum V. (2009) Diagnosis of dental caries in populations with different levels of dental fluorosis. *Eur. J. Oral Sci.*;1117:161-168.

Onetto J.E., Flores M.T., and Garbarino M.L. (1994) Dental trauma in children and adolescents in Valparaiso, Chile. *Endod Dent. Traumatol.*;10:223-227.

Oredugba F.A. (2006) Use of oral health care services and oral findings in children with special needs in Lagos, Nigeria. *Spec. Care Dentist*;26:59-65.

Ostapiuk B. (2006) Tongue mobility in ankyloglossia with regard to articulation. *Ann Acad Med. Stetin.*;52 Suppl 3:37-47.

Oulis C.J., Berdouses E.D. (1996) Dental injuries of permanent teeth treated in private practice in Athens. *Endod Dent. Traumatol*;12:60-65.

Oyejide C.O., Aderikonun, G.A. (1991) Teething myths in Nigerian rural Yoruba communities. *Afr. Dent. J.*;5:31-34.

Oyelami O.A. (1993) Traditional Uvulectomy among preschool children in the far North. Eastern Nigeria. *Journal of Tropical paediatric*;39: 314-315.

Parhar G., Yoon R.K., Chussid S. (2009) Maternal child oral health behaviours and caries experience in the child. *J. Clin. Pediatric Dentistry*; 34: 135-139.

Parisotto T.M., Steiner- Oliveira C., Peres R.C., Rodrigues L.K., Nobre-dos-Santos M. (2010) Relationship among microbiological composition and presence of dental plaque, sugar exposure, social factors and different stages of early childhood caries. *Arch. Oral Boil.*, Epub; 55; 365-373.

Peretz B., Ram D., Hermida L., Otero M.M. (2003) Systemic manifestations during eruption of primary teeth in infants. *ASDC J. Dental Child*;70:170-173.

Petrovic B., Marković D., Peric T., Blagojevic D. (2010). Factors related to treatment and outcomes of avulsed teeth. *Dent Traumatol*; 26:52-59.

Petti S., Tarsitani G. (1996) Traumatic injuries to anterior teeth in Italian schoolchildren: prevalence and risk factors. *Endodontics Dental Traumatology*;12:294-297.

Pindborg J.J. (1969) Dental mutilation and associated abnormalities in Uganda. *Amer S. Phys. Anthop*;31:383.

Post E.D., Rupert A.W., Schulpen T.W. (2010) Problematic breastfeeding due to a short frenulum. *Ned. Tijdschr Geneeskd.* 2010;154:A918.

Prual A., Gamatie Y., Djakounda M., Huguet D. (1994) Traditional uvulectomy in Niger: a public health problem? *Soc Sci Med*; 39: 1077-1082.

Rai S.B., Munshi A.K. (1998) Traumatic injuries to the anterior teeth among South Kamara school children - a prevalence study. *J. Indian Soc. Pedod Prev. Dent.*; 16 : 44 – 51.

Ramar-Gomez F.J., Huang G.F., Masouredis O.M. (1996) Prevalence and treatment costs of infant caries in Northern Califonia. *J. Dent. Child*; 2:108-111.

Ramirez O., Planells P., Batberia E. (1994) Age and order of eruption of primary teeth in Spanish children. *Community Dent. Oral Epidemiol.*;22:56-59.

Rebelo M.A., Lopes M.C., Vieira J.M., Parente R.C. (2009) Dental caries and gingivitis among 15 to 19 year-old students in Manaus, AM, Brazil. *Braz. Oral Res*;23:248-254.

Reisine S., Tellez M., Willem J., Sohn W., Ismail A. (2008) Relationship between caregiver's and child's caries prevalence among disadvantaged African Americans. *Community Dent. Oral. Epidemiol.*;36:191-200.

Rocha M.J.C., Cardoso M. (2001) Traumatized permanent teeth in Brazilian children assisted at the Federal University of Santa Catarina, Brazil. *Dental Traumatology*;17:245-249.

Rodd H., Davidson L.E. (2000) "Ilko dacowo:" canine enucleation and dental sequelae in Somali children. *Int. J. Paediatr. Dent.*;10:290-297.

Roder D.M. (1970) The South Australian school canteen programme: an interim report. *Austral Dent. J.;*15:324-328.

Rosenblatt A., Zarzar P. (2004) Breast feeding and early childhood caries. Assessment among Brazilian infants. *Int. J. Paediatr. Dent.*; 14: 439-445.

Rugarabamu P.G.N., Poulsen S., Masalu J.R.P. (2002) A longitudinal study of occlusal caries among school children in Tanzania. *Community Dent. Oral Epidemiol.*;30:37-51.

Sarrell E.M., Horev Z., Cohen Z., Cohen H.A. (2005) Parents' and medical personnel's beliefs about infant teething. *Patient Educ. Couns*; 57:122-125.

Savani S., Kahabuka F.K. (2008) Risk factors of early childhood caries among Dar es Salaam children. *Tanzania Medical Jo*urnal; 23:15-18.

Schwarz E. (2006) Access to oral health care - an Australian perspective. Community *Dent. Oral Epidemiol.*;34:225-231.

Shulham J.D., Peterson J. (2004) The association between incisor trauma and occlusal characteristics in individuals 8-50 years of age. *Dental Traumatology*;20:67-74.

Silk H., Douglass A.B., Douglass J.M., Silk L. (2008) *Oral health during pregnancy. Am Fam Physician.* 15;77:1139-1144.

Tan A.E. (2009) Periodontal maintenance. *Aust Dent. J.*:54 Suppl 1:S110-117.

Teles R.P., Teles F.R. (2009) Antimicrobial agents used in the control of periodontal biofilms: effective adjuncts to mechanical plaque control. *Braz Oral Res*; (23 Suppl)1:39-48.

Traebert J., Almeida I.C., Marcenes W. (2003) Etiology of traumatic dental injuries in 11 to 13-year-old schoolchildren. *Oral Health Prev. Dent*;1:317-323.

Traebert J., Bittencourt D.D., Peres K.G., Peres M.A., de Lacerda J.T., Marcenes W. (2006) Aetiology and rates of treatment of traumatic dental injuries among 12-year-old school children in a town in southern Brazil. *Dent Traumatol*;22:173-178.

van Palenstein W.H., Mabelya L., van't Hof M.A., König K.G. (1997) Two types of intraoral distribution of fluorotic enamel. *Community Dent. Oral Epidemiol.*; 25:251-255.

van Palenstein-Helderman W., Soe W., Van't Hof M.A. (2006) Risk factors of early childhood caries in Southeast Asian population. *J. Dent. Res.*; 85: 85-88.

Vanderas A.P., Papagiannoulis L. (1999) Incidence of dentofacial injuries in children:a 2-year longitudinal study. *Endod Dent Traumatol*;15:235-238.

Wake M., Hesketh K., Allen M. (1999) Parent beliefs about infant teething: A survey of Australian parents. *J. Paediatr. Child Health*; 35:446 – 449.

Welbury R.R., Nunn J.H., Gordon P.H., Green-Abate C. (1993) "Killer" canine removal and its sequelae in Addis Ababa. *Quintessence International*;24:323-327.

Wilson P.H., Mason C. (2002) The trouble with teething—misdiagnosis and misuse of a topical medicament. *Int. J. Paediatr. Dent*;12:215-218.

Wind J. (1984) Cross culture and anthropological reflections on Africa Uvulectomy Lancet.; 12:1267-1268.

World Health Organization. (2002) Global Oral Health Data Bank. Geneva: World Health Organization.

Wright J.E. (1995) Tongue-tie. *J. Paediatr Child Health*;31:276-278.

www.ada.org/goto/jada (2005) Tooth eruption. The primary teeth, For the Dental patient November:1619.

www.endoexperience.com (2003) Recommended guidelines of the American Association of Endodontics for the treatment of traumatic dental injuries.

www.mchoralhealth.org/openwide/media/flash/eruption-flash.htm (Accessed February 2010) Tooth eruption and exfoliation charts.

www.who.int/water sanitation_health/publications/fluoride drinking water (2006) *Fluoride in Drinking-water. World Health Organization.* pp. 5–27.

Wyne A., Darwish S., Adenubi J., Baltata S., Khan N. (2001) The prevalence and pattern of nursing caries in Saudi pre-school children. *Int. J. Paediatr. Dent.*;11:361-364.

Xavier A.C., Silva I.N., Costa Fde O., Corrêa D.S. (2009) Periodontal status in children and adolescents with type 1 diabetes mellitus. *Arq. Bras. Endocrinol. Metabol*;53:348-354.

Yoder K.M., Mabelya L., Robison V.A., Dunipace A.J., Brizendine E.J., Stookey G.K. (1998) Severe dental fluorosis in a Tanzanian population consuming water with negligible fluoride concentration. *Community Dent. Oral Epidemiol.*; 26: 382-393.

Zadik Y. (2007) Oral trauma and dental emergency management recommendation of first-aid text-books and manuals. *Dental Traumatol.*; 23: 304-306.

Zerman N., Cavalleri G. (1993) Traumatic injury to permanent incisors. *Endod Dent. Traumatol.*;9:61-64.

In: Oral Health Care for Socially Disadvantaged Communities   ISBN: 978-1-62948-287-3
Editors: F.K. Kahabuka, E.N. Kikwilu and I. Anderson © 2013 Nova Science Publishers, Inc.

Chapter VII

Management of Orthodontic Conditions in Socially Disadvantaged Communities

Emeria A. Mugonzibwa and Matilda Mtaya-Mlangwa
School of Dentistry, Muhimbili University of
Health and Allied Sciences

7.1. Introduction

Orthodontic conditions are irregularities of the teeth or malrelationship of the dental arches beyond the accepted range of normal also referred to as malocclusion(s). Orthodontics is a dental clinical specialty involving supervision, guidance and correction of the growing or mature dentofacial structures including those conditions that require movement of the teeth or correction of malrelationships and malformations of their related structures and the adjustment of relationships between and among teeth and facial bones by the application of forces and/or the stimulation and redirection of functional forces within the craniofacial complex (Daskalogiannaskis, 2000).

The frequency of orthodontic conditions in children varies among and between populations and the occurrence has no racial or geographical boundaries as indicated in tables 7.1 and 7.2. Whereas orthodontic treatment is objectively needed by most people affected by malocclusions, the challenge to the oral health professionals is to provide the quality orthodontic care in all socioeconomic backgrounds. Provision of quality orthodontic treatment in socially disadvantaged settings where finance, optimum oral health human resource, communication infrastructure, maintenance of equipment, restricted supplies of materials and possibilities of sophisticated investigations is still a huge challenge (Karaiskos et al., 2005; Martin et al, 2008). In cases of Sub-Saharan countries, limited access to orthodontic care is partly due to low priority given to orthodontic concerns (Otuyemi, 2001). Preventive and early interceptive orthodontics procedures that aim at eliminating or reducing the need for later comprehensive orthodontic treatment in permanent dentition, are presented as affordable alternatives that do reintroduce a salvation in the orthodontic care system in socially disadvantaged settings (Karaiskos et al., 2005; Kerosuo et al., 2008; Keski-Nisula et al., 2008). It is generally accepted that prevention and early orthodontic intervention attempts are successful in minimizing some inherited and environmentally acquired orthodontic conditions (Popovich and Thompson, 1975; Hiles, 1985; Pirttiniemi et al., 1990; Al Nimri and Richardson, 2000; Hesse et al., 1997; Nguyen et al., 1999; Kluemper et al., 2000; Westwood et al., 2003; Artun et al., 2005; Kerosuo et al., 2008; Keski-Nisula et al., 2008). Treatment in the early mixed dentition with or without the eruption guidance appliance is an effective method to restore normal occlusion, eliminates the need for further orthodontic treatment, and only a few spontaneous corrective changes can be expected without active intervention (Chung and Kerr, 1987; Al Nimri and Richardson, 2000; Vakiparta et al., 2005; Keski-Nisula et al., 2008).

Significant barriers exist to ensuring the socially disadvantaged communities receive basic oral health care including orthodontic treatment. Amongst these are poverty, ignorance, inadequate financial resources, travel distance, shortage of educated and trained oral health care human resource, restricted supplies of materials, deficiencies in and poor maintenance of equipment (Ntabaye et al., 1998). Due to aforementioned barriers, need for orthodontic services are usually not accessed by all who have both the subjective and objective orthodontic treatment. This leads to a situation in which large segments of the population receive inadequate or completely lack orthodontic care.

Malocclusions are not life threatening, but are important public health issues (Sheiham, 1993) as most can be prevented or intercepted (Ricketts and Robert, 1979). They are conditions that affect people's well being and quality of life creating a burden on top of other diseases which continue to inflict many socially disadvantaged communities. It has been reported that patients are motivated to seek orthodontic care due to the physical, psychological and social effects of malocclusion (Bowling, 1997; Zhang et al., 2006). It is advocated that every government especially in developing economy countries should campaign for considering preventive and interceptive programmes, because sophisticated orthodontic treatment by orthodontic specialists is almost impossible for individuals who absolutely require orthodontic treatment. Hence, supervision of occlusion development, prediction and prevention of malocclusion in the primary and early mixed dentitions is essential especially in socially disadvantaged communities.

At the end of this chapter, the reader must be able to understand the epidemiology, aetiology, prevention of malocclusions, concept and modalities of early interceptive orthodontics for specific orthodontic conditions and challenges of providing orthodontic care in socially disadvantaged settings.

7.2. Epidemiology of Malocclusions

Many studies on the prevalence of malocclusions in developed, well to do and socially disadvantaged communities have been reported. The reported prevalence of malocclusions ranges from 13% to 76% in deciduous dentition (Table 7.1). Malocclusions in the permanent dentition have been reported to range from 39% to 98% in children (Table 7.2). Divergence in the prevalence figures may depend on ethnic differences, wide ranges in number, as well as in the age range of subjects examined. Moreover, the criteria for the recorded items (registration methods) seem to play an important role for the variation in the prevalence figures (Thilander et al., 2001). The temptation is to conclude that, most of the classic malocclusions occur among children worldwide but the prevalence differs.

Table 7.1. The prevalence of malocclusion in deciduous dentition in different populations

Authors	Population	Age	Prevalence (%)
Visković et al. (1990)	Croatian	3-6	47.5
Kerosuo (1990)	Tanzanian	3-4	18
Jones et al. (1993)	USA	3-4	13
Kabue et al. (1995)	Kenyan	3-6	51
Trottman and Elsbach (1996)	USA	2-5	49.8
Chevitarese et al. (2002)	Brazilian	4-6	75.8
Stahl and Grabowski (2003)	Germany	4½	42
Mugonzibwa et al. (2004a)	Tanzanian	3½-5	19.8
Katz et al. (2004)	Brazilian	4	49.7
Grabowski et al. (2007)	Germany	4½	74.7
Robke (2008)	Germany	2-6	75.1
Mtaya (2008)	Tanzanian	3-5	32.5

Table 7.2. The prevalence of malocclusion in permanent dentition in different populations

Authors	Population	Age in years	Prevalence (%)
Thilander and Myrberg (1973)	Swedish	13	73.8
al-Emran et al., (1990)	Saudi Arabian	14	62.4
Kerosuo et al., (1991)	Finnish	12-18	88
Kerosuo et al., (1991)	Tanzanian	11-18	45
Lew et al., (1993)	Chinese	12-14	92.9
Ng'ang'a et al., (1996)	Kenyan	13-15	72
Silva and Kang, (2001)	American-Latino	12-18	93
Thilander et al. (2001)	Colombian	13-17	88
Mugonzibwa et al. (2004)	Tanzanian	3½-16	Up to 51
Onyeaso (2004)	Nigerian	12-17	76
Abu Alhaija et al. (2005)	Jordanian	13-15	92
Behbehani et al. (2005)	Kuwaiti	13-14	86
Ciuffolo et al. (2005)	Italian	11-14	93
Gábris et al. (2006)	Hungarian	16-18	70.4
Rwakatema et al. (2006)	Tanzanian	12-15	97.6
Dhar et al. (2007)	Indian	11-14	38.9
Mtaya et al. (2009)	Tanzanian	12-14	63.8
Murshid et al., (2010)	Saudi Arabia	13-14	91

7.3. Aetiology of Malocclusions

It is generally acknowledged that genetics and the environment are aetiological factors for the development of malocclusion (Proffit et al., 2005). Combinations of both factors have often been found in the same individual. While it is suggested that malocclusions are predominantly genetically determined (Chung et al., 1972; Chung and Niswander, 1975; Smith and Bailit, 1977; Saunders et al., 1980; Nakasima et al., 1982; Peck et al., 1998, Proffit et al., 2005), the importance of environmental influence is widely acknowledged (Lombardi and Bailit, 1972; Niswander, 1975; Corrucini and Potter, 1980).

The concept of polygenic factors where both genetic factors and environmental influence have a role to play in development of malocclusions has also been supported (Harris and Smith, 1980, 1982). On the other hand, the dominance of environmental influences over genetic factors among monozygous and dizygous twins in the dental and/or alveolar area has been reported (Lobb, 1987). Genetic factors have influence mainly on dental and skeletal growth abnormalities. Besides heredity, sucking habits involving the fingers, lips or tongue, impaired nasal breathing, atypical swallowing, premature loss of deciduous teeth largely due to caries in the primary molars are considered to be important factors in the aetiology of malocclusion (Melsen et al., 1979; Behlfelt et al., 1989; Kurol and Berglund, 1992; Larsson et al., 1992; Korpar et al., 1994; Øgaard et al., 1994; Thilander and Lennartsson, 2002; Proffit et al., 2005). Also, the association between poor nutrition and impaired growth and development of facial bones leading to development of some malocclusions has been reported (Gulati et al., 1991; Weissman et al., 1994; Thomaz and Valenca, 2009; Thomaz et al., 2010).

7.3.1. Premature Loss of Deciduous Teeth

Untreated carious primary teeth create a risk for malocclusion by shortening the dental arch either through breakdown of interproximal surfaces or loss of these teeth (Haavikko and Rahkamo, 1977). Premature loss of primary teeth is regarded as the most common local factor leading to a malocclusion. When young children live with unattended severely decayed deciduous molars, loose deciduous teeth prematurely due to caries, there can be an impact on the position of the permanent teeth as they emerge into the oral cavity (Richardson, 1965; Love and Adams, 1971; Ngan et al., 1999). Various forms of individual teeth occlusal irregularities and malocclusions such as crowding, shifting of the midline and changing of the molar relationship may occur.

7.3.2. Sucking Habits

As a general rule, sucking habits during the primary dentition phase, have little long-term effects. However, the role of sucking habits in the aetiology of malocclusions has been investigated by Melsen et al. (1979), Larsson (2000), and Øgaard et al. (1994). These cross-sectional studies on the effects of prolonged sucking habits indicated that irreversible malocclusions will be produced if the sucking persisted beyond 4 years of age (Lindsten et al., 1996). Prolonged sucking habits may lead to malocclusions depending on frequency, length and intensity of sucking (Hellman 1914; Backlund, 1963; Bowden, 1966; Tewari, 1970; Larson, 1972, 1978, 1987; ; Melsen et al., 1979; Lindner and Modeer, 1989; Estripeaut et al 1989; Garattini et al 1990; Warren et al., 2001, Warren and Bishara, 2002; da Costa et al 2002). The malocclusions include: (1) reduced vertical growth of the frontal parts of alveolar process which creates an anterior open bite [Fiure 1]; (2) proclination and protrusion of the maxillary incisors as a result of the horizontal force created by the digit; (3) a lengthening of the maxillary arch; (4) anterior displacement of the maxilla; (5) a unilateral and bilateral postnormal molar relationship that is often associated with finger sucking. Other published effects of prolonged sucking are proclination or retroclination of the lower incisors, which seems to be due to the strength of the tightness of the lower lip and tongue activity during sucking (Ravn 1976, Estripeaut et al., 1989; Larsson 1994). The characteristic malocclusions associated with sucking habits arise from a combination of direct pressure on the teeth and an alteration in the pattern of resisting cheek and lip pressures. The extent of teeth displacement usually correlates well with the number of sucking hours per day than with the magnitude of the pressure.

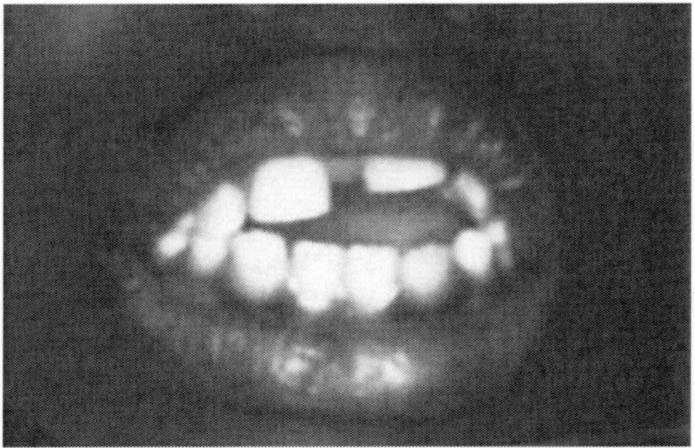

Figure 7.1. Open bite (Courtesy of F. K. Kahabuka).

There are mainly four different forces generated by sucking habits that work on various components of orofacial system:

1) Lingual tipping forces on the mandibular incisors cause linguoversion.
2) The cheek pressures are the greatest around the corners, explaining the V-shaped maxillary arch, while the posterior cross bite could be related to the buccinator's force in the posterior region.
3) The interposed thumb directly impedes the incisor eruption, and the lowering forces on the mandible can allow over eruption of the posterior teeth leading to anterior open bite.
4) The tongue applies force against the thumb, which is transferred to the premaxillary area. The nose floor does not descent to its expected position and a narrow nose floor and high palate can be expected. The tongue pressure is decreased on the posterior teeth due to the lowered position of the tongue.

Hence, the consequences of sucking habits to the maxillary and mandibular arches are conditions such as: spaced and protrusive maxillary anterior teeth; posterior cross bite; short and hypotonic upper lip; accentuated curve of Spee; lingually tilted mandibular anterior teeth;

mentalis muscle hyperactivity; retrusion and clockwise rotation of the mandible; anterior open bite; tongue-thrush development; narrow nose floor and high palate associated with speech interferences.

7.3.3. Tongue Thrusting

Tongue thrust swallowing is defined as placement of the tongue tip forward between the incisors during swallowing. The reason for tongue thrust to create an oral seal. The consequences of tongue thrusting include speech distortion; anterior open bite; posterior or lateral open bite; Angle's class II, deep bite and class III malocclusions (Proffit et al., 2005).

7.3.4. Mouth Breathing

Mouth breathing is an abnormal respiratory pattern also called 'Adenoid facies'. Individuals with this condition may present with irregularities in the maxillary dental arches, a long facial profile, proclined maxillary and mandibular incisors, tendence towards posterior cross bite and toward anterior open bite (Linder-Aronson, 1979; Hesby et al., 2006). Causes of mouth breathing may be among the following: enlarged tonsils and adenoids; swollen nasal mucosa; deviation of the nasal septum; narrow airway; allergic conditions and nasal polyps. The consequences of mouth breathing to the developing occlusion are: narrowed maxillary arches; protrusion of the maxillary arch; supraversion of the mandibular incisors; poor vertical development of the premolar and molar areas; the mandibular Class II tendency; short, poorly developed upper lip; underdeveloped external nares and poor muscle tone of the facial muscles (Melsen et al., 1987; Lessa et al., 2005; Proffit et al., 2005).

7.4. Prevention and Management of Orthodontic Conditions

For socially disadvantaged communities, preventive and early interceptive orthodontics are thought to be the procedures of choice aiming at eliminating or reducing the need for later comprehensive orthodontic treatment in the permanent dentition and affordable alternatives. The orthodontic preventive and interceptive measures have the advantage of being simple and affordable provided that they are applied at appropriate critical stages of development of occlusion. They are the procedures that can be carried out by the general dental practitioners after undergoing short and follow-up professional development orthodontic courses.

7.4.1. Prevention of Orthodontic Conditions

Preventive orthodontics is a procedure to promote the development of a normal occlusion and aid in preventing malocclusion from developing (Ricketts, 1979). Preventive measures for orthodontic conditions may sometimes be made already in the primary and/or early mixed dentition phases, when the signs of developing occlusal anomalies can be detected. In socially disadvantaged communities where there are limited resources and facilities, inadequate or no orthodontic specialists and no organized school oral health programmes with orthodontic component, children may have little opportunities to receive preventive and interceptive orthodontic management. In order preventive and interceptive orthodontic measures to play a significant part in meeting the need and demand for orthodontic care, screening of the children is essential. Screening of children would not only be beneficial in the prevention and interception of various orthodontic conditions but would also help to identify children with absolute need for orthodontic treatment. Although it has been reported that early orthodontic treatment may benefit only 15-20% of those needing treatment (Proffit et al., 2005), the proportions are still substantial for socially disadvantaged communities with inadequate or without orthodontic services infrastructure at all. Therefore, it is strongly suggested that in socially disadvantaged communities, oral health policies and training curricula should incorporate components on preventive and interceptive orthodontic management coupled with organized regular oral health screening programmes in elementary and primary schools. Furthermore, in communities where oral health insurance schemes exist, insurance companies have to be encouraged to direct a proportion of their corporate social responsibility budgets to support oral health screening in schools; and preventive and interceptive orthodontic programmes.

7.4.1.1. Premature Loss of Deciduous Teeth

Space loss occurring after the premature loss of primary second molars has the potential to influence crowding and arch length significantly (Northway et al., 1984). Hence, organized regular school and community oral health programmes comprising of oral health education, oral hygiene instructions and caries treatment involving children, teachers, parents and/or caretakers need to be seriously advocated in socially disadvantaged communities. This is crucial for prevention of premature loss of deciduous teeth that often lead to preventable malocclusions in the emerging permanent dentition. Many orthodontic cases involving crowding and lack of space in the permanent dentition could have been prevented or the severity of the problems alleviated if tooth loss was prevented or the practitioner had maintained adequate space during the initial treatment of the mixed dentition (Choonara, 2005). General Dental Practitioners and trained oral health Clinicians (Dental Assistsants/Dental Therapists and Assistant Dental Officers) available in Tanzania and some oral health care systems in various countries can use space maintainers provided they have clinical experience, good judgment and knowledge of the principles of orofacial growth and development (Gianelly, 1995; Terlaje and Donly, 2001).

7.4.1.2. Space Maintenance

Treatment planning guidelines for very early loss of a deciduous tooth are as follows:

Deciduous tooth lost	Treatment Guidelines
Loss of a deciduous incisor	Space maintenance is not necessary since the eruption of the permanent incisors will probably be delayed if a deciduous incisor is lost at a very early age.
Loss of a deciduous canine	Space maintenance may be attempted because the incisor teeth tend to shift laterally into this space, creating a midline deviation and dental asymmetry

(Continued).

Deciduous tooth lost	Treatment Guidelines
Loss of a deciduous first molar	Space maintenance may be attempted because the early loss of a deciduous first molar might lead to asymmetry within the arch and space loss is possible.
Loss of a deciduous second molar	The deciduous second molar not only reserves space for the permanent second premolars but its distal root also guides the erupting permanent first molar into position. If the primary second molar is lost prematurely, the permanent first molar will usually migrate mesially within the bone even before it emerges into the oral cavity. A space-maintaining device is needed that will both guide eruption of the permanent first molar before its emergence and then hold the first molar in proper position after occlusion is established.

7.4.1.3. Oral Habits

Often malocclusions associated with sucking habits including anterior open bite will correct spontaneously (self-correcting) after breaking the responsible habit in time (Larsson 1986a, b; 1987). Therefore, early habit breaking should be encouraged (Levine 1999). It is advised that in the deciduous dentition phase of development, positive encouragement to stop oral habits should be instituted. Although many children manage to give up sucking habits spontaneously, some would need professionals to help them stop. In such cases, a habit breaker appliance may assist in breaking the habit. Occlusal anomalies that may be prevented by habit breaking are anterior open bite, posterior cross bite, increased overjet and anterior cross bite. Nowadays, there are also special dummy designs (e.g. flat teat) to reduce effects of dummy sucking.

7.4.1.4. Anteroposterior Molar Malocclusions

Prevention of the development of anteroposterior molar malocclusion due to environmental factors can be achieved through caries management, space maintenance and habit breaking.

7.4.1.5. Anterior Open Bite

Anterior open bite (AOB) occurs when there is no vertical overlap of the incisors. This type of malocclusion is more common in individuals of African origin than in Caucasians. A strong indication exists in the literature that habits such as thumb-sucking may cause anterior open bites (de Muelenaere, 1997). Early elimination of sucking habits before seven years, will allow spontaneous correction of the occlusion.

7.4.1.6. Lateral Cross Bite

Lateral cross bite also termed posterior cross bite is a transverse malocclusion which occurs when one or more buccal cusps of the maxillary premolars and/or molars occlude lingually to the buccal cusps of the mandibular antagonists (Daskalogiannaskis, 2000). Lateral cross bite may be unilaterally or bilaterally. There may be maxillary, mandibular, buccal, lingual and accompanied by a lateral functional shift of the mandible in particular in the cases of unilateral cross bites. Aetiology can be local factors for instance sucking habits and/or skeletal factors for example wider mandible occluding with a narrower maxilla.

Thus, occurrence of a lateral cross bite can be prevented by preventive measures such as early termination of sucking habits.

7.4.2. Management of Orthodontic Conditions

Interceptive orthodontics are procedures to restore a normal occlusion once a malocclusion has started to develop (Ricketts, 1979). Although orthodontic treatment can be accomplished at any age, growth modification is the backbone of orthodontic practice. The younger the individual the more ideal is the orthodontic treatment outcome. The objectives of preventive and interceptive orthodontic management are to provide information about and intercept the harmful effects of oral habits; prevent and/or correct the skeletal discrepancy between the maxilla and the mandible; to achieve Angle's class I molar relationship; to create ideal overjet and overbite; to maintain space from early loss of deciduous teeth; to correct the crowding and rotation of maxillary and mandibular incisors; to manage arch length and width for emergence of permanent canines and premolars; to improve the facial profile; and to eliminate any perioral muscular function. In the primary dentition, usually there are less occlusal disorders than in the mixed and permanent dentitions. Treatment of some malocclusions should be started in the primary and early mixed dentition stages, as it is generally believed that the status of the primary occlusion affects the development of the permanent occlusion (Far č nik et al., 1985, 1988; Kurol and Berglund, 1992; Trottman and Elsbach, 1996; Ovsenik et al., 2004; Kurol, 2006; Proffit, 2006). Posterior crossbites have been reported to be one of the most prevalent malocclusions of the primary dentition in children, and if left untreated, may lead to craniofacial asymmetry (Pirttiniemi et al. , 1990; Kurol and Berglund, 1992; Sonnesen et al. , 2001; Thilander and Lennartsson, 2002; Ovsenik et al., 2004). It has also been suggested that the later these crossbite malocclusions are treated, the greater the risk of damage to the temporomandibular joint (Pirttiniemi et al., 1990; Sonnesen et al., 2001; Kurol, 2006). It is therefore, considered important to treat incorrect orofacial functions and functional malocclusions as early as possible (Far č nik et al., 1988; Kurol and Berglund, 1992; Thilander and Lennartsson, 2002; Ovsenik et al., 2004; Kurol, 2006).

7.4.2.1. Anteroposterior Molar Malocclusion

The antero-posterior plane of the occlusion is determined by the first permanent molar relationship and usually classified as Angle's Class I, Class II (with divisions 1 and 2) and Class III. In Class I malocclusions, the skeletal pattern is usually Class I but there are discrepancies such as crowding, spacing, displaced teeth, vertical discrepancies, transverse discrepancies and incisor proclination. Class II molar relationship is the deviation of at least one half cusp widths mesial to Class I, while, a Class III molar relationship occurs when there is at least one half cusp width displacement distally. Early orthodontic treatment of Class II and Class III malocclusions in socially disadvantaged settings is possible and should be considered, provided that there is no severe skeletal pattern discrepancy and there is favourable amount of future growth. Furthermore, the degree of crowding in each arch should be well thought-out. When premolars and canines are emerging in the oral cavity, it is the best time to intervene. This is often also the time of the onset of the pubertal growth spurt. For Class II malocclusions, treatment can be done easily by a general dental practitioner using functional appliances such as 'the activator'. The activator is an acrylic appliance adapted to both upper and lower arches, which is in itself passive. The mechanism of action of an activator is through altering functional pattern, at the same time stimulating muscular activities. Treatment of Class III malocclusion can begin in the deciduous dentition, by doing occlusal grinding. In the mixed dentition, dento-alveolar discrepancies can be treated by using removable appliances namely the retractor and function regulator. Treatment of Class II and Class III malocclusions with severe skeletal pattern discrepancies and unfavourable amount of future growth, remain a challenge for general dental practitioners in socially disadvantaged communities without orthodontic specialization referral infrastructure.

7.4.2.2. Increased Overjet

Overjet is defined as the distance from the most labial point of the incisal edge of maxillary central incisor to the most labial surface of the corresponding mandibular incisor. According to the Index of Orthodontic Treatment Need (IOTN), an overjet of more than 3.5 is considered increased while 6 millimeters or more should be considered for treatment (Richmond et al. 1992). Studies have reported that the prevalence of dental trauma increases with increasing overjet (Jarvinen, 1978; Baus et al., 2004; Shulham and Peterson, 2004; Kahabuka and Mugonzibwa, 2009) justifying prevention where possible and early management of the malocclusion. It is generally suggested that in cases with good arch alignment (neutral occlusion) and spacing, removable appliances can be easily utilized in the management of increased overjet in socially disadvantaged communities. If pubertal growth spurt is timed for treatment, functional appliances can also be used to reduce an increased overjet.

7.4.2.3. Open Bite

Diagnosis and treatment of open bite malocclusion challenges oral health practitioners who attempt to intercept this malocclusion at an early age. Patients with open bite malocclusion can be diagnosed clinically and using radiographs where the facility is available. However, diagnosis should be viewed in the context of the skeletal and dental aetiology. Accurate classification of this malocclusion requires experience and training. Simple open bite during the exchange of deciduous to permanent dentition usually resolves without treatment. Complex open bites that extend further into the premolar and molar regions, and those that do not resolve by the end of the mixed dentition years may require orthodontic and/or surgical intervention. Vertical malocclusion develops as a result of the interaction of many different etiologic factors including thumb and finger sucking, lip and tongue habits, airway obstruction, and true skeletal growth abnormalities (Larsson, 1987; Melson et al., 1979; Lindner and Modeer, 1989; Estripeaut et al., 1989; Garattini et al., 1990; de Muelenaere, 1997; Warren et al., 2001, Warren and Bishara, 2002; da Costa et al 2002). Treatment for open bite ranges from observation or simple habit control to complex surgical procedures. Successful identification of the etiology improves the chances of treatment success. Vertical growth is the last dimension to be completed, therefore treatment may appear to be successful at one point and fail later. Some treatment may be prolonged, if begun early. Various removable appliances can be used in socially disadvantaged communities to correct open bite, particularly before cessation of the arch growth. An open bite due to localized failure of development (for example due to cleft of the lip) and habitual mouth breathing (for example due to chronic nasal obstruction), can be managed in conjunction with other disciplines such as Ear Nose and Throat (ENT) specialists and Paediatric Surgeons for surgery.

7.4.2.4. Anterior Cross Bite

Anterior crossbite also termed reverse overjet or mandibular overjet (Figure 7.2 and 7.3) is a situation in which one or more primary or permanent mandibular incisors are labial to their antagonists (or one or more maxillary incisors are lingual to their antagonists) in normal occlusion (Daskalogiannakis, 2000). In most situations anterior crossbites occur together with angle's Class III molar relationship. Anterior crossbite has been reported in 1-12% of the children (Mugonzibwa et al., 2004b; Karaiskos et al., 2005; Mtaya et al., 2008). It occasionally occurs in the primary dentition because of incisor interferences that cause an anterior shift of the mandible. If this occurs it should be corrected in an effort to avoid hypertrophy of facial muscles that can contribute to facial soft tissue asymmetry. Usually this correction can be made merely by removing the interference, by either occlusal grinding or extracting the primary incisors if it is already near exfoliation (Proffit et al., 2005). Anterior crossbites should be treated as soon as they are detected, because a purely dental malocclusion may lead to growth problems and skeletal deviations if left untreated (Faber, 1981).

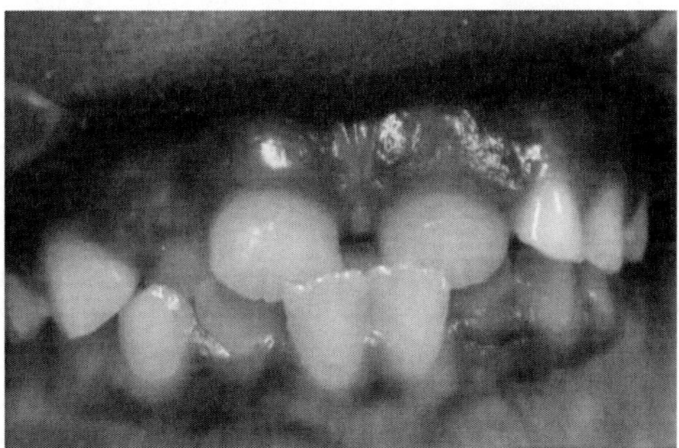

Figure 7.2. Anterior cross bite in the early mixed dentition (Courtesy of E. A. Mugonzibwa).

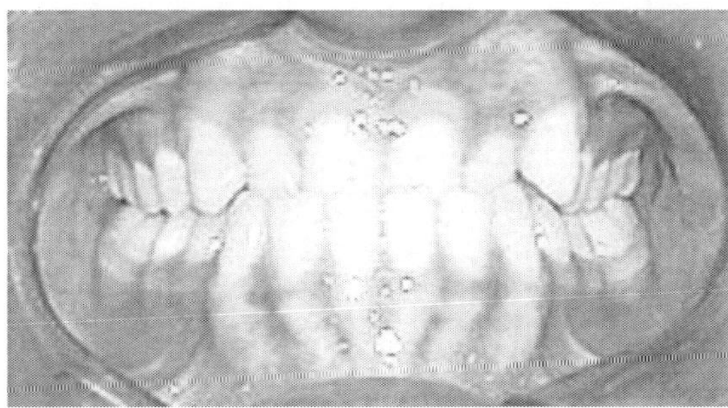

Figure 7.3. Anterior cross bite in the permanent dentition (Courtesy of E. A. Mugonzibwa).

They are best treated at an early age, because the upper incisor may traumatically occlude with the lower incisor, potentially giving rise to adverse periodontal problems, mobility and fracture (Richardson, 1982). In planning treatment for anterior crossbites, it is critically important to differentiate skeletal problems of deficient maxillary or excessive mandibular growth from cross bites due only to displacement of teeth (Ngan et al., 1997). If the etiologic factor is truly dental and space is available, the problem should be corrected when encountered. Anterior cross bites diagnosed after the incisors have erupted and overbite is established require appliance therapy for correction. The diagnostic evaluation should determine whether tipping will provide appropriate correction. If teeth are tipped when bodily movement is required, stability of the result is questionable. Many of these cross bites, especially single-tooth cross bites, could be successfully intercepted with removable appliances (z-spring appliance) (Figures 7.5a, b and c). As with any anterior cross bite correction, the teeth should be stabilized for 1 to 2 months after tooth movement and can then be released without further retention if the overbite is sufficient. Although some anterior cross bites can be treated with removable appliances, a fixed appliance is more effective and is required to correct severely displaced incisors. When anterior cross bite of 1.1-3.5 millimeters characterized with masticator and speech difficulties can also be considered for treatment in a similar manner using removable or functional appliances.

7.4.2.5. Lateral Cross Bite

Spontaneous correction of lateral cross bite has been reported in the literature (Faber, 1981) but it is rare. Lateral cross bites should be treated as soon as they are detected, because a purely dental malocclusion may lead to growth problems and skeletal deviations if left untreated (Faber, 1981). This is especially true in posterior cross bites caused by a functional shift. These cross bites should be corrected as soon as they are discovered, even in the deciduous dentition (Proffitt, 2000) and can be accomplished in the mixed dentition stage. Removable screw appliance with a buccal capping aiming at expanding the upper arch can readily be used. Treatment of lateral cross bites involving a single tooth can be achieved by the use of cross elastics. Without early intervention, a more expensive form of treatment with fixed appliances may be required.

7.4.2.6. Space Discrepancies

Inadequate space for the teeth in the arch is termed as crowding and the excess space is known as spacing. From the professional view in oral health, spacing of teeth is not considered as a malocclusion. However, in several societies worldwide spacing is perceived and considered as an anomaly, significantly disliked and clients demand orthodontic closure of the spaces between teeth (Helm et al, 1986; Kerosuo et al., 1995). On the other hand, crowding is the most common malocclusion placing patients in the highest orthodontic treatment need and demand for orthodontic care in all settings (Mugonzibwa et al., 2004a,b), in many socially disadvantaged communities spacing closure is rarely demanded for unless if lacking a whole anterior tooth. Moreover, correction of spacing in socially disadvantaged communities is a difficult task, since it involves the use of sophisticated fixed appliances and an orthodontist expertise that is often not accessible or available.

From the Tanzanian experience that may be similar to most oral health systems in sub-Saharan African settings/region, developing countries and many socially disadvantaged communities, there is no organized regular screening for orthodontic problems in the elementary and primary schools. Patients demanding crowding intervention often report to the oral health practitioner when the permanent canines emerge or erupt in the buccal aspect of either the mandible, the maxilla or both arches with severe crowding like in figures 7.4 a, b and c. At this stage, the opportunity for guided occlusion development is no more.

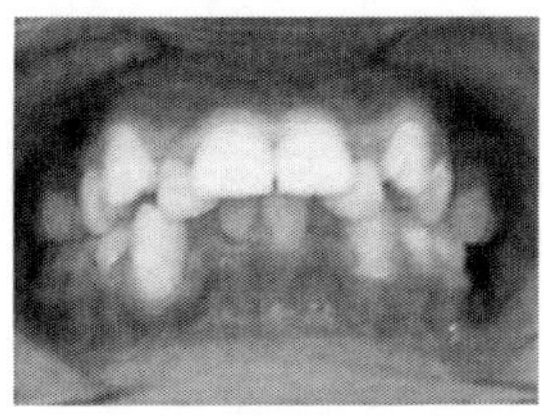 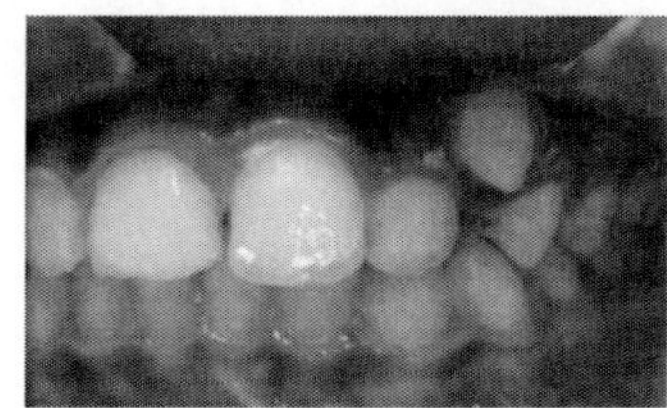 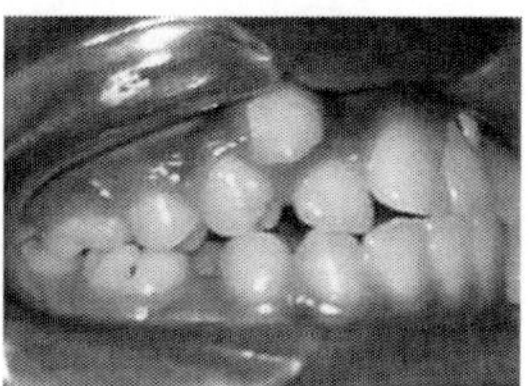

Figure 7.4a   Figure 7.4b   Figure 7.4c

Figure 7.4a, b and c. Late presentation of severe crowding (Courtesy of E. A. Mugonzibwa).

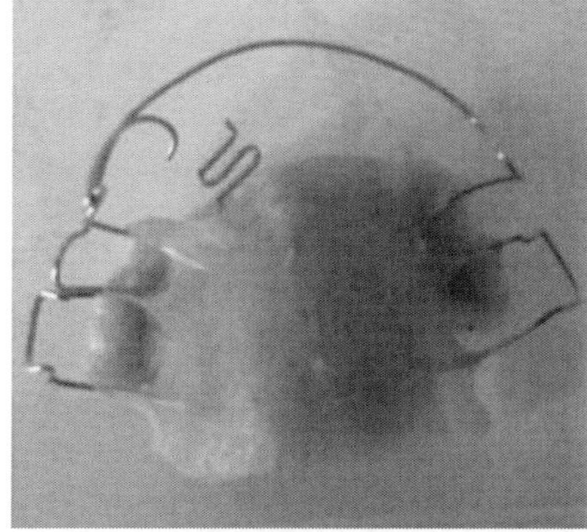

Figure 7.5a. Maxillary removable appliance with Adam's clasps, an active and/or passive labial bow(s), z spring and a canine retractor. (Courtesy of E. A. Mugonzibwa).

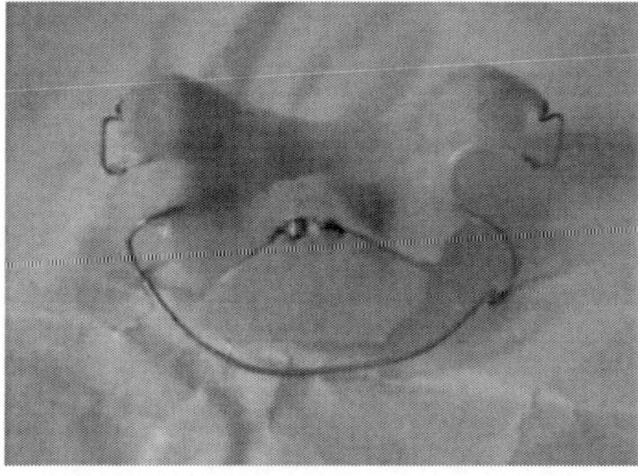

Figure 7.5b. Maxillary removable appliance with Adam's clasps, an active and/or passive labial bow(s) and expansion screw(s) . (Courtesy of E. A. Mugonzibwa).

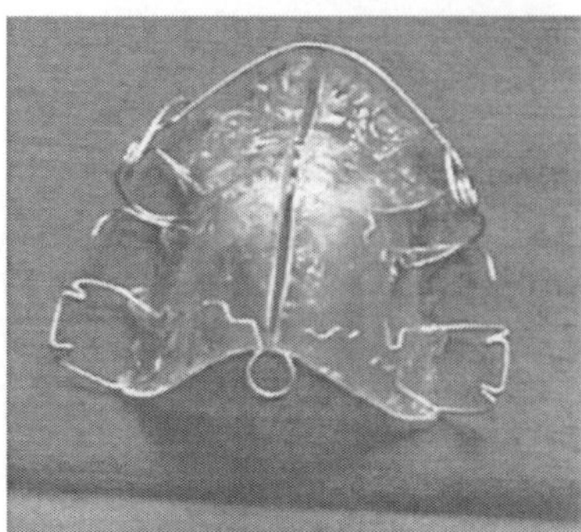

Figure 7.5c. Maxillary removable appliances with Adam's clasps, an active and/or passive labial bow, canine retractor(s) and expansion screw. . (Courtesy of F. Mdoe).

Treatment of crowding is indicated in case of displacement of teeth of greater than 4 millimeters. Preventive and early interceptive measures are particularly emphasized, because they are cheap and effective for socially disadvantaged groups in low income communities. In early intervention of crowding, the use of serial extraction concept which provides space while guiding a permanent tooth into the desired eruption path is advised. Serial extraction steps include extraction of deciduous canines (at about 7-8 years) to provide space for the permanent incisors, extraction of deciduous first molars (10-11 years) to speed up first premolars emergence and extraction of first premolars (10-12 years) to provide space for the permanent canines.

After relieving the crowding, a degree of natural spontaneous movement may take place. This will be greater in a growing a child, or when extractions are carried out just prior to emergence of the adjacent teeth, or where adjacent teeth are favourably positioned and where there are no occlusal interferences.

The mentioned ages work well in Caucasian children populations whereas permanent teeth in African black children often emerge in the oral cavity at earlier ages (Mugonzibwa et al., 2002). Therefore, when planning orthodontic treatment in particular serial extraction for different populations as well as for individuals, ethnic background and the emergence stage of the dentition need to be considered.

7.5. Advantages and Disadvantages of Preventive and Interceptive Orthodontics

7.5.1. Advantages of Preventive and Interceptive Orthodontics

Addressing malocclusions in the deciduous and mixed dentition offers several benefits. First, children at this age are often more attentive and cooperative than adolescent patients (de Muelenaere and Wiltshire 1995).

Second, early treatment of harmful habits, such as digit sucking and tongue thrusting, is recommended after 8 years of age as it can simultaneously improve speech impediments due to the open bite, which often develops as a result of oral habits (Varrela and Alanen, 1995). Also, at 8 years, the first permanent molars are fully erupted, facilitating removable appliance therapy, which is also better tolerated at this age.

7.5.1.1. Improved Treatment Outcomes

Preventive and early orthodontic interceptions at young age make patients more adaptive to the changes and lessen post orthodontic treatment relapses.

For example early interceptions of the narrowing of maxillary and mandibular arches that result into the inadequacy of the transverse growth help to optimize the patients' facial appearance and harmony. On the other hand, expansion of the dental arches creates additional space for emergence of the permanent teeth reducing the likelihood of crowding and extraction of the teeth.

7.5.1.2. Improved Cooperation

While younger children are enthusiastic about following instructions than adolescent patients, both children and their parents are often more enthusiastic about orthodontic treatment resulting into improved cooperation.

7.5.1.3. Less Pain and Discomfort

Due to lower resistance of bones and teeth to orthodontic movement, younger children have a tendency to have higher pain threshold and therefore experiencing minimal discomfort during early orthodontic interceptions.

7.5.1.4. Reduce Treatment Time

In young children, tissues adaptation and turnover occur at a higher rate leading to bones and teeth moving faster. Generally preventive and early orthodontic interceptions take shorter time compared to full orthodontic treatment in adolescents.

7.5.1.5. Minimal Side Effects

Moving teeth in younger patients using preventive and early orthodontic interceptive approaches involves more guidance and less force with fewer occurrences of orthodontic treatment side effects. The most common orthodontic treatment side effects including root resorption and gum recession are dramatically reduced.

7.5.1.6. Lower Costs

The costs for preventive and early orthodontic interceptions are significantly less than that of full orthodontic treatment.

7.5.2. Disadvantages of Preventive and Interceptive Orthodontics

7.5.2.1. Inadequate Oral Care

Many of the young children have not acquired the necessary skills to independently, properly brush and floss their teeth. Supervision from parents or guardians is needed in order for the young children to keep their teeth and appliances clean particularly during any kind of orthodontic treatment.

7.5.2.2. Possibility of Further Orthodontic Treatment

Usually preventive and early orthodontic interceptions are completed before completion of the permanent dentition phase of development. On completion of the permanent dentition, further orthodontic treatment may be required although of a short duration and relatively less expensive in terms of cost and time.

Also the additional treatment may comprehensive and too expensive to be incurred by disadvantaged communities.

7.6. Challenges for Provision of Quality Orthodontic Services in Socially Disadvantaged Communities

7.6.1. Health Services Utilization

Due to very limited budgets and other multiple factors, oral health services are not always directed to those most in need. These lead to situations in which large segments of the population have limited or no access to oral health care, and hence continue to suffer. Most patients in socially disadvantaged communities report to oral health facilities for relief of pain often with already formed dental abscesses rather than for comprehensive care or prevention (Mosha and Scheutz, 1993; Ntabaye et al., 1998;). Inability to pay for oral health services, travel distance, inadequate or lack of human resource and fear for dental are some of the reported barriers to oral health services utilization (Ntabaye et al., 1998;). This situation calls for considering oral health including orthodontic challenges as a public health priority and for establishment and implementation of the essential basic oral health care protocol that is feasible and affordable within the prevailing health infrastructures of remote communities within the framework of primary health care (PHC) delivery. PHC aims at providing basic curative and preventive care for all at a cost that communities and country can afford.

7.6.2. Materials and Equipment

In socially disadvantaged communities, oral health systems infrastructure is usually not the best. Dental materials are often in limited supply, when available may be sub standard and sometimes expired. Dental equipment is often not adequate, not repaired adequately and timely and sometimes dilapidated.

7.6.3. Human Resource

Many countries and communities both developed and developing are experiencing shortages of skilled health workers. These shortages which tend to be more severe in remote, rural areas and especially in socially disadvantaged communities reduce capacity to provide good quality health services to their populations. Some countries are responding to the problem by systematically recruiting health care workers from other countries, in particular from developing countries. This helps some recipient countries, to overcome their staff and skills shortages, while it deprives source countries of knowledge, skills, and expertise for which large amounts of resources have been spent. Although emigration from health sector provides many involved health workers with opportunities to develop their careers, gain valuable experience, and improve living conditions for themselves and their families, it also results in negative experiences for the source. Health workers within communities are also moving from clinical to public health sectors and rural to urban areas.

Emigration results from a combination of push factors (in source sectors and/or countries) and pull factors (in recipient sectors and/or countries). The reasons for scientific researchers failing to return to their home countries after training abroad include: inadequate or lack of research funding; poor research facilities; limited career structures; poor intellectual stimulation; threats of violence; lack of good education for children (WHO, 2006) and lack of the evidence-based decision-making culture, leading to lack of recognition of potential contribution of researchers to national health development. The key push factors driving out health workers include: weak health systems; insecurity including violence at the workplace; poor living conditions; low remunerations; lack of professional development opportunities (e.g. continuing education or training); lack of clear career development paths (WHO, 2005) and risk of HIV infection due to lack of appropriate protective gear when handling specimens, blood and blood products; nepotism in recruitment and promotion; political unrest/civil wars; widespread poverty; poor governance; and case overload. Some of the factors that pull professionals to developed countries may include: availability of information, easy access to communication and technology, making it easy to find jobs or complete visa applications and process; aggressive targeted recruitment to fill vacancies in richer countries; availability of employment opportunities; better remunerations and working conditions (McCoy et al.,, 2008) secure and conducive living conditions; and opportunities for intellectual growth (e.g. refresher courses, access to Internet and modern library facilities). The push and pull factors in tandem have led to brain drain of health professionals from rural to urban, health to non health sectors, country to country and African countries to developing and developed countries. This has exacerbated the already weak national and district health systems, making it extremely difficult for countries in the Region to achieve the United Nations Millennium Development Goals (MDGs) (WHO; 2006, UNDP, 2009). The pay and income of health workers varies widely, whether between countries, by comparison with cost of living, or between the public and private sectors. To optimise the distribution and mix of health workers, policy interventions to address their pay and incomes are needed. Financial constraints to increased salaries might need to be overcome in many socially disadvantaged settings, and non-financial incentives improved (Habte et al, 2004; McCoy et al., 2008).

The unmet need for oral health human resource including dental specializations especially in socially disadvantaged communities is immeasurable. While there is shortage of trained oral health human resource, the majority of the few skilled oral health human resources work in large cities and towns leaving facilities in the rural areas seriously understaffed and most of the socially disadvantaged citizens unattended. For socially disadvantaged communities, interested general dental practitioners and allied oral health workers should be empowered to practice preventive and early interceptive orthodontic treatment.

7.6.4. Health Systems

Socially disadvantaged communities are found in every society worldwide with wide range of levels of deprivation. Those found in developing economies are the most severely socially disadvantaged communities with, inadequate or no oral health policies in place. Where oral health policies are available, not all oral health specialties are addressed adequately. For example organized sustainable comprehensive school oral health programmes in a number of developing economies, are either in development stages or lacking. On the other hand, people in the socially disadvantaged communities particularly in developing economies are not able to access oral health insurance schemes to support the expensive general oral health and orthodontic care bills. Reasons for not accessing the oral health insurance schemes are often because they cannot afford and/or the insurance scheme are not available in their settings.

Conclusion

Potential prevention and significant reduction of the need for orthodontic treatment in the permanent dentition by employing preventive and interceptive orthodontic measures are widely acknowledged. World Health Organization in collaboration with governments, other oral health international organizations, professional associations and interested corporate fraternity should consider partnership in developing policies to train and empower interested general dental practitioners and allied oral health workers to plan and practice preventive and early interceptive orthodontic treatment in socially disadvantaged communities and continuing education sessions. On the other end, development and deployment of an appropriate and motivated oral health human resource, and the environment necessary for the workforce to perform optimally are advocated as these are basic critical determinants of the improved oral health status of children in socially disadvantaged communities worldwide.

References

Abu Alhaija E.S., Al-Khateeb S.N., Al-Nimri K.S. (2005) Prevalence of malocclusion in 13 – 15 year-old North Jordanian school children. *Community Dent Health* 22 : 266 – 271.

Al Nimri K., Richardson A. (2000) Interceptive orthodontics in the real world of community dentistry. *Int. J. Pediatr. Dent.* 10:99-108.

al-Emran S., Wisth P.J., Bøe O.E. 1990 Prevalence of malocclusion and need for orthodontic treatment in Saudi Arabia . *Community Dent. Oral Epidemiol.* 18 : 253 – 255.

Årtun J., Behbehani F., Al-Jame B., Kerosuo H. (2005). Incisor trauma in an adolescent Arab population: prevalence, severity, and occlusal risk factors. *Am. J. Orthod. Dentofacial Orthop.* 128:347-352.

Backlund E. (1963) Facial growth and the significance of oral habits, mouth breathing and soft tissues for malocclusion. *Acta Odontol. Scand.*;21:55-73.

Baus O., Rohling J., Schwestka-Polly R. (2004) Prevalence of traumatic injuries to the permanent incisors in candidates for orthodontic treatment. *Dent. Traumatol*; 20:61-6.

Behlfelt K., Linder-Aronson S., McWilliam J., Neander P., Laage-Hellman J. (1989) Dentition in children with enlarged tonsils compared to control children. Eur. J. Orthod. 11:416-429.

Behbehani F., Årtun J., Al-Jame B., Kerosuo H. (2005) Prevalence and severity of malocclusion in adolescent Kuwaitis . *Med. Principles and Pract.* 14 : 390 – 395.

Bowden B.D. (1966) A longitudinal study of the effects of digit and dummy-sucking. *Am. J. Orthod.*; 52:887-901.

Bowling A. (1997) Measuring Health: a review of quality of life measuring scales. 2nd Edition. Backingham. Open University Press. XI. 159s.

Chevitarese AB, Della Valle D, Moreira TC (2002) Prevalence of malocclusion in 4-6 year old Brazilian children. *J. Clin. Pediatr. Dent..* ;27:81-85.

Choonara S.A. (2005) Orthodontic space maintenance: a review of current concepts and methods. *South Afr. Dent. J.;* 60:113, 115-117.

Chung C.K. Kerr W.J. (1987) Interceptive Orthodontics: application and outcome in a demand population. Br. Dent. J. 162:73-76.

Chung C.S., Niswander J.D. (1975) Genetic and epidemiologic studies of oral characteristics in Hawaii's schoolchildren: V. Sibling correlations in occlusion traits. *J. Dent. Res.* ;54:324-329.

Chung C.S., Niswander J.D., Runck D.W., Bilben S.E., Kau M.C. 1972 Genetic and epidemiologic studies of oral characteristics in Hawaii's school children: dental anomalies. *Am. J. Phys. Anthropol.* ;36:427-433.

Chung C.S., Niswander J.D., Runck D.W., Bilben S.E., Kau M.C.W. (1971) Genetic and epidemiologic studies of the oral characteristics in Hawaii's school children. II. Malocclusion. *Am. J. Human. Genet.* 23: 471-495.

Ciuffolo F., Manzoli L., D'Attilio M., Tecco S., Muratore F., Festa F., Romano F. (2005) Prevalence and distribution by gender of occlusal characteristics in a sample of Italian secondary school students: a cross-sectional study. *Eur. J. Orthod.* ;27:601-6.

Corruccini R.S., Potter R.H. (1980) Genetic analysis of occlusal variation in twins. *Am. J. Orthod.* ;78(2):140-154.

da Costa O.O,, Orenuga O.O. (2002) Dent facial anomalies related to the digit sucking habit. *Afr. J. Med. Sci.*; 3:239-42.

Daskalogiannakis J. (2000) Glossary of orthodontic terms. *Quintessence Publishing Co,* Inc Paris.

de Muelenaere K.R. (1997) Possibilities for prevention of malocclusions in South African children. *J Dent Assoc S Afr;* 52(1):9–14.

de Muelenaere K.R., Wiltshire W.A. (1995) The status of the developing occlusion of 8 – 9 year old children from a lower socio-economic group in a developing country. *J. Dent. Assoc. S. Afr.*; 50(3):113–118.

Dhar V., Jain A., Van Dyke T.E. , Kohli A. (2007) Prevalence of gingival diseases, malocclusion and fluorosis in school-going children of rural areas in Udaipur district . *J Indian Soc. Pedod. Prev. Dent.* 25: 103 – 105.

Estripeaut L.E., Henriques J.F., de Almeida R.R. (1989) Thumb sucking and malocclusion-presentation of a clinical case. *Rev. Odontol. Univ. Sao Paulo.*; 3:371-376.

Faber R.D. (1981) The differential diagnosis and treatment of crossbites. *Dent. Clin. North Am*; 25:53–68.

Far č nik F., Korpar M., Premik M., Zorec R. (1988) An attempt at numerically evaluating dysgnathias in the deciduous dentition. *Stomatologie DDR* 38: 386 – 391.

Far č nik F., Korpar M., Premik M., Zorec R. (1985) Numerical evaluation of malocclusion in study models of the mixed dentition. *Zobozdravstveni Vestnik* 40 : 169 – 176.

Gábris K., Márton S., Madléna M. (2006) Prevalence of malocclusions in Hungarian adolescents. *Eur. J. Orthod.* 28 : 467 – 470.

Garattini G., Crozzoli P., Valsasina A. (1990) Role of prolonged sucking in the development of dento skeletal changes in the face. Review of literature. *Mondo Orthod.*; 15:539-50.

Gianelly A.A. (1995) Leeway space and the resolution of crowding in the mixed dentition. *Semin. Orthod.* 1:188-194.

Graber T.M., Vanarsdall, Jr. (1994) Orthodontics: Current Principles and Techniques . 2nd Edition W B Sunders Company, Philadelphia.

Grabowski R., Kundt G., Stahl F. (2007) Interrelation between occlusal findings and orofacial myofunctional status in primary and mixed dentition: Part III: Interrelation between malocclusions and orofacial dysfunctions. *J. Orofac. Orthop.*; 68:462-476.

Gulati A., Taneja J.R., Chopra S.L., Madan S. (1991) Inter-relationship between dental, skeletal and chronological ages in well-nourished and mal-nourished children. *J. Indian Soc. Pedod. Prev. Dent.* 81:19-23.

Gulati A., Taneja J.R., Chopra S.L., Madan S. (1991) Inter-relationship between dental, skeletal and chronological ages in well-nourished and mal-nourished children. *J. Indian Soc. Pedod. Prev. Dent.* 81:19-23.

Haavikko K, Rahkamo A. (1977) Changes in the dental arches induced by premature extraction of deciduous molars. *Proc. Finn. Dent. Soc.*; 73:14–20.

Habte D., Dussault G., Dovlo D. (2004) Challenges confronting the health workforce in sub-Saharan Africa. *World Hosp. Health Serv.*;40:23-6, 40-41.

Hellman H. (1914) A study of some etiological factors of malocclusion. *Dent. Cosmos*; 56:1017-1031.

Helm S., Petersen P.E., Kreiborg S., Solow B. (1986) Effect of separate malocclusion traits on concern for dental appearance. *Community Dent. Oral Epidemiol..* 14:217-220.

Hesby R.M., Marshall S.D., Dawson D.V., Southard K.A., Casko J.S., Franciscus R.G., Southard T.E. (2006) Transverse skeletal and dentoalveolar changes during growth. Am. *J. Orthod Dentofacial Orthop.* ; 130:721-731.

Hesse K.L., Årtun J., Joondeph D.R., Kennedy D.B. (1997). Changes in condylar position and occlusion associated with maxillary expansion for correction of functional unilateral posterior crossbite. *Am. J. Orthod. Dentofac. Orthop.* 111:410-418.

Hiles A.M. (1985) Is orthodontic screening of 9-year old school children cost effective? Br. Dent. J. 159; 41-45.

Jarvinen S. (1978) Incisal overjet and traumatic injuries to upper permanent incisors. *Acta Odontol Scand*; 36:359-62.

Jones M.L., Mourino A.P., Bowden T.A. (1993) Evaluation of occlusion, trauma, and dental anomalies in African-American children of metropolitan Headstart programs. *J. Clin. Pediatr. Dent..* l;18:51-54.

Kabue M.M., Moracha J.K., Ng'ang'a P.M. (1995) Malocclusion in children aged 3-6 years in Nairobi, Kenya. *East Afr. Med. J.*; 72:210-212.

Kahabuka F.K.A., Mugonzibwa E.A. (2009) Risk Factors for Injuries to Upper Lip and Maxillary Incisors among School Children in Dar es Salaam, Tanzania. *Int. J. Paediatr. Dent.*;19:148-54.

Karaiskos N., Wiltshire W.A., Odlum O., Brothwell D., Hassard T.H. (2005) Preventive and interceptive orthodontic treatment needs of an inner-city group of 6- and 9-year-old Canadian children. *J. Can Dent. Assoc.* 71:649.

Karaiskos N., Wiltshire W.A., Odlum O., Brothwell D., Hassard T.H. (2005) Preventive and interceptive orthodontic treatment needs of an inner-city group of 6- and 9-year-old Canadian children. *J. Can. Dent. Assoc* ;71:649.

Katz C.R., Rosenblatt A., Gondim P.P. (2004) Nonnutritive sucking habits in Brazilian children: effects on deciduous dentition and relationship with facial morphology. *Am. J. Orthod. Dentofacial. Orthop.*;126:53-57.

Kerosuo H. (1990) Occlusion in the primary and early mixed dentition in a group of Tanzanian and Finnish children. *ASDC J. Dent. Child*;57:293-8.

Kerosuo H., Hausen H., Laine T., Shaw W.C. (1995) The influence of incisal malocclusion on the social attractiveness of young adults in Finland. *Eur. J. Orthod.* 17:505-512.

Kerosuo H., Laine T., Kerosuo E., Ngassapa . , Honkala E. (1988) Occlusion among a group of Tanzanian urban schoolchildren . *Community Dent. Oral Epidemiol.* 16 : 306 – 309.

Kerosuo H., Laine T., Nyyssonen V., Honkala E. (1991) Occlusal characteristics in groups of Tanzanian and Finnish urban schoolchildren . *Angle Orthod* 61 : 49 – 56.

Kerosuo H., Väkiparta M., Nyström M., Heikinheimo K. (2008) The seven-year outcome of an early orthodontic treatment strategy *J. Dent. Res.* ;87:584-588.

Keski-Nisula K., Hernesniemi R., Heiskanen M., Keski-Nisula L., Varrela J. (2008) Orthodontic intervention in the early mixed dentition: a prospective, controlled study on the effects of the eruption guidance appliance. *Am. J. Orthod. Dentofacial. Orthop.* ;133:254-260.

Kluemper GT, Beeman CS, Hicks EP (2000) Early orthodontic treatment: what are the imperatives? *J. Am. Dent. Assoc.* ;131:613-20.

Korpar M. , Far č nik F. , Premik M. , Zorec R. (1994) Changes in the orofacial system between the 3rd and the 9th years of age . In: Far č nik F (ed). Preventive and interceptive orthodontics. Book of Proceedings, Slovenian Orthodontic Society, Rantovi dnevi , Ljubljana , pp. 41 – 47.

Kurol J. (2006) Impacted and ankylosed teeth: why, when, and how to intervene . *Am. J. Orthod. Dentofacial. Orthop* 120 : S50 – S54.

Kurol J., Berglund L. (1992) Longitudinal study and cost-benefi t analysis of the effect of early treatment of posterior cross-bites in the primary dentition . *Eur. J. Orthod.* 14 : 173 – 179.

Larsson E. (1986a) Effect of dummy-sucking on the prevalence of posterior cross-bite in the permanent dentition. *Swed Dent. J.;*10:97-101.

Larsson E. (1986b) The effect of dummy-sucking on the occlusion: a review. *Eur. J. Orthod.*;8:127-130.

Larsson E. (1987) The effect of finger sucking on occlusion: A review. *Eur. J. Orthod*; 9:279-282.

Larsson E. (1994) Artificial sucking habits: etiology prevalence and effect on occlusion. *Int. J. Orofacial Myology.* ;20:10-21.

Larsson E. (2000) Sucking, chewing, and feeding habits and development of crossbite: a longitudinal study of girls from birth to 3 years of age . *Angle Orthodontist* 71 : 116 – 119.

Larsson E. , Øgaard B. , Lindsten R. (1992) Dummy- and fi nger-sucking habits in young Swedish and Norwegian children . *Scand J. of Dent. Res.* 100 : 292 – 295.

Lessa FC., Enoki C., Feres M.F., Valera F.C., Lima W.T., Matsumoto M.A. (2005) Breathing mode influence in craniofacial development. *Braz. J. Otorhinolaryngol.*; 71:156-160.

Levine RS. (1999) Briefing paper: oral aspects of dummy and digit sucking. *Br. Dent. J.* 13;186:108.

Lew K.K., Foong W.C., Loh E. (1993) Malocclusion prevalence in an ethnic Chinese population . *Australian Dent. J.* 38 : 442 – 449.

Linder-Aronson S. (1979) Respiratory function in relation to facial morphology and the dention. *Br. J. Orthod.* 6:59-71.

Lindner A, Modeer T. (1989) Relationship between sucking habits and dental characteristics in preschool children with unilateral posterior crossbite. *Scand. J. Dent* Res;97:278-83.

Lindsten R. , Larsson E. , Øgaard B. (1996) Dummy sucking behaviour in 3- year old Norwegian and Swedish children . *Eur. J. Orthod* 18 : 205 – 209.

Lobb W.K. (1987) Craniofacial morphology and occlusal variation in monozygous and dizygous twins. *Angle Orthod.* ;57:219-233.

Lombardi A.V., Bailit H.L. (1972) Malocclusion in the Kwaio, a Melanesian group on Malaita, Solomon Islands. *Am. J. Phys. Anthropol.* ;36:283-93.

Lombardi A.V., Bailit H.L. (1972) Malocclusion in the Kwaio, a Melanesian group on Malaita, Solomon Islands. *Am. J. Phys. Anthropol.* ;36:283-93.

Love W.D., Adams R.L. (1971) Tooth movement into edentulous areas. *J. Prosthet Dent.*; 25:271-278.

Martin C.A., McNeil D.W., Crout R.J., Ngan P.W., Weyant R.J., Heady H.R., Marazita M.L. (2008) Oral health disparities in Appalachia: orthodontic treatment need and demand. *J. Am. Dent Assoc.*;139:598-604.

McCoy D., Bennett S., Witter S., Pond B., Baker B., Gow J., Chand S., Ensor T., McPake B. (2008) Salaries and incomes of health workers in sub-Saharan Africa. *Lancet.* 23;371(9613):675-81.

Melsen B., Attina L., Santuari M., Attina A. (1987) Relationships between swallowing pattern, mode of respiration, and development of malocclusion. *Angle Orthod.* ;57:113-120.

Melson B., Stensgaard K., Pedersen J.(1979) Sucking habits and their influence on swallowing pattern and prevalence of malocclusion. *Eur. J. Orthod*;1:271-280.

Mosha H.J., Scheutz F. (1993) Perceived need and use of oral health services among adolescents and adults in Tanzania. *Community Dent. Oral. Epidemiol.*;21:129-132.

Mtaya M., Astrom A.N., Brudvik P. (2008) Malocclusion, psycho-social impacts and treatment need: A cross-sectional study of Tanzanian primary school-children. *BMC Oral Health.* 6;8:14.

Mtaya M., Brudvik P., Astrøm A.N. (2009) . Prevalence of malocclusion and its relationship with socio-demographic factors, dental caries, and oral hygiene in 12- to 14-year-old Tanzanian schoolchildren. *Eur. J. Orthod.* ;31(5):467-76.

Mugonzibwa E.A., Eskeli R., Kuijpers-Jagtman A.M., Laine-Alava M.T., van ' t Hof M.A. (2004a) Occlusal characteristics during different emergence stages of the permanent dentition in Tanzanian Bantu and Finnish children . *Eur. J. Orthod* 26 : 251 – 260.

Mugonzibwa E.A., Kuijpers-Jagtman A.M., Laine-Alava M.T., Van 't Hof M.A. (2002) Emergence of permanent teeth in Tanzanian children. *Community Dent. Oral Epidemiol.*; 30:455-462.

Mugonzibwa E.A., Kuijpers-Jagtman A.M., Van 't Hof M.A., Kikwilu E.N. (2004b) Need for Orthodontic Treatment need among Tanzanian Children. *East Afr. Med. J.;* 81:10-15.

Mugonzibwa E.A., Kuijpers-Jagtman A.M., Van't Hof M.A., Kikwilu E.N.(2004c) Demand for Orthodontic Treatment demand among 9-18-year-old children seeking dental care in Dar es Salaam, Tanzanian. *East Afr. Med. J.;* 81:3-9.

Murshid Z.A., Amin H.E., Al-Nowaiser A.M. (2010) Distribution of certain types of occlusal anomalies among Saudi Arabian adolescents in Jeddah city. *Community Dent Health.* 27:238-41

Nakasima A., Ichinose M., Nakata S., Takahama Y. (1982) Hereditary factors in the craniofacial morphology of Angle's Class II and Class III malocclusions. *Am. J. Orthod.* ;82:150-156.

Ng'ang'a P.M., Ohito F., Øgaard B., Valderhaug J. (1996) The prevalence of malocclusion in 13- to 15-year-old children in Nairobi, Kenya . *Acta Odontol. Scand.* 54 : 126 – 130.

Ngan P., Alkire R.G., Fields H. Jr. (1999) Management of space problems in the primary and mixed dentitions. *J. Am. Dent Assoc.* ;130:1330-1339.

Ngan P., Fields H.W. (1997) Open bite: a review of etiology and management. *Pediatr. Dent..* ;19:91-98.

Ngan P., Hu A.M., Fields H.W. Jr. (1997) Treatment of Class III problems begins with differential diagnosis of anterior crossbites.*Pediatr. Dent..*;19:386-395.

Nguyen Q.V., Bezemer P.D., Habets L., Prahl-Andersen B. (1999). A systematic review of the relationship between overjet size and traumatic dental injuries. *Eur. J. Orthod* 21:503-515.

Niswander J.D. (1975) Genetics of common dental disorders. *Dent. Clin. North Am.* ;19:197-206.

Niswander J.D. (1975) Genetics of common dental disorders. *Dent. Clin. North Am.* ;19:197-206.

Northway W.M., Wainright R.L., Demirjian A. (1984) Effects of premature loss of primary molars. *Angle Orthod.*;54:295-329.

Ntabaye M.K., Scheutz F., Poulsen S. (1998) Household survey of access to and utilization of emergency oral health care services in rural Tanzania. *East Afr. Med. J;* 75:649-653.

Øgaard B., Larsson E., Lindsten R. (1994) The effect of sucking habits, cohort, sex, intercanine arch widths, and breast or bottle feeding on posterior crossbite in Norwegian and Swedish 3-year-old children . *Am. J. Orthod. Dentofacial. Orthop.* 106 : 161 – 166

Onyeaso C.O. (2004) Prevalence of malocclusion among adolescents in Ibadan, Nigeria. *Am. J. Orthod. Dentofacial. Orthop.* 126: 604 – 607.

Otuyemi O.D. (2001) Orthodontics in Nigeria: journey so far and the challenges ahead. J. Orthod. 28:90-92.

Ovsenik M., Far č nik F., Verdenik I. (2004) Comparison of intra-oral and study cast measurements in the assessment of malocclusion. *Eur. J. of Orthod.* 26: 273 – 277.

Peck S., Peck L., Kataja M. (1998) Class II Division 2 malocclusion: a heritable pattern of small teeth in well-developed jaws. *Angle Orthod.* 68:9-20.

Pirttiniemi P., Kantomaa T., Lahtela P. (1990) Relationship between craniofacial and condyle path asymmetry in unilateral cross-bite patients. *Eur. J. Orthod* 12: 408 – 413.

Popovich F., Thompson G.W. (1979) Maxillary diastema: indications for treatment. *Am. J. Orthod.* ;75:399-404.

Proffit W.R. (2006) The timing of early treatment: an overview. *Am. J. Orthodontics Dentofacial Orthopedics* 120 : S47 – S49.

Proffit W.R., Fields H.W., Ackerman J.L., Bailey J.L., Tulloch J.F.C. (2005) Contemporary Orthodontics. 3rd edition Philadelphia.

Proffitt W.R. (2000) Treatment planning for preadolescents (early mixed dentition). In: Contemporary orthodontics, 3rd edition. St. Louis: Mosby Year Book; p. 218–28.

Ravn J.J. (1976) Sucking habits and occlusion in 3-year old children. *Scand. J. Dent. Res.*;84:204-209.

Richardson A. (1965) The relationship between the relative amount of space present in the deciduous dental arch and the rate and degree of space closure to the extraction of a deciduous molar. *Dent. Pract. Dent. Rec.*;16:111-118.

Richardson A. (1982) Interceptive orthodontics in general practice. Part 1 —Early interceptive treatment. *Br. Dent. J.;* 152(3):85–89.

Richmond, S., O'Brien, K., Buchanan, I. and Burden, D. (1992) An introduction to occlusal indices. Bradford: Ortho-care (UK) Ltd.

Ricketts R.M. (1979) Ricketts on early treatment: part 1 and 2. *J. Clin. Orthod.*; 8:23–28, 115–127.

Robke F.J. (2008) Effects of nursing bottle misuse on oral health. Prevalence of caries, tooth malalignments and malocclusions in North-German preschool children. *J. Orofac. Orthop.*;69:5-19.

Rwakatema D.S., Ng'ang'a P.M., Kemoli A.M. (2006) Prevalence of malocclusion among 12-15-year-olds in Moshi, Tanzania, using Bjork's criteria . *East Afr. Med. J.* 83 : 372 – 379.

Saunders S.R., Popovich F., Thompson G.W. (1980) A family study of craniofacial dimensions in the Burlington Growth Centre sample. *Am. J. Orthod.* ;78:394-403.

ShulhAm. J..D., Peterson J. (2004) The association between incisor trauma and occlusal characteristics in individuals 8-50 years of age. *Dent. Traumatology*;20:67-74.

Sidlauskas A., Lopatiene K. (2009) The prevalence of malocclusion among 7-15-year-old Lithuanian schoolchildren. *Medicina* (Kaunas).;45:147-52.

Silva R G., Kang D.S. (2001) Prevalence of malocclusion among Latino adolescents . *Am. J. Orthod. Dentofacial. Orthop.* 119 : 313 – 315.

Smith R.J., Bailit H.L. (1977) Variation in dental occlusion and arches among Melanesians of Bougainville Island, Papua New Guinea. I. Methods, age changes, sex differences and population comparisons. *Am. J. Phys. Anthropol.* ;47:195-208.

Sonnesen L., Bakke M., Solow B. (2001) Bite force in pre-orthodontic children with unilateral crossbite . *European Journal of Orthodontics* 23 : 741 – 749.

Stahl F., Grabowski R. (2003) Orthodontic findings in the deciduous and early mixed dentition--inferences for a preventive strategy. *J Orofac. Orthop.* ;64(6):401-416.

Terlaje R.D., Donly K.J. (2001) Treatment planning for space maintenance in the primary and mixed dentition. *ASDC J Dent Child*; 68:109-114, 180.

Tewari A. (1970) Abnormal oral habits: Relationship with malocclusion and influence on anterior teeth. *J. Indian Dent. Assoc.*;42:81-4.

Thilander B. , Myrberg N. (1973) The prevalence of malocclusion in Swedish schoolchildren . *Scand. J. Dent. Res.* 81 : 12 – 21.

Thilander B., Lennartsson B. (2002) A study of children with unilateral posterior crossbite, treated and untreated, in the deciduous dentitionocclusal and skeletal characteristics of significance in predicting the long-term outcome. *J. Orofacial Orthop.* 63: 371 – 383.

Thilander B., Pena L., Infante C , Parada S.S., de Mayorga C. (2001) Prevalenceof malocclusion and orthodontic treatment need in children and adolescentsin Bogota, Colombia. An epidemiological study related to different stages of dental development. *Eur. J. Orthod* 23 : 153 – 167.

Thomaz E.B., Cangussu M.C., da Silva A.A., Assis A.M .(2010) Is malnutrition associated with crowding in permanent dentition? *Int. J. Environ. Res. Public Health*;7:3531-3544.

Thomaz E.B., Valença A.M. (2009) Relationship between childhood underweight and dental crowding in deciduous teething. *J. Pediatr.* (Rio J). ;85:110-116.

Thomaz E.B., Valença A.M. (2009) Relationship between childhood underweight and dental crowding in deciduous teething. *J. Pediatr.* (Rio J). ;85:110-116.

Trottman A., Elsbach H.G. (1996) Comparison of malocclusion in pre-school black and white children . *Am. J. of Orthod and Dentofacial Orthopedics* 110 : 69 – 72.

Tschill P., Bacon W., Sonko A. (1997) Malocclusion in the deciduous dentition of Caucasian children. *Eur. J. Orthod.*;19:361-7.

United Nations Development Program. Human Development Report 2009. Fact Sheets Indonesia and Philippines. New York: UNDP.

Väkiparta M.K., Kerosuo H.M., Nyström M.E., Heikinheimo K.A. (2005) Orthodontic treatment need from eight to 12 years of age in an early treatment oriented public health care system: a prospective study. *Angle Orthod.* ;75:344-349.

Varrela J, Alanen P. (1995) Prevention and early treatment in orthodontics: a perspective. *J. Dent. Res.*; 74:1436–1438.

Visković R., Vujanović M., Brcić V. (1990) [Prevalence of orthodontic anomalies, analysis and evaluation of dental health in three groups of pre-school children in Zadar]. *Acta Stomatol. Croat.* 24:271-280.

Warren J.J., Bishara S.E. (2002) Duration of nutritive and nonnutritive sucking behaviors and their effects on the dental arches in the primary dentition. *Am. J. Orthod. Dentofacial. Orthop.*;121:347–356.

Warren J.J., Bishara S.E., Steinbock K.L., et al. (2001) Effects of oral habits duration on dental characteristics in the primary dentition. *J. Am. Dent. Assoc*;132:1685–1693.

Weissman A.M. (1994) Preventive health care and screening of Latin American immigrants in the United States. *J. Am. Board Fam. Pract.* ;7:310-323.

Westwood P.V., McNamara J.A. Jr, Baccetti T., Franchi L., Sarver D.M. (2003). Long-term effects of Class III treatment with rapid maxillary expansion and facemask therapy followed by fixed appliances. *Am. J. Orthod. Dentofacial. Orthop.* ;123:306-320.

World Health Organization. Country health systems fact sheet – Nigeria. Brazzaville: WHO, 2006. World Health Organization. Statistical information system. Geneva, WHO, 2005.

World Health Organization. The World Health Report: working together for health. Geneva, WHO; 2006.

Zhang, M, McGrath C, Hagg U. 2006 The Impact of Malocclusion and its treatment on quality of life: a literature review. *Int. J. Paediatr. Dent.* 16:381-387.

In: Oral Health Care for Socially Disadvantaged Communities   ISBN: 978-1-62948-287-3
Editors: F.K. Kahabuka, E.N. Kikwilu and I. Anderson © 2013 Nova Science Publishers, Inc.

Chapter VIII

Oral Health Care for the Elderly

Irene A. Kida[1] and Anne N. Astrom[2]
[1] School of Dentistry, Muhimbili University of Health and Allied Sciences
[2] Department of Odontology-Community Dentistry, University of Bergen

8.1. Introduction

8.1.1. Definition of the Elderly Person

It is important to note that the chronological and biological age in the elderly may differ immensely. There is no consensus reached as to what represents the elderly age. In most developed countries, chronological age of 65+ years has been accepted as the age defining an elderly. In developing countries though, this has not been a straight forward solution, hence, different approaches have been utilized in order to classify an elderly person including: chronology, retirement age, life expectancy at birth, change in social role and change in capability   (http://www.who.int/healthinfo/survey/ageingdefnolder/en/index.html,   Allen, 2002). In this chapter therefore, an elderly person will be classified as a person aged sixty (60) years and above, the pensionable age used more often by governments.

8.1.2. Changing Global Demography

A considerable change in the global demography has been noted, referred to as the aging population. Thus, population ageing occurs globally and by 2050 people older than 80 years will comprise 20% of the world's elderly population (United Nations 2002). This has been attributed to a decrease in fertility rates and increased longevity in the developed countries. Since most of the populations in the developing countries maintain high to moderate fertility levels, and due to a gradual shift in disease patterns towards non communicable diseases, it is projected that most of the elderly people will live in the developing part of the world despite setbacks from the HIV/AIDS epidemic (Petersen and Yamamoto, 2005). This situation might create tremendous challenges to health and social policy planners. In developing countries, the situation is worsened by the still existing communicable diseases.

8.1.3. The Elderly as the Socially Disadvantaged Community

Globally, it has been observed that quality of life deteriorates with age. A study in Great Britain, among 'the third age' group, (defined as a period during which people are freed from work and family constraints and have time to pursue a good quality of life) revealed that advancing years lead to deterioration of quality of life (Wiggins et al., 2004). The study reported increased odds for poor quality of life with disadvantages in health, housing and pension provision experienced by an elderly, as well as a recent life event and stress. On the other hand, the study reported a raised quality of life among the elderly, when having people around whom; make them happy, give them support and encouragement, accept them as they are, care for them and make them feel important (Wiggins et al., 2004).

In most of the countries in the developing part of the world, elderly people have a significant role to play in the communities in which they live. They are viewed as a respected group of the population, expected to make wise decisions. Additionally, in the era of HIV / AIDS, older people have contributed a lot in the care of their bereaved grand children who have lost their parents due to HIV / AIDS (Ntozi and Mukiza-Gapere, 1995; Sefasi, 2010). Regrettably, the majority of elderly people belong to the poorest and most vulnerable groups of the population. This situation is more severe in rural areas, where older people face difficulties in meeting their basic needs and have limited access to general and oral health care services (Kikwilu et al,. 2009[b]). Elderly people are also burdened by other systemic conditions that may affect their quality of life such as hypertension, diabetes and cancers to name the few. This situation might create a vicious cycle as seen in figure 8.1. Since physical deterioration due to old age and financial debility (step 1) may impair an elderly from being productive to meet basic needs (such as required nutrition, shelter and clothing) and / or to be able to attend to health care facility (step 2), and hence end up being poor and unhealthy (step 3) and the cycle continues (Figure 8.1).

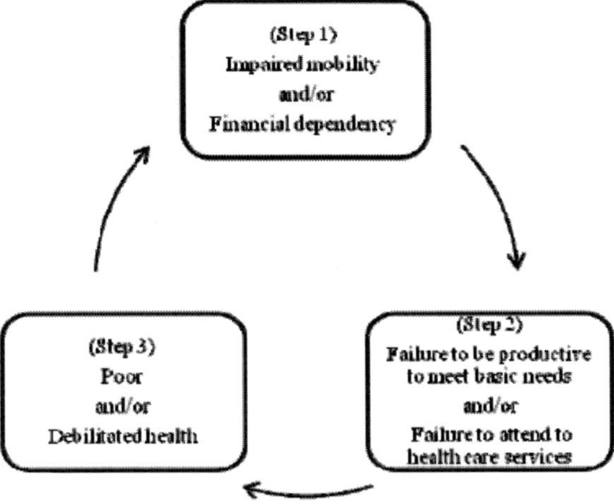

Figure 8.1. A vicious cycle of the elderly as underprivileged group of the population (Courtesy of I.A. Kida).

Moreover, the elderly have been discriminated and subjected to abuse in some cultures in the society due to a number of issues; firstly, witchcraft beliefs, where the elderly have been accused to be witches and therefore harmed. Secondly, elderly people have not been receiving the required hospital care since they are simply 'too old'. The notion that an elderly dentition can not be endodontically treated is inaccurate. Therefore, treatment plan for an elderly should not be based on age, but on general and local factors (Allen, 2002).

8.2. Oral Health Situation of the Elderly

8.2.1. Oral Health Status

Globally, deterioration of oral health with increasing age has been reported among the elderly in terms of poor oral hygiene, high levels of teeth lost, high prevalence of dental / root caries and periodontal disease (Kumar et al., 2009, Du et al., 2009). Accumulated experiences with oral problems and tooth loss might make older people more likely to report poor oral health related quality of life (Ekback et al., 2010).

Studies in developing countries report poor oral health situation among the elderly especially those residing in rural areas. They have been observed to have high levels of plaque and untreated oral diseases (dental caries and mobile teeth), reported to significantly affect their quality of life (Kida et al., 2006[a], Kida et al., 2006[b]). Apart from deteriorating oral health, elderly people have been reported to be at risk of a number of chronic, non-communicable diseases. Many major non-communicable ailments are lifestyle related and have risk factors common with those of the two major oral diseases i.e. dental caries and periodontal disease in terms of tobacco use, heavy drinking and poor dietary choices (Sheiham and Watt, 2000).

8.2.1.1. Dental Caries

A number of epidemiological studies done, globally, to assess the level of dental caries report an increasing prevalence of the disease with ageing. Dental caries has been reported to be the main reason of tooth loss even at old age (Thorstensson and Johansson, 2009). In most parts of the developed countries where extractions are not the norm of caries management, most elderly are more likely to retain their teeth and hence will require increased dental services. In these populations the F- component of the mean decayed, missing and filled teeth (DMFT) is high, which might increase need for complicated dental care at old age.

Studies done to determine the dental caries status and treatment need, in some parts of the African continent reported the mean DMFT scores to be high among the elderly, with M and D -components increasing with age (Milstein and Rudolph, 2000; Adegbembo et al., 2000). Contrary, the F-component is reported to decrease with age and this is thought to be due to increasing number of missing teeth. Furthermore, in most of these developing countries, the F-component is documented to be negligible (Sarita et al., 2004). The low rates of restorative care are reported to be mostly attributable to: lack of advice from dentists regarding alternative dental treatment available and poor knowledge of restorative care (Kikwilu et al., 2009[a]). Other barriers to restorative care documented, also include lack of access to dental care and personal / individual perceptions (Kikwilu et al., 2009[a]). The increase in caries experience with age might be attributable to the cumulative tendency of this disease and the limited dental health care facilities in many African countries.

8.2.1.2. Root Caries

Globally, elderly people exhibit a higher prevalence of root caries than their younger counterparts. This is attributable to exposure of root surfaces after gingival recession when teeth are retained into old age. Elderly who are at risk of developing root caries are reported to be of older age, having low education, chronic diseases, poor oral hygiene, consume fermentable carbohydrates, tobacco use of different forms and are irregular dental clinic attendants. They are also reported to be those who have gingivitis and loss of attachment. Furthermore, those living in rural areas are reported to have high Root Caries Index (RCI) than those living in the cities (Du et al., 2009)

8.2.1.3. Periodontal Disease

With regard to periodontal health, oral hygiene has been seen to decrease on ageing (Kumar et al., 2009). A number of studies show that almost all elderly are in need of oral hygiene instructions (Milstein and Rudolph, 2000). The fact that plaque control is found to be more difficult to maintain with aging, might create a significant danger to oral health.

Conversely, in some studies, done in developing countries, a slow periodontal progression to attachment loss with increasing age has been reported. These studies report a high prevalence of plaque, calculus and gingivitis, but a low prevalence of severe periodontal disease (Baelum et al., 1986; Darout et al., 2000). However, presence of calculus, gingival recession and deep probing depth are reported to be higher among older age groups, males and people residing in the rural areas. Periodontal destruction is not frequently present, but this is seen to be a problem for a small group of the population, who are mostly at older age.

8.2.1.4. Tooth Wear

Clinically, attrition as well as abrasion and erosion have been seen to be associated with increasing age. Attrition means occlusal wear due to muscular activity; abrasion involves cervical wear due to mechanical influences such as tooth brushing and erosion of teeth is due to chemical influences (Kaidonis et al., 2003). Studies conducted among adults in rural and urban areas of the Eastern Africa; report an increase in tooth wear with increasing age. This increase in tooth wear is more common among older adults aged 40 years and above, and mostly among those with reduced posterior support (Sarita et al., 2003).

8.2.1.5. Edentulousness

Loss of teeth (tooth mortality) is generally the result of disease processes and it may, therefore, be classified as an oral problem (Berk 1984). However, the most common oral diseases, dental caries and periodontal disease, have been seen not to be the sole cause of edentulousness. Other factors such as attitudes, behaviour, dental attendance and characteristics of health care system, and socio-economic factors, play an important role in the probability of becoming edentulous (Zarb and Schmit, 1997). There is, therefore, a large geographical variation in percentage of the elderly (65 years and more) who are edentulous (Trulsson et al., 2002, Mark et al, 2004 and Shah et al., 2004). Globally, studies show an increase in the percentage edentulousness with increasing age (Kida et al., 2006[b], Astrom et al., 2010). However, in some developed countries, edentulousness has been reported to decrease owing to improved oral health and dental awareness, hence most elderly prefer retaining their natural teeth to extraction (Jokstad, 2002). A reduction in the rates of tooth loss with time has occurred in many industrialized countries (Muller et al., 2007). Repeated cross-sectional studies have shown that the proportions of dentate Swedes aged 65–74 increased from 45% in 1975 to 85% in 1996/97 (Østerberg et al., 2006). A recent review suggests that the annual incidence of persons losing one or more teeth varies from 1.3% for a 1 year birth cohort of young adults in Dunedin to 13.7% in the Piedmont 65+ Dental Study in the U.S. (Haugejorden et al., 2008). Nevertheless, edentulousness is still associated with the lower socio-economic groups of the world population (Ettinger, 1993).

In many developing African countries though, the prevalence of edentulousness is less than 1%. Inaccessibility to oral health services might be the reason for the low prevalence since a high percentage of untreated caries are reported among these populations (Figure 8.2), and the treatment needs for such population groups are mainly palliative (Manji et al., 1988, Ntabaye et al., 1998).

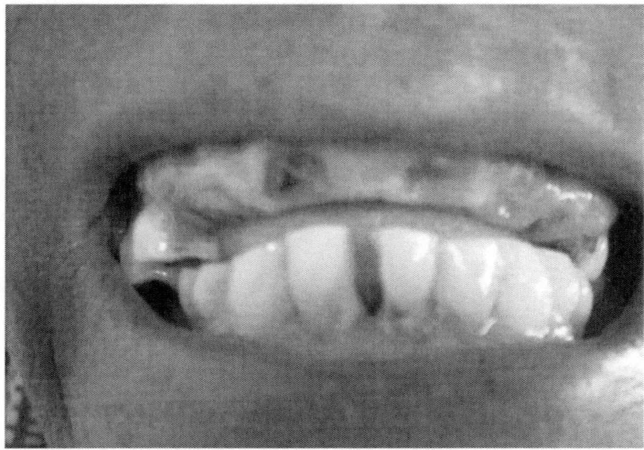

Figure 8.2. An elderly with untreated caries. (Courtesy of I.A. Kida).

8.2.1.6. Oral Health Related Quality of Life

Oral health is related to general health as documented in a number of studies (Kandelman et al., 2008). Oral diseases have been reported to impact on individuals' physical, psychological, and social dimensions of daily living. This person centered approach has gradually been accepted as a new public health paradigm that has replaced the traditional professional approach (Adulyoanon et al., 1996; Srisilapanan and Sheiham, 2001).

Studies, both in developed and developing countries, report higher prevalence of impact among the disadvantaged groups of the population (Adulyoanon et al., 1996; Srisilapanan and Sheiham, 2001). As portrayed among older adults in a study in a sub-Saharan African country, a higher proportion of rural populations have been reported to have their daily performances affected by their oral health when compared to their urban counterparts (Kida et al., 2006[a]). In the later study, more rural subjects rated their oral health as poor and had clinically detected poor oral health in terms of decayed and mobile teeth; and reduced anterior and posterior occluding units; which might affect their daily performances, more than urban subjects (Kida et al., 2006[a], Kida et al., 2006[b]).

Furthermore, poor oral health may interfere with efficiency of oral function in terms of ability to chew (Kim et al., 2009). Being able to bite and chew is considered to be particularly important in older people and might influence their nutritional status. Moreover, oral conditions, such as dry mouth and discomfort / pain associated with dental caries and periodontal disease may affect chewing ability. Impaired masticatory function has been reported to be one of the factors that influence food choices and consequently have detrimental effects on health, due to reduced intake of some key nutrients from foods perceived as difficult to chew (Akpata et al., 2011; Sheiham and Steel, 2001). Furthermore, inefficient chewing ability may increase the likelihood of over preparing / cooking of foods in an effort to make consumption practical, while in the process, a number of nutrients are lost (Anastassiadou and Heath, 2002) (Figure 8.3).

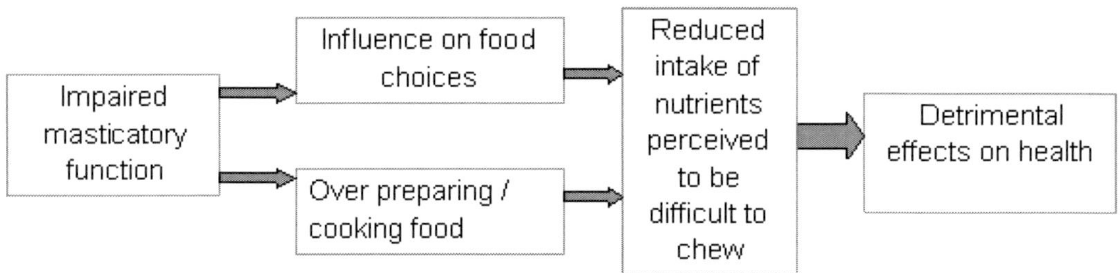

Figure 8.3. Oral health status and nutritional deficiency (Courtesy of I.A. Kida).

8.2.2. Oral Health Knowledge, Attitudes and Practice of the Elderly

Behavioral choices have been considered to be the most prominent domain influencing a person's view of health. In order to practice behaviors conducive to oral health, it is beneficial to have a good knowledge on the causes of diseases affecting oral health, how to prevent them and also be in an environment that will facilitate individuals' performance of a lifestyle conducive to oral health.

In the western world, studies report on improved oral health owing to improved peoples' awareness and change of attitude towards losing teeth, hence they seek treatment to retain their teeth (Jokstad, 2002).

On the contrary, elderly people in developing countries have been reported to have poor knowledge on causes and prevention of oral diseases, the situation being worse among those from the rural areas (Lin et al., 2001). Furthermore, most elderly and the communities in which they live, as well as some traditional health care providers do believe that tooth loss is inevitable with age. This belief coupled with lifestyle related factors such as poor dietary choices, tobacco use in different forms, excessive alcohol consumption and poor oral hygiene; contribute significantly to the deterioration of their oral health.

Despite the poor knowledge on oral health issues, older adults have been reported to have a positive attitude towards oral health, providing an opportunity for oral health promotion interventions (Lin et al., 2001).

Regarding oral hygiene practice, most elderly in these community report to brush their teeth at least once a day (Lin et al., 2001; Kida et al., 2006[b]). Mechanical oral hygiene is reported to be advantageous in prevention of oral diseases as well as other systemic conditions, such as pneumonia and respiratory tract infections among elderly people (Sjogren et al., 2008). In most of these underserved communities poor oral hygiene among the elderly is reported to be high despite the reported high frequency of tooth brushing, indicating the need for promoting proper mechanical oral hygiene practices (Kida et al., 2006[b]).

8.2.3. Access to Oral Health Care

Access and utilization of oral health services is generally low among the elderly (Kumar 2009). In the developed countries, elderly people have been reported to be the least likely of any age group to utilize dental services. However this evidence is not equivocal. Higher rates of dentate subjects and an aging population imply that the elderly population's need of dental healthcare services becomes increasingly prominent. Nationwide Swedish surveys have demonstrated time lag period differences in terms of large increases in utilization rates in middle- and older age groups between 1968 and 2000. Whereas 20% of 70-year-old Swedes reported regular annual dental attendance in 1971, the corresponding figure was 80% in 2001 (Østerberg et al., 2006).

Atchison et al., (1993) suggested identifying factors associated with use of dental health care services for preventive reasons, and comparing them with factors associated with illness related utilization of this service. In a recent study of community dwelling older Japanese people, Ohi et al (2009) found regular dental attendance to be associated with a higher number of teeth, younger age, higher educational level and presence of systemic diseases, whereas non compliances with treatment recommendations were associated with tooth loss and smoking status.

Studies have shown that barriers to dental health service utilization were related to the presence of teeth and financial status. Conversely, in some studies of these communities of the developed world, the costs of treatment, fear of dentistry, functional independence and poor general health, have been seen to be of little significance in explaining the low utilization patterns.

Others have posed that perceived need for treatment is the strongest predictor of the elderly to utilize dental health services. Regular dental attendance has been reported to be most prevalent in higher socio-economic status groups and is also associated with better oral health outcomes. Attitudes and perceptions influence dental attendance patterns such as anxiety, cost of dental care, availability and organization of dental health care services and beliefs regarding the importance of teeth and regular dental care. Recent findings based on the 1998 Community Health Assessment Project (CHAP) and the behavioral Risk factor Surveillance System (BRFSS) revealed that socio-demographics in terms of race (whites more likely to visit the dentist), income (higher income most likely to visit the dentist), education (higher education more likely to visit the dentist) and marital status (married most likely to visit the dentist) are the most important determinants of dental visiting habits in the general US population (Donaldsson et al., 2008, Seirawan, 2008).

Likewise, in the developing part of the world for instance in Sub-Saharan African countries, most studies report low levels of dental attendance in the population, especially among the elderly (Kikwilu et al., 2009[b]). Oral disability has been reported to be prevalent in developing countries, and that this poor dental status reflects insufficient dental care and limited access to oral health services (Petersen et al., 2010). This low level of dental attendance has been reported to be attributed to inaccessibility of health services and absence or limited health care resources.

Furthermore, majority of dental health care services are located in the higher levels of health care hierarchy, that is in regional and district hospitals, making it difficult for the elderly, especially in rural areas, to access (Petersen, 2005). In the majority of these countries, dental treatment for the elderly is reported to be exempted (Kikwilu et al., 2009[b]). Regrettably, these clinics have shortage of instruments and facilities (such as gloves, syringe, and local anaesthesia) hence, patients, including the elderly, are obliged to purchase these, in order to receive treatment (Matee et al., 2000).

8.3. Oral Health Care for the Elderly

8.3.1. Prevention

Due to the increasing number of the elderly in the developed world, a number of strategies have been worked out to promote their health as well as oral health. These strategies include not only treatment of oral diseases and conditions but also increased focus on the prevention of oral disease and condition to enhance oral health status and quality of life (McGrath et al., 2008). Measures utilized to prevent and control oral diseases in developed countries, have shown a significant positive impact to oral health of populations of different age groups. These include but not limited to adequate exposure to fluorides, improvement of oral health care system and increased dental awareness. As a result most elderly nowadays prefer restoration and conservation of their teeth to extraction. In addition, favorable dental insurance systems in these countries have also contributed significantly to this improvement.

In contrast, oral health care for the elderly has not been addressed much in the developing countries of the world. In most of these countries, structured oral health care systems for the elderly are lacking. Oral health care programs have been focusing on school children and rarely among the elderly despite the high burden of disease in this population segment. Adapting the western methods of controlling oral diseases has been considered futile in these underserved communities, due to high demand for resources (both human and financial). Community water fluoridation would be unrealistic in places where access to safe water is a problem. Fluoride rinses and application are expensive.

The reported high prevalence of oral diseases, low awareness and lack of access to oral health services entails an action towards improvement of oral health of the elderly. Further, the fallacy that older people will not benefit from health education and preventive measures, conspire to deprive the elderly of essential oral care.

Strengthening dental preventive and promotion services among this underserved group of the population would, therefore, be beneficial. According to the (WHO oral health report, 2003), oral health is the fourth most expensive ailment to treat in most industrialized countries. In most of the developing countries, a very limited budget is allocated for oral and dental care. Targeting specifically on oral health prevention and promotion activities for the elderly is not being considered a priority. In view of the fact that the elderly are also at risk of other lifestyle related illnesses i.e. chronic / non-communicable diseases other than oral diseases; adoption of the common risk factor approach would be feasible. This entails promoting general health, rather than oral health specific approaches, by controlling a small number of risk factors and hence a major impact on a large number of diseases while utilizing less resources (Sheiham and Watt, 2000). Oral health prevention and promoting activities should aim at modifying common risk factors such as dietary habits, hygiene, smoking and alcohol consumption, while collaborating with other agencies and professionals. It signifies that to improve oral health of the elderly, oral health promotion and disease prevention should be integrated with non-communicable and chronic disease prevention. Studies have shown that health promotion intervention programs have been successful in changing lifestyles in terms of tooth cleaning and change in dietary habits and other health behavior (McGrath et al., 2008).

8.3.2. Management

8.3.2.1. At the Dental Clinic

In the western world, the elderly are classified into those who are self living or independent and the dependant or frail – mostly living in the institutions (homes). Care of the elderly is anticipated as a challenge among dental practitioners due to the increase in life expectancy and retention of teeth needing complex procedures. In these communities, older adults no longer believe that tooth loss is an unavoidable consequence of ageing (Allen, 2002). It has been emphasized that old age is not a contraindication to treatment, and that oral health practitioners should be prepared to provide the best evidence based care. It is imperative to note that, despite the improvement in oral health and oral health care systems in these countries, oral diseases still exist among the underserved groups of these populations.

In most communities of developing countries, resources for conventional oral health care are relatively scarce. Most oral health facilities are inaccessible to the underserved communities (Kikwilu et al., 2009[b]). Furthermore, the ratio of dentist to patient is very low. It necessitates increasing the dentist to population ratio and formulating means to retain dentists; so that dental practitioners could reach at the lower levels of health systems. In addition, utilization of non-dental personnel (task shifting), located closer to the community to provide oral health education and promotion activities and simple procedures aiming at alleviating discomfort and preserving teeth would reduce oral impacts on quality of life of the elderly in these groups of population. The basic package of oral care (BPOC) and the concept of shortened dental arch (SDA) should be tested and applied in these communities; as they have proven to be a practical way of managing oral diseases in a number of studies among underserved communities (Frencken et al., 2002, Kumar et al,. 2009)

The BPOC constitutes three main components that have proven effective, acceptable, feasible and affordable for most disadvantaged communities. The first component is *Oral Urgent Treatment (OUT)* which involves relief of pain by removing badly decayed and mobile teeth under local anesthesia, provision of first aid for oral infections and dental-alveolar trauma, and referring complicated cases. In view of the fact that, untreated oral diseases have been reported to be prevalent among the elderly especially in the rural communities, OUT could facilitate improvement of oral health and quality of life of the elderly in these communities. A study to assess satisfaction with oral urgent care among adults in the developing country, Tanzania, revealed that the participants had moderate levels of satisfaction. The two main aspects of oral urgent care that were reported to be the least satisfactory were cost of treatment and explanation of treatment by health care provider (Kikwilu et al., 2009[b]). *Affordable Fluoride Toothpaste (AFT)* that is, brushing teeth using toothpaste containing optimum amount of fluoride is the second component and has been proven an effective preventive measure against dental caries. Most elderly report to brush their teeth at least once a day. Educating the elderly and making fluoridated toothpaste reasonably priced would help reduce the burden of dental caries among elderly. Lastly, is the *Atraumatic restorative treatment (ART)*; which is a novel approach to management of dental caries and does not require the conventional dental restorative equipments and materials. The procedure has been developed for use in rural areas where electrical power is unavailable or unstable. It has shown a significant improvement in individuals' satisfaction with oral health and good survival rate in some studies among elderly who were provided treatment in their home (Honkala and Honkala, 2002).

Shortened dental arch (SDA), defined as a dentition with reduction of teeth starting from posterior, is a concept that aims to provide a functional rather than a complete dentition. It has been advocated that having 20 well distributed teeth is enough to satisfy biting and chewing ability. As the major reason for tooth loss has been reported to be dental caries and the most affected part of the dentition being the molar region; the concept would be advantageous as resources for treatment are directed at preserving the less affected and easy to treat part of dentition (anterior and premolar teeth).

8.3.2.2. Home Based / Out-Reach Care

Frail elderly in most developed countries are institutionalized and therefore benefit from oral health care provided at their institutions (Bourgeois et al., 1998). Staffs at the nursing homes are usually trained to care for oral health of the elderly as part of general care. Complicated cases are usually referred to the dental clinic for further management. Contrary, in most developing countries, elderly are usually cared for by their relatives at home, making it difficult for them to access health and oral health care facilities. Outreach programs have proven fruitful as reported in a number of studies. Training of non-dental personnel who are accessible to the community in early diagnosis and referral of cases on oral as well as other chronic diseases would, therefore, be beneficial. Furthermore, educating the elderly on the importance of leading a lifestyle conducive to general and oral health would be beneficial.

Conclusions and Recommendations

The Common Risk Factor Approach

The elderly are classified as socially disadvantaged group in the community. They have been seen to be burdened by untreated oral diseases, as well as other chronic diseases such as hypertension, diabetes and the like, most of which are lifestyle related sharing common risk factors (Sheiham and Watt, 2000, Dounis et al., 2010).

The goal while managing elderly, should be to improve function, maintain independence, promote disease prevention and enhance quality of life (Dounis et al., 2010). It is therefore, advocated that oral health preventive and promotion strategies should utilize the common risk factor approach. This approach entails promotion of general health by controlling a small number of risk factors, in order to have a large impact on a larger number of diseases at a lower cost, great efficiency and effectiveness (Grabauskas, 1987). Current oral health education and promotion methods that target diseases separately have been seen to be ineffective and expensive in terms of money and human resources. This scarcity has been seen in both developed and developing countries. Furthermore, oral health problems have not been given much priority when it comes to health care interventions in most developing countries. There is a sizeable gap between resources allocated and population needs (Petersen et al., 2010). This is due to the existence infectious / communicable diseases in these communities, hence, very little of the available resources is budgeted for oral / dental interventions despite the high burden of oral diseases in populations. Therefore, health promotion interventions that also include other sectors of health are advantageous in that: they avoid duplication; increase effectiveness and efficiency; reduce isolation; and reach the deprived / socially excluded populations that carry the greatest burden of oral diseases (Sheiham and Watt, 2000). The existing policies should therefore be reviewed in order to include the elderly people, (who are disadvantaged in many health issues in developing countries) in planning of national and international oral health care strategies that will bring about improvement in oral health and quality of life of this disadvantaged group of population.

References

Adegbembo A.O., Adeyinka A, George M.O., Aihveba N., Danfillo I.S., Thorpe S.J., Enwonwu C.O. (2000) National pathfinder survey of dental caries prevalence and treatment need in The Gambia. *South African Dental Journal*, 55: 77-81.

Adulyanon S., Vourapukjaru J. and Sheiham A. (1996) Oral impacts affecting daily performance in a low dental disease Thai population. *Community Dentistry and Oral Epidemiology*, 24(6):385-389.

Akpata E., Otoh E., Enwonwu C., Adeleke O., Joshipur2011) Tooth loss, chewing habits, and food choices among older Nigerians in Plateau State: a preliminary study. *Community Dent Oral Epidemiol doi:10.1111/j.1600-0528.2011.00612.x*

Allen, P.F. (2002) Teeth for life for older adults. *Quintessentials of Dental Practice-7.*

Anastassiadou V., Heath M.R. (2002) Food choices and eating difficulty among elderly edentate patients in Greece. *Gerodontology* 19: 17-24.

Astrom A.N., Ekback G, Ordell S and Unell L. (2010) Socio-behavioral predictors of changes in dentition status: a prospective analysis of the 1942 Swedish birth cohort. *Community Dentistry and Oral Epidemiology,.* 1-11.

Atchison K.A., Mayer-Oakes S.A., Schweitzer S.O., Lubben J.E., De Jong F.J., Matthias R.E (1993) The relationship between dental utilization and preventive participation among a well-elderly sample. *Journal of Public Health Dentistry.* 53(2): 88-95.

Baelum V., Fejerskov T. and Karring T. (1986) Oral hygiene, gingivitis and periodontal breakdown in adult Tanzanians. *Journal of Periodontal Research*, 21(3): 221-232.

Bourgeois D., Nihtila A. and Mersel A. (1998) Prevalence of caries and edentulousness among 65-74-year-olds in Europe. *Bulletin of the World Health Organization*, 76, 413.

Darout I.A., Albandar J.M and Skaug N. (2000) Periodontal status of adult Sudanese habitual users of miswak chewing sticks or toothbrushes. *Acta Odontol Scand*, 58(1): 25-30.

Donaldson A.N., Everitt B., Newton T., Steel J., Sherriff M., Bower E. (2008) The effects of social class and dental attendance on oral health. *Journal of Dental Research*, 87(1): 60-64.

Dounis G., Ditmyer M., McClain M., Cappelli D. and Mobley C. (2010) Preparing the dental workforce for oral disease prevention in an aging population. *Journal of Dental Education*, 74; 10.

Du M.Q., Jiang H., Tai., B.J., Zhou Y., Wu B., Bian Z. (2009). Root caries patterns and risk factors of middle-aged and elderly people in China. *Community Dentistry and Oral Epidemiology*, 37: 260-266.

Ekback G., Astrom A.N., Klock K., Ordell S. and Unell L. (2010) Satisfaction with teeth and life-course predictors: a prospective study of a Swedish 1942 birth cohort. *European Journal of Oral Sciences*, 118:66-74.

Ettinger R.L. (1993) Demography and dental needs, an international perspective. Gerodontology, 10, 3-9.

Frencken J.E. and Holmgren C.J. (1999) How effective is ART in the management of dental caries? *Community Dentistry and Oral Epidemiology*, 27, 423.

Frencken J.E., Holmgren C.J. and van Palestein Helderman W.H. (2002) Basic package of oral care. WHO Collaborating Center for Oral Health Care.

Grabauskas V. (1987) integrated program for community health in non-communicable disease (Interhealth). In: Leparski E, editor. The prevention of non-communicable diseases: experiences and prospects. Copenhagen: WHO Regional office for Europe. 285-310.

Haugejorden O., Klock K.S., Astrom A.N., Skaret E., Trovik T.A. (2008). Socio-economic inequality in the self-reported number of natural teeth among Norwegian adults- an analytical study. *Community Dentistry and Oral Epidemiology* 36(3): 269-278.

Honkala S. and Honkala E. (2002) Atraumatic dental treatment among Finnish elderly persons. *Journal of Oral Rehabilitation*, 29; 435-440.

Jokstad A. (2002) Oral prosthetics from a Nordic perspective. *International Journal of Prosthodontics*. 15; 145-153.

Kaidonis J.A., Gratiaen J., Bhatia N., Richards L.C., Townsend G.C. (2003)-Tooth wear prevention: a quantitative and qualitative in vitro study. *Australian Dental Journal*, 48(1): 15-19.

Kandelman D., Petersen P.E. and Ueda H. (2008) Oral health general health, and quality of life in older people. *Special Care Dentistry* 28(6): 224-236.

Kida I.A., Astrom A.N., Strand G.V. and Masalu J.R. (2006[b]) Clinical and social-behavioral correlates of tooth loss: a study of older adults in Tanzania. *BMC Oral Health*, 6:5

Kida I.A., Astrom A.N., Strand G.V. and Masalu J.R. (2007) Chewing problems and dissatisfaction with chewing ability: a survey of older Tanzanians. *European Journal of Oral Sciences* 115: 265-274.

Kida I.A., Astrom A.N., Strand G.V., Masalu J.R. and Tsakos G. (2006[a]) Psychometric properties and the prevalence, intensity and causes of oral impacts on daily performance (OIDP) in a population of older Tanzanians. *Health and Quality of Life Outcomes*, 4:56.

Kikwilu E.N., Frencken J.E., Mulder J., Masalu J.R. (2009[a]) Barriers to restorative care as perceived by dental patients attending government hospitals in Tanzania. *Community Dent Oral Epidemiol;* 37, 35-44.

Kikwilu E.N., Kahabuka F.K., Masalu J.R. and Senkoro A. (2009[b]) Satisfaction with urgent oral care among adult Tanzanians. *Journal of Oral Sciences* 51(1): 47-54.

Kim H.Y., Jang M.S., Chung C.P., Paik D.I., Park Y.D., Patton L.L., Ku Y. (2009). Chewing function impacts oral health-related quality of life among institutionalized and community-dwelling Korean elders. *Community Dentistry and Oral Epidemiology*, 1-9.

Kumar T.S., Dagli R.J., Mathur A., Jain M., Balasubramanyam G., Prabu D., Kulkarni S. (2009). Oral health status and practices of dentate Bhil adult tribes of Southern Rajasthan, India. *International Dental Journal*, 59; 133-140.

Lin H.C., Wong M.C.M., Wang Z.J., Lo E.C.M. (2001) Oral health knowledge attitudes and practices of Chinese adults. *J Dent Res* 80(5): 1466-1470.

Mack F, Mojon P, Budtz-Jorgensen E, Kocher T, Splieth C, Schwahn C, Bernhardt O, Gesch D, Kordass B, John U, et al., (2004) Caries and periodontal disease of the elderly in Pomerania Germany: results of the study of Health in Pomerania. *Gerodontology*, 21; 27.36.

Manji F, Baelum V and Fejerskov O. (1988) Tooth mortality in an adult rural population in Kenya. *Journal of Dental Research*, 67, 496-500.

Matee I.M., Simon E.N and Kalyanyama B. (2000) Utilization of dental services in Tanzania before and after the introduction of cost sharing. *International Dental Journal*, 50: 69-72.

McGrath C., Zhang W. and Lo E.C. (2008) A review of the effectiveness of oral health promotion activities among elderly people. *Gerodontology;* 26:85-96.

Milstein L. and Rudolph M.J. (2000) Oral health status in an institutionalized elderly Jewish population. *South African Dental Journal*, 55: 302-306.

Muirhead V.E., Quinonez C., Figueiredo R., Locker D. (2009) Predictors of dental care utilization among working poor Canadians. *Community Dent Oral Epidemiol* 37: 199-208.

Ntabaye M.K, Scheutz F. and Poulsen S. (1998) Household survey of access to and utilization of emergency oral health care services in rural Tanzania. *East African Medical Journal*, 75;649.53.

Ntozi J.P. and Mukiza-Gapere J. (1995) Care for AIDS orphans in Uganda: findings from focus group discussions. *Health Transition Review*, Vol 5 suppl. 245-252.

Ohi T., Sai M., Kikuchi M., Hattori Y., Tsuboi A., Hozawa A., Ohmori-Matsuda K., Tsuji I., Watanabe M. (2009) Determinants of the utilization of dental services in a community-dwelling Elderly Japanese population. *Tohoku Journal of Exp. Medicine.*, 218: 241-249.

Osterberg T., Johanson C., Sundh V., Steen B., and Birkhed D. (2006) Secular trend of dental status in five 70-year-old cohorts between 1971-2001. *Community Dentistry and Oral Epidemiology*, 34: 446-454.

Petersen P.E. and Yamamoto T. (2005) Improving the oral health of older people: the approach of the WHO Global Oral Health Programme. *Community Dentistry and Oral Epidemiology*, 33(2): 81-92.

Petersen P.E., Bourgeois D., Ogawa H., Estupinan-Day S., Ndiaye C. (2005) The global burden of diseases and risks to oral health. *Bulletin of the World Health Organization* 83 (9): 661-669.

Petersen P.E., Kandelman D., Arpin S. and Ogawa H. (2010) Global oral health of older people – call for public health action. *Community Dental Health*, 27 (Suppl 2), 1-11.

Sarita P.T., Kreulen C.M., Witter D. and Creugers N.H. (2003) Signs and Symptoms associated with TMD in adults with shortened dental arches. *International Journal of Prosthodontics*, 16; 265-70.

Sarita P.T., Witter D.J., Kreulen C.M., Matee M.I., van't Hof M.A. (2004) Decayed/ Missing/Filled teeth and shortened dental arches in Tanzanian adults. *Int J Prosthodont*; 17, 224-230.

Sefasi A.P. (2010) Impact of HIV and AIDS on elderly: A case study of Chiladzulu district. *Malawi Medical Journal*, 22(4): 101-103.

Seirawan H. (2008) Parsimonious prediction model for the prevalence of dental visits. *Community Dentistry and Oral Epidemiology*, 36(1): 401-408.

Shah N, Parkash H. and Sunderam K.R. (2004) Edentulousness, denture wear and denture needs of the Indian elderly: a community baed study. *Journal of Oral Rehabilitation*, 31, 467-476.

Sheiham A. and Steele J. (2001). "Does the condition of the mouth and teeth affect the ability to eat certain foods, nutrient and dietary intake and nutritional status amongst older people?" *Public Health Nutr*, 4(3): 797-803.

Sheiham A. and Watt R.G. (2000) The Common Risk Factor Approach: a rational basis for promoting oral health. *Community Dent Oral Epidemiol*; 28: 399-406.

Sjögren P., Nilsson E., Forsell M., Johansson O., Hoogstraate J. (2008) A systematic review of the preventive effect of oral hygiene on pneumonia and respiratory tract infection in elderly people in hospitals and nursing homes: effect estimates and methodological quality of randomized controlled trials. *J. Am. Geriatr. Soc.*; 56: 2124-2130.

Srisilapanan P. and Sheiham A. (2001) The prevalence of dental impacts on daily performances in older people in Northern Thailand. *Gerodontology*, 18, 102-8.

Thorstensson H. and Johansson B. (2009) Why do some people lose teeth across their lifespan whereas others retain a functional dentition into old age? *Gerodontology;* 1-7.

Trulsson U., Engstrand P., Berggren U., Nannmark U., Branemark P.J. (2002) Edentulousness and oral rehabilitation: experiences from the patients' perspective. *European Journal of Oral Sciences*, 110(6), 417-424.

United Nations, (2002). World Population Ageing 1950-2050, population division, Department of Economic and Social Affairs, New York. United Nations.

WHO, Definition of older or elderly person. http://www.who.int/healthinfo/ survey/ageingdefnolder/en/index.html. Accessed 01/12/09.

Wiggins R.D., Higgs P.D., Hyde M. and Blane D.B. (2004) Quality of life in the third age: key predictors of the CASP-19 measure. *Aging and Society* 24: 693-708.

Zarb G. and Schmitt A. (1997) Clinical decision-making in implant prosthodontics. *Ont Dent;* 74, 21-23.

In: Oral Health Care for Socially Disadvantaged Communities   ISBN: 978-1-62948-287-3
Editors: F.K. Kahabuka, E.N. Kikwilu and I. Anderson © 2013 Nova Science Publishers, Inc.

Chapter IX

Management of Oral Lesions Associated with HIV/AIDS

Omar J. M. Hamza[1] and Andre J. A. M. van der Ven[2]
[1] Muhimbili National Hospital
[2] Department of General Internal Medicine, Radboud University Nijmegen

9.1. Introduction

The Human Immunodeficiency Virus (HIV), which is the cause of the Acquired Immunodeficiency Syndrome (AIDS), globally has infected about 33 million (30 million–36 million) people up to the year 2007 (UNAIDS, 2008). Most of the HIV-infected individuals are from low-income countries especially Sub-Saharan Africa that accounts for over 70% of the world's HIV cases. Sub-Saharan Africa's epidemics vary significantly from country to country in both scale and scope. Adult national HIV prevalence is below 2% in several countries of West and Central Africa, as well as in the horn of Africa, but in 2007 it exceeded 15% in seven southern African countries (Botswana, Lesotho, Namibia, South Africa, Swaziland, Zambia, and Zimbabwe), and was above 5% in seven other countries, mostly in Central and East Africa (Cameroon, the Central African Republic, Gabon, Malawi, Mozambique, Uganda, and the United Republic of Tanzania) (UNAIDS, 2008). HIV/AIDS is currently the leading cause of death in Africa and the fourth leading cause of death worldwide. HIV-related deaths and illnesses have crippled economic growth and strained the health care systems of several countries especially those in Sub-Saharan Africa.

HIV is a lentivirus, subfamily of retroviruses. HIV has a lipid envelope that has specific glycoproteins that attach to the CD4 protein on the cell surface. HIV needs the CD4 receptor (as well as some co-receptors, such as CCR5 and CXCR4) to attach. The CD4 receptor is expressed by CD4- positive lymphocytes, monocytes, macrophages, microglial cells, and langerhan's cells in skin. Disturbances in number and function of CD4 cells underlie the immunodeficiency and related opportunistic conditions.

Oral diseases are common manifestations of HIV infection, with up to 90% of HIV-seropositive patients developing oral lesions through the course of their HIV-infection

(Schiodt et al., 1990, Samaranayake et al., 2000). Oral lesions such as oral candidiasis and oral hairy leukoplakia are among the early clinical features of HIV-infection and may as such not only function as a marker of an HIV-infection but may predict the progression to AIDS as well (Schiodt et al., 1990, Greenspan et al. 1997, Singh et al., 2003). Oral lesions are generally used in staging and classification systems and can serve as entry or end-points in therapy and vaccine trials (WHO (AIDS) 1990, CDC 1999). Furthermore, oral lesions may give an indication to start HAART while the development of oropharyngeal candidiasis in a patient taking HAART may point to a failing regiment. Fungal, bacterial and viral opportunistic oral infections as well as malignancies of the oral cavity and non-specific presentations such as aphthous ulcerations and salivary gland disease are common in HIV/AIDS patients (Schiodt et al., 1990, Greenspan et al. 1997, Samaranayake et al., 2000, Singh et al., 2003, Hamza et al., 2006). A key but not exclusive basis for the pathogenesis involves reduced numbers and function of CD4+ T-lymphocytes, the resultant decrease in systemic and mucosal immune integrity is in turn associated with an increased frequency of oral lesions (Matee et al., 2000, Campo et al., 2002). Other factors that predispose to HIV-related oral lesions include high plasma HIV-RNA levels (greater than 3000 copies/mL), poor oral hygiene, xerostomia, smoking, ethnicity, nutritional status socio-economical status and concurrent endemic diseases (Campo et al., 2002).

HAART therapy has decreased the prevalence of several but not all HIV-associated oral lesions (Patton et al., 2000, Schmidt-Westhausen et al., 2000, Tappuni et al., 2001). Overall, the use of HAART reduced the incidence of candidiasis, Kaposi's sarcoma, oral hairy leukoplakia, and necrotizing ulcerative periodontitis (Patton et al., 2000, Schmidt-Westhausen et al., 2000, Shetty et al., 2000, Ramirez-Amador et al., 2003). However, as a consequence of HAART, the increase in CD4+ T-lymphocytes numbers and renewed ability to mount an inflammatory response, sometimes referred as the immune reconstitution syndrome, may lead to increased frequency of selected oral lesions such as Human Papilloma Virus (HPV) associated oral warts and salivary gland diseases (Schmidt-Westhausen et al., 2000, Shetty et al., 2000, King et al., 2002, Ramirez-Amador et al., 2003).

The presence of oral lesions may have a significant impact on health-related quality of life since HIV-associated orofacial lesions alter facial appearance, impair speech and make swallowing difficult, which may lead to significant weight loss and pain (Coulter et al., 2002).

This emphasizes the need to assess the oral cavity during routine care by health care personnel that is trained to diagnose and treat HIV-associated oral lesions while at the same occasion, voluntary counseling and testing and/or HIV care can be provided (Cruz et al., 1996).

Patients need to be referred elsewhere if the latter services cannot be provided. Oral health care is important for most patients with HIV/AIDS and these services need to be integrated in more general comprehensive HIV/AIDS care. This will also greatly improve access to care, especially for deprived and socially disadvantaged communities where services are already limited. The strategies for the prevention and control of common HIV-related orofacial disease are poorly documented in social disadvantaged communities in low income countries where expensive pharmacotherapy is unavailable (Hodgson et al., 2006), and more efforts should go to establish protocols for management, prevention and control of these lesions.

By the completion of this chapter the reader will be able to:

- Understand and identify specific lesions associated with HIV/AIDS.
- Diagnose specific lesions associated with HIV/AIDS.
- Describe basic treatments for oral lesions associated with HIV infection.
- Determine need for consultation and referral related to HIV infection.

9.2. Classification of Oral Lesions Associated with HIV/AIDS

The oral lesions associated with HIV/AIDS can be classified according to the underlying pathophysiological process (Table 9.1) and/or the frequency that these lesions develop during HIV-infections (Table 9.2 and 9.3) (EC-Clearinghouse/WHO classification 1993). The presence of one or more lesions requires that HIV infection be considered as a possible underlying cause.

However, no particular lesion is uniquely associated with HIV infection. Oral candidiasis and oral hairy leukoplakia are so strongly associated with HIV infection that they have been incorporated in "the Center for Disease Control clinical classification and staging of HIV disease" (CDC 1999).

Table 9.1. Classification of the oral lesions associated with HIV/AIDS based on pathophysiological process (EC-Clearinghouse/WHO classification 1993)

1.	Infections	
	Fungal	Oral candidiasis, Cryptococcus, histoplasmosis, aspergillos
	Viral	Oral hairy leukoplakia, Herpes simplex virus infection, Human papilloma virus, Cytomegalovirus, Varicella-zoster virus infection, Moluscum contagiosum.
	Bacteria	Periodontal diseases, *Mycobacterium avium-intracellulare*, *Mycobacterium tuberculosis, Actinomyces israelii, Esterichia coli, Klebsiella pneumoniae*
2.	Neoplasm	
		Kaposi's sarcoma, non-Hodgkin's lymphoma
3.	Immune-mediated	
		Recurrent aphthous ulcers, necrotizing stomatitis
4.	Other	
		Xerostomia, salivary gland disease, pain syndromes, ulcerations not otherwisw specified

Table 9.2. EC-Clearinghouse classification of the oral lesions associated with HIV/AIDS in adults (EC-Clearinghouse/WHO classification 1993)

Group 1: lesions strongly associated with HIV infection		
Candidiasis		
	Erythematous	
	Pseudomembranous	
Hairy leukoplakia		
Kaposi's sarcoma		
Non-Hodgkin's lymphoma		
Periodontal diseases	Linear gingival erythema	
	Necrotizing (ulcerative) gingivitis	
	Necrotizing (ulcerative) periodontitis	
Group 2: lesions less commonly associated with HIV infection		
Bacterial infections	*Mycobacterium avium-intracellulare*	
	Mycobacterium tuberculosis	
Melanotic hyperpigmentation		
Necrotizing (ulcerative) stomatitis		
Salivary gland disease	Dry mouth due to decreased salivary flow rate	
	Unilateral or bilateral swelling of major salivary glands	
Thrombocytopenia purpura		
Ulceration NOS (not otherwise specified)		
Viral infections	Herpes simplex virus	
	Human papilloma virus (warty-like lesions)	Condyloma acuminatum
		Focal epithelial hyperplasia
		Verruca vulgaris
	Varicella zoster virus	Herpes zoster
		Varicella
Group 3: lesions seen in HIV infection		
Bacterial infections	*Actinomyces israelii*	
	Escherichia coli	
	Klebsiella pneumoniae	
Cat-scratch disease		
Drug-reactions	Ulcerative,	
	Erythema multiforme	
	Lichenoid	
	Toxic epidermolyis	
Epitheloid (bacillary) angiomatosis		
Fungal infections other than candidiasis	*Cryptococcus neoformans*	
	Geotrichum candidum	
	Histoplasma capsulatum	
	Mucoraceae (mucurmycosis, zygomycosis)	
	Aspergillus flavus	
Neurologic disturbances	Facial palsy	
	Trigeminal neuralgia	
Recurrent aphthous stomatitis		
Viral infections	Cytomegalovirus	
	Molluscum contagiosum	

Table 9.3. EC-Clearinghouse and WHO classification of the oral lesions associated with HIV/AIDS in children (Ramos-Gomez et al. 1999)

Group 1: lesions commonly associated with pediatric HIV infection		
Candidiasis	Erythematous	
	Pseudomembranous	
	Angular cheilitis	
Herpes simplex virus infection		
Linear gingival erythema		
Parotid enlargement		
Recurrent aphthous ulcers	Minor	
	Major	
	Herpetiform	
Group 2: lesions less commonly associated with pediatric HIV infection		
Seborrheic dermatitis		
Bacterial infections of oral tissues	Necrotizing (ulcerative) stomatitis/Noma	
Periodontal diseases	Necrotizing (ulcerative) gingivitis	
	Necrotizing (ulcerative) periodontitis	
Viral infections	Cytomegalovirus	
	Human papilloma virus	
	Molluscum contagiosum	
	Varicella zoster virus	Herpes zoster
		Varicella
Xerostomia		
Group 3: lesions strongly associated with HIV infection but rare in children		
Neoplasms	Kaposi's sarcoma	
	Non-Hodgkin's lymphoma	
Oral hairy leukoplakia		
Tuberculosis-related ulcers		

9.3. General Diagnosis of Oral Lesions Associated with HIV/AIDS

Primary health care workers or dental practioners may be the first to recognize the signs and symptoms of a HIV-infection. In social disadvantaged communities where oral health care for HIV-infected patients is hindered by shortage of oral health personnel, primary health care workers may be trained to take a dental history, examine the oral cavity and surrounding tissues as well as to diagnose and treat oral lesions. This is very relevant since it has been shown that proper management of oral lesions reduces morbidity and increase survival. In addition, early diagnosis of oral lesions related to HIV/AIDS can be useful for recruiting cases for voluntary counseling and testing (VCT) services as the key entry point for care and treatment services.

9.3.1. Medical History and Clinical Examination

A full medical and dental history should be taken. Specific information related to the orofacial complaint should include details of site, onset, relieving and exacerbating factors. Clinical examination should include both extra-oral and intra-oral examination. Initially an overall assessment should be made and then depending on signs and symptoms a more detailed examination of a particular area will be required.

9.3.2. Special Investigations

The type of investigations depends on the oral lesions and includes tissue biopsy, microbiologic, hematologic and salivary gland investigations. Tissue biopsy should be done in case of oral Kaposi's sarcoma, squamous cell carcinoma, non-Hodgkin's lymphoma or other tumors.

Microbiologic investigations can consist of a smear or plain swab. Smears are obtained by spreading material scraped from lesion onto a glass slide which can subsequently be examined for presence of bacteria or fungi. Plain swabs can be cultured in specialized media to detect bacteria, fungi and viruses.

9.4. Management of Oral Lesions Associated with HIV/AIDS

Oral lesions may occur at varying degrees of immune-deficiencies. Oropharyngeal candidiasis for instance may occur while CD4 cell counts are still high and can therefore be managed with anti-fungal treatment only. Recurrent oropharyngeal candidiasis may indicate more severe immune-deficiency while concurrent esophageal complaints always indicate severe immune-depression. In these cases, candidiasis does not only require anti-fungal treatment but recurrence can only be prevented by reversal of the immunodeficiency by initiation of HAART. Potent antiretroviral therapy has also been shown to be the single best intervention to reduce the incidence of oral lesions. Apart from that, strategies for management of oral lesions associated with HIV-infection using the available cheap drugs are warranted. The management of specific oral lesions associated with HIV-infection is hereby discussed.

9.4.1. Fungal Infections

9.4.1.1. Oral Candidiasis

Oral candidiasis is the most prevalent fungal infection in HIV-infection, and is the most common HIV-related oral lesion (Schiodt et al., 1990, Greenspan et al. 1997, Samaranayake et al., 2000, Matee et al., 2000, Singh et al., 2003, Hamza et al., 2006). Oral candidiasis is caused by *Candida* species predominantly due to *Candida albicans.* Other *Candida* species have been isolated in HIV-infected patients such as *C.glabrata, C.tropicalis, C.krusei, C.parapsilosis, C.guilliermondii* and *C.dubliniensis. Candida* species are however also isolated from 30-50% of the oral cavities of healthy adults, making it a constituent of the normal oral flora, but clinical oral candidiasis rarely occurs in healthy patients (Brawner et al., 1989). Adhesion of *Candida* to the oral mucosal surface is the vital prerequisite for successful colonization and subsequent infection by this yeast.

Oral candidiasis occurs in up to 90% of HIV/AIDS patients, with a higher prevalence in low-income countries (Schiodt et al., 1990, Samaranayake et al., 2000, Singh et al., 2003). As mentioned above, candidiasis affects mainly the oral mucosa in the early stages of HIV-infection while the esophageal mucosa is also being affected in more advanced stages of HIV disease. Recurrent candidiasis has been associated with low CD4+ T-lymphocytes count and high HIV viral load. Oral candidiasis has also been associated with a more frequent progression to AIDS, and it has been used as a marker to define severity of HIV-infection.

Based on clinical appearance, oral candidiasis can appear as one of four distinct clinical entities; pseudomembranous, erythematous, hyperplastic and angular cheilitis. In all cases, the infection is superficial. Despite the frequency of mucosal candidiasis, disseminated or invasive infections with *Candida* are uncommon.

Pseudomembranous candidiasis is the most common clinical presentation (Schiodt et al., 1990, Samaranayake et al., 2000, Hamza et al., 2006). It appears as creamy white or yellowish patches that can be wiped off leaving a red, raw or a bleeding surface (Figure 9.1). Pseudomembranous candidiasis appears on any oral mucosal surface as well as in the oropharynx and although it can be seen at various levels of CD4 cell counts, it appears significantly more with CD4 cell counts below 200 cells/mm^3.

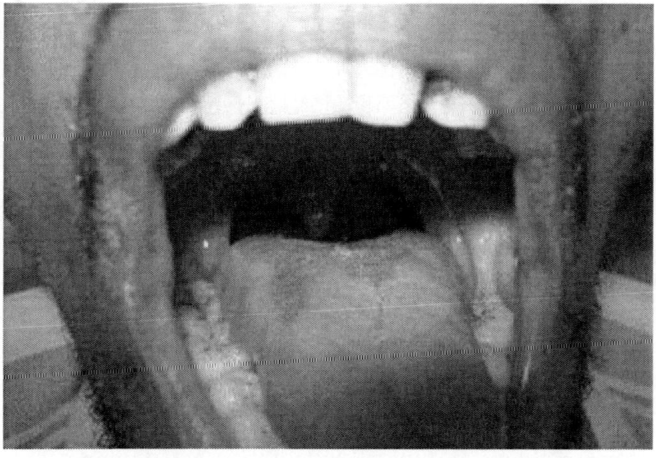

Figure 9.1. Pseudo membranous candidiasis (a courtesy of O. Hamza).

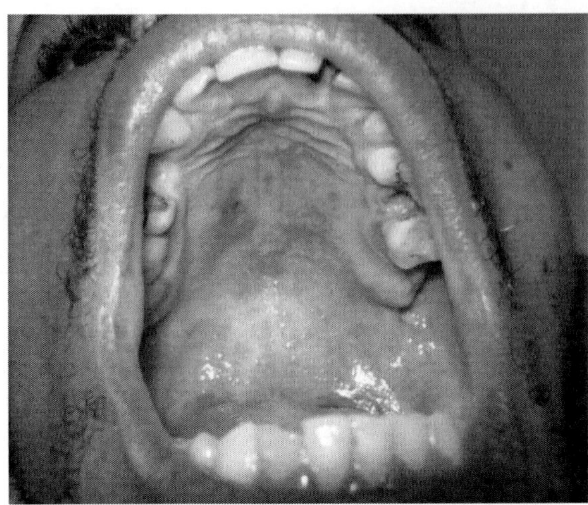

Figure 9. 2. Erythematous candidiasis (a courtesy of O. Hamza).

Erythematous candidiasis may be the most underdiagnosed and misdiagnosed oral manifestation of an HIV-infection (Reznik, 1999). The condition presents as a red velvet lesion, most commonly on the palate, buccal mucosa and dorsum of the tongue and is more frequent in the early stages of HIV infection when CD4 cell counts are above 200 cells/mm^3 (Figure 9.2). Hyperplastic/chronic candidiasis appears as a white non-removable plaque/usually adherent to the tissue in any oral mucosa surface. These lesions usually occur at later stages of HIV-infection and are associated with severe immunosuppression/long standing disease. Hyperplastic candidiasis can persist for an extensive period of time if left untreated and is associated with an increased risk for malignant transformation.

Finally, angular cheilitis presents as cracks or fissures from the corners of the mouth, sometimes covered with pseudomembranes. It can occur with or without erythematous or pseudomembranous candidiasis and mixed infections with gram-positive cocci are frequently seen.

Burning pain, altered taste sensation, difficulty in swallowing liquids and solids are symptoms related to oral candidiasis although many patients may have lesions without any complaint. Diagnosis of oral candidiasis is made mainly on clinical appearance especially in social disadvantaged communities in low income countries where laboratory facilities may be limited. The diagnosis can however easily be confirmed by microscopic examination of 10% potassium hydroxide (KOH) slide preparation of a scraping of an active lesion. Pseudohyphae and yeasts are characteristic findings. Culture is usually not necessary unless the lesions fail to clear with antifungal therapy.

Treatment of oral candidiasis is determined by the clinical type, distribution, and severity of infection. A wide variety of agents are effective for the treatment of oral candidiasis (Table 9.4). Important factors that determine clinical response, besides the choice of antifungal agent, include the extent and severity of disease, patient adherence, as well as pharmacokinetics and pharmacodynamics. Classes of antifungal agents include polyenes, azoles (imidazoles and triazoles), Candines, pyrimidines synthesis inhibitors and cyclic lipopeptides. Polyenes (nystatin and amphotericin B) bind to ergosterol in the fungal cell membrane and induce osmotic instability and loss of membrane integrity.

Azoles, including the imidazoles (clotrimazole, miconazole) and triazoles (ketoconazole, itraconazole, fluconazole, voriconazole, ravuconazole and posaconazole), inhibit fungal cytochrome P450-dependent enzymes, resulting in the impairment of ergosterol biosynthesis and depletion of ergosterol from the fungal cell membrane. Pyrimidines synthesis inhibitors, including 5-fluorocytosine, inhibit DNA and RNA synthesis in fungal organisms and newer agents like the candins (caspofungin and V-echinocandins), cyclic lipopeptides that inhibit beta-1:3 glucan synthase, an enzyme involved in fungal wall biosynthesis.

Topical therapy is effective for limited and accessible lesions and is effective for mild to moderate episodes. Clotrimazole troches and creams, nystatin pastilles and oral suspensions, miconazole creams are effective for mild to moderate oral candidiasis. Systemic therapy for oral candidiasis involves the use of triazole antifungal medications. These anti-fungal agents should be used in case of severe or recurrent oral candidiasis and in case of a (concurrent) esophageal candidiasis. Fluconazole is available in suspension, tablet, and parenteral form. It is more completely absorbed than itraconazole or ketoconazole and absorption is not dependent on gastric acidity or food intake. Fluconazole has a long half-life (30 hours) and is therefore administered once a day or even as a single dose. The use of single high dose fluconazole (750 mg) has namely been shown to be as effective (>95%) for the treatment of oropharyngeal candidiasis in patients with HIV-infection as a 14 days course of fluconazole while resistance development was not different in the two treatment arms (Hamza et al., 2008). Moreover, the single dose has the advantage of simplicity and is less costly, and seems therefore a rational choice especially in social disadvantaged communities. The candins are only available in parenteral forms and are therefore mostly reserved for severe azole resistant candidiasis.

Topical therapies with antifungal agents have minimal side effects since it's not absorbed. However these remedies have the disadvantage that they should be administered many times in a day and patients should be instructed to keep the solution in the oral cavity for some minutes. The general profile of side effects of ketoconazole, itraconazole, fluconazole, posaconazole, and voriconazole are similar, the more common being headache, dyspepsia, diarrhea, nausea, vomiting, hepatitis and skin rash. The frequency at which these side effects occur may however be different: ketoconazole is for instance mostly associated with hepatitis while fluconazole is usually well tolerated. Each drug may also induce specific adverse effects: voriconazole for instance is known to cause visual disturbances and the occurrence is dose related. The wide spread introduction of oral azoles, most notably fluconazole, has led to the increased incidence of azole resistant *Candida albicans* as well as the emergence of non-albicans species such as *Candida glabrata*, which are inherently resistant to this class of drug (Cartledge et al., 1999, Fichtenbaum et al., 2000). Factors that increase the probability of azole resistant strains of Candida presenting in the oral cavity include previous exposure to azoles, low CD4 cell count and the presence of non-albicans species.

To minimize the risk of resistance, topical therapies should be considered for first-line treatment of initial cases of mild to moderate oral candidiasis and systemic therapies should be utilized for moderate to severe cases.

Clinicians should realize that relapse of oral candidiasis after successful treatment is common when the underlying immune deficiency persists. As stated above, HAART restores immune function and prevents thereby the development of new oral lesions. Management of these patients becomes very difficult when no HAART is available. Some remedies have been advocated but their effects have not well been studied. Chlorhexidine for instance is an inexpensive mouthrinse with antifungal activity that may be used after successful treatment of the oral candidiasis to prolong the time to recurrence.

Rinsing the mouth with home-made salt water may be another option to reduce oral *Candida* levels, and provide mechanical cleansing effect to decrease the chance in adhering of the organism to the mucosal surfaces, which is the most critical step of the infection. These remedies can be used in social disadvantaged communities to minimize risk of recurrence after successful treatment of oral candidiasis.

Treatment options for oropharyngeal candida infections are summarized in table 9.4. Mild infections may be treated with topical treatment but severe infections, including esophageal candidiasis should be treated with systemic treatment. If treatment response to fluconazole is not satisfactory (for example if resistance to fluconazole) develops, a higher dose of fluconazole may be tried. Ideally, a resistance test should be done to explore the activity of the other azoles and/or other anti-fungal drugs. In social disadvantaged communities these tests may not available, therefore, worse clinical responses will determine change of antifungal therapy.

Treatment of oral candidiasis in social disadvantaged communities in low income countries will depend primarily on availability of affordable antifungal agents in the hospital pharmacy. In Tanzania for example, the present guidelines for management of candidiasis include miconazole ointment, clotrimazole oral troches, 2% sodium benzoate solution, gentian violet solution, nystatin oral suspension, ketoconazole and fluconazole (MOH, 2005).

9.4.1.2. Other Fungal Infections

Several other opportunistic fungal infections have been reported in HIV infected patients, but majority of these infections have been reported in AIDS patients and with very low CD4 cell counts (below 200 cells/mm^3) (Manfredi et al., 1994, Ampel 1996, Hicks et al., 1997). Cryptococcosis, histoplasmosis, aspergillosis, geotrichosis and mucormycosis are well known systemic mycotic infections caused by *Cryptococcus neoformans*, *Histoplasma capsulatum*, *Aspergillus flavus*, *Geotricum candidum* and *Phycomycetes*. After candidiasis, cryptococcosis is the most frequently observed fungal infection in AIDS patients and has been reported in both developing and developed world including Sub-Saharan Africa (Ampel 1996). However mucormycosis, histoplasmosis, aspergillosis, and geotrichosis are rarely reported in Africa and occur in areas where these fungi are endemic such as southwestern United States and Central and South America (Ampel 1996). These deep seated fungal infections can affect the lung, central nervous system, skin, esophagus, maxillary sinuses and occasionally oral cavity and perioral regions of patients with HIV disease (Manfredi et al., 1994, Ampel 1996, Hicks et al., 1997).

Intraoral lesions of these systemic fungal infections present as single or multiple, deep oral lesions with the potential for considerable local tissue destruction. Intraoral lesions associated with cryptococcosis, histoplasmosis, and aspergillosis have been reported as being ulcerative, nodular, or necrotic in nature, whereas geotrichosis lesions are described as being pseudomembranous. Since oral lesions of this category are nonspecific, definitive diagnosis requires histological examination.

Treatment of these infections is generally by systemic antifungal therapy and surgical debridement of the infected and necrotic tissues. Treatment of choice depends on the condition and what may be available at low-income settings. Some drugs are very expensive and may not be available, like Caspofungin while others, like Amphotericin B, are less costly and can be offered.

Treatment is generally on the hands of physicians, amphotericin B followed by maintance therapy with fluconazole may be used in social disadvantaged communities (Ampel 1996). Due to its renal toxicity, parental Amphotericin B should be reserved for invasive fungal infections and oropharyngeal and esophageal candidiasis resistant to azole antifungal agents.

Table 9.4. Treatment options for oral Candida infections in HIV infected patients (Modified from: David A. Sirois (1998), Oral manifestations of HIV disease. 66: 322-332)

Antifungal agent	Route	Indication	Dose
Nystatin pastille	topical	erythematous and pseudomembranous	200,000 IU, 1 pastille 4 times daily for 14 days
Nystatin suspension	topical	erythematous and pseudomembranous	500,000 IU/5ml 4 times daily for 14 days
Clotrimazole troche	topical	erythematous and pseudomembranous	10 mg, 1 troche 5 times daily for 14 days
Miconazole cream 2%	topical	erythematous,	apply to affected area 4 times daily for 14 days
Clotrimazole cream 1%	topical	pseudomembranous and angular cheilitis	apply to affected area 4 times daily for 14 days
Amphotericin B	topical	erythematous and pseudomembranous	50 mg in 500 ml, rinse and spit out 3-6 times daily
Ketoconazole	Tablet	erythematous and pseudomembranous	100 mg once daily after meals for 14 days
Fluconazole	Tablet Parental	all intra-oral types or If no response to topical	150 mg once daily for 7-14 days or 750 mg Single dose
Itraconazole	Tablet Parental	fluconazole resistance	200 mg capsules once daily after a full meal
Voriconazole	Tablet Parental	fluconazole and itraconazole resistant	200 mg tablets twice daily for 7-14 days
Amphotericin B	systemic IV	no response to above therapy Invasive fungal infections	app. 0.3 mg/kg per day for 14 days

9.4.2. Viral Infections

9.4.2.1. Oral Hairy Leukoplakia

Oral hairy leukoplakia (OHL) is a white lesion found predominantly on the lateral margins of the tongue of HIV-infected individuals, induced by Epstein-Barr virus (EBV). OHL also has been reported on the floor of mouth or the buccal mucosa in AIDS patients. The loss of langerhan's cells has been reported to be important for its development. The occurrence of OHL is associated with moderately reduced CD4 cell numbers, and more frequent among homosexual or bisexual men. Clinically, it appears as a well-demarcated, corrugated white lesion varying from flat, plaque-like to papillary-villous which does not rub off and it is frequently confused with hyperplastic oral candidiasis. The lesion is asymptomatic. However, patients may complain of appearance and fuzzy feeling and sometimes can get super infected with bacteria that may cause a burning sensation. Diagnosis is mainly clinically; if the lesion is not apparent clinically biopsy may be indicated. Sometimes Candida infection is superimposed to OHL, which will complicate the diagnosis.

This asymptomatic lesion has no malignant potential and does not require treatment. However, for cosmetic purposes, some patients may request treatment. Several treatment options are available including systemic acyclovir. Also, topical applications of 25% podophyllum resin or 0.05% retinoids and surgical removal have all been reported as successful treatments as well. Recurrences are common. Studies have reported that the frequency of OHL decreases with the use of HAART. Patients on HAART that present with new OHL lesion may therefore be suspected for failing HIV treatment, although OHL have been documented in the context of an immune reconstitution inflammatory syndrome as well.

9.4.2.2. Herpes Simplex Infection (Orolabial Herpes)

Oral manifestations of herpes simplex virus type 1 (HSV-1) and type 2 (HSV-2) are found in both immunocompetent and immunodeficient individuals. However, HSV infections among immunocompromised individuals can present with more severe and extensive lesions than what is noticed in immunocompetent patients. HSV-1 is by far, the most common cause of the oral Herpes lesions, although HSV-2 that primarily occurs in the genital area can also cause recurrent lip and oral mucosal lesions. However, the diagnosis and treatment of these types do not differ. Individuals are usually exposed to HSV before puberty, generally during infancy or childhood. Once infected, the virus remains in a latent form in regional ganglia indefinitely. Later, Herpes simplex virus (HSV) infection is due to reactivation of latent HSV in regional ganglia.

Gingivostomatitis and pharyngitis are the most frequent clinical manifestations of first-episode HSV-1 infections whereas reactivations of HSV-1 often presents with recurrent herpes labialis. The primary oral HSV infection in immunocompetent individuals results in multiple, small, shallow ulcerations which usually coalesce to form a large ulcer, which heals uneventfully in 7-10 days. Reactivation of HSV in HIV-infected subjects may present with herpes labialis but also with intraoral lesions whereby the typical labial and intraoral lesions are more severe and last longer compared to immunocompetent patients.

Diagnosis is mainly clinically, but the diagnosis can be confirmed by viral culture and/or examination of a cytologic smear using immunohistochemistry. Herpetic ulcerations are often self-limiting, although use of antiviral medication is sometimes necessary to control the infection. Oral HSV infection responds well to systemic acyclovir. Acyclovir 200 - 400 mg orally three times daily for 7 days is indicated for mild and moderate cases of HSV and for severe and recurrent HSV higher dosages of acyclovir is recommended. Famciclovir and Valacyclovir are prodrugs with better bioavailability than acyclovir and that are converted into acyclovir after resorption. The patient may also need supportive care with antipyretic analgesics such as paracetamol or diclofenac.

9.4.2.3. Herpes (Varicella) Zoster (HZV) Infection

Hepes (Varicella) zoster infection is not specifically related to HIV but is also commonly observed among non-HIV infected individuals. In the latter group, Herpes Zoster usually involves only one dermatome that is not crossing the midline while in HIV-infected subjects multiple dermatomes may be involved. Intraoral ulcerations and facial manifestations (Orofacial) of HZV have been reported in patients with HIV/AIDS. Orofacial herpes zoster results from the reactivation of Varicella zoster virus of one of the divisions of the trigeminal nerve. No consistent associations have been documented between the appearance of these lesions and HIV disease progression. The diagnosis is usually established by clinical features of sudden onset, fever, pain, and the unilateral distribution of skin and mucosal lesions. Clinically, it is characterized by the appearance of clusters of vesicles that later become ulcerated; they are located along the distribution of a nerve branch. Intra- and extra-oral lesions may be present simultaneously and are particularly painful and serious in HIV-infected patients.

Given the higher rate of postherpetic neuralgia, recurrence and other complications such as spread to the ophthalmic branch of trigeminal nerve, systemic anti-herpes zoster therapy should be initiated as soon as possible. Involvement of the ophthalmic branch can be suspected if the tip of the nose or eyes has lesions as well. Systemic antiviral such as acyclovir or valaciclovir is the treatment of choice. Acyclovir 800 mg five times per day for 7 days may be used for uncomplicated herpes zoster. For disseminated HZV infection or ophthalmic nerve involvement, intravenous/ oral acyclovir 10 mg/kg/day 8 hourly for 7 days is used. In case of pain and post-herpetic pain analgesics such as amitryptiline 25-50 mg taken at night is indicated, also paracetamol or diclofenac. Long-term administration of anti-herpes drugs to prevent recurrences of herpes zoster is not routinely recommended in AIDS patients. VZV can also present as immune recovery inflammatory syndrome after HAART initiation and is therefore not a sign of failing regimen. Post-zoster neuropathy can significantly alter the quality of life.

9.4.2.4. Human Papilloma Virus

Intraoral and perioral warts in HIV patients are caused by Human Papilloma Virus (HPV). The most common HPV genotypes found in the mouth of patients with HIV infection are 2, 6, 11, 13, 16 and 32. HPV can be transmitted through oral sex with infected partner (oral-genital contacts). HPV causes focal epithelial and connective tissue hyperplasia, forming an oral wart. The wart-like growths are called condyloma tissues. Condyloma tissue appears like a small, cauliflower-type growth on the skin or mucosa. These growths are usually painless, but can cause some irritation, itching, or burning. The incidence of oral warts has increased in the HAART era (Greenspan et al., 2001). Oral warts are associated with increased CD4 cell counts in patients on antiretroviral therapy and its development may be related to immune reconstitution inflammatory syndrome. Clinically 3 types of warts are seen in HIV; cauliflower, spiky and flat (Greenspan et al., 1997). Most commonly the lesions are multiple, covering areas of the gingival, palate, buccal mucosa, the inside of the lips, and the skin surrounding the lips. The diagnosis is mainly made by history and clinical appearance.

Treatment of warts consists of surgical removal by excision for lesions that interfere with function or are of esthetic concern. Also, cryotherapy or Carbon dioxide laser may also be used but in underprivileged societies where facilities are lacking such therapy may not be available. Recurrences are common hence posing a significant challenge.

9.4.2.5. Cytomegalovirus (CMV) Infection

CMV is an uncommon cause of intraoral ulceration in HIV/AIDS patients. Oral lesions of CMV infection are associated with severe immune suppression with CD4 cell counts below 100 cells/mm^3. Oral CMV appears as solitary, without preceding vesicles, chronic deep ulceration most often involving the buccal and labial mucosa. These ulcers are painful and tend to heal poorly. Such lesions may represent early sign of disseminated CMV infection, which must be diagnosed as early as possible because of the serious nature of its sequelae, including retinitis and meningitis. Clinically, it is indistinguishable from other nonspecific ulcerations. Thus for definitive diagnosis viral culture, biopsy and histological examination are essential. Histologically shows basophilic intranuclear inclusions of CMV. Since oral lesions of CMV may be associated with disseminated disease, once an oral diagnosis is confirmed, the patient needs to be referred to an ophthalmologist for evaluation of CMV retinitis, which is a common cause of impaired vision in HIV-infected patients.

Systemic antiviral with gancyclovir is a treatment of choice. Gancyclovir may increase HAART toxicity (zidovudine) and therefore the combination of these agents demands considerable caution.

9.4.3. Bacterial Infections

Isolated cases of oral infection with *Klebsiella pneumoniae*, *Enterobacter cloacae*, *Actinomyces israelii*, *Escherichia coli* and *Mycobacterium avium intracellulare* have been reported in patients with HIV infection. However, the most common oral lesions associated with bacterial infection are periodontal diseases and followed by syphilis and bacillary epithelioid angiomatosis.

9.4.3.1. Periodontal Diseases (PD)

In HIV associated periodontal disease (PD) the bacterial flora is not differ from the flora of a non-immune compromised individual with PD. The clinical lesions in HIV associated PD are however manifestations of an altered immune response and include; linear gingival erythema (LGE), necrotizing ulcerative gingivitis (NUG) and necrotizing ulcerative periodontitis (NUP). LGE has been associated with a CD4 cell count of less than 200 cells/mm^3 but not with high viral loads, while NUG and NUP diseases are not associated with low CD4 cell counts or high viral loads. Apart from HIV induced immunosuppression, other habits such as tobacco smoking and poor oral hygiene also play a role in its etiology.

9.4.3.2. Linear Gingival Erythema (LGE)

LGE can be the early sign of HIV infection and is clinically characterized by distinctive red line (erythema) (1-3 mm wide) at the free gingival margin, often with petechiae. It is typically associated with no symptoms or only mild gingival bleeding and mild pain.

LGE differs from ordinary gingivitis in that it can be seen even with excellent oral hygiene and little or no plaque accumulation. The erythema in LGE unlike in ordinary gingivitis often persists following simple dental prophylaxis. Its treatment includes periodontal debridement by a dental professional; twice-daily rinses with a 0.12% chlorhexidine gluconate suspension for 2 weeks, and improved home oral hygiene.

9.4.3.3. Necrotizing Ulcerative Gingivitis (NUG) and
Necrotizing Ulcerative Periodontitis (NUP)

Several microorganisms are implicated as causative agents in this condition, especially anaerobic bacteria. The term, necrotising gingivitis refers to rapid soft tissue destruction, whereas the term, necrotising periodontitis refers to hard tissue destruction. These conditions are therefore jointly discussed as necrotising periodontal diseases (NPD). Both NUG and NUP are characterized by rapid, progressive destruction of periodontal tissues with sphacelus, loss of interdental papillae, intense pain, significant erythema that is often associated with spontaneous bleeding and a putrid odour. It follows an acute, rapidly progressive course, to the point of exposing bone and tooth loss when the periodontal structures are significantly destroyed. The clinical presentations in HIV-infected patients may resemble the lesions as seen in immune competent subjects but a more aggressive course with severe pain has been noticed as well. The destruction is not self-limiting and can result in loss of the entire alveolar process in the involved area.

NPD is an indicator of immunosuppression, but other factors such as poor oral hygiene, pre-existing periodontal status and smoking are involved in its etiopathogeny.

Treatment is built upon the foundation of four pillars:

1. Mechanical removal of necrotic tissue, plaque and calculus.
2. Oral antiseptics such as twice-daily rinses with a 0.12% chlorhexidine gluconate suspension for 2 weeks.
3. The use of broad-spectrum antibiotics, such as metronidazole (400 mg orally three times daily for 7 days), amoxicillin (500 mg orally three times daily for 7 days) or clindamycin.
4. Adhering to strict oral hygiene measures must be adhered to.

9.4.3.4. Syphilis

Syphilis is caused by the spirochete *Treponema pallidum* that is mainly transmitted by sexual contact. There are three stages following infection, primary, secondary, and tertiary and in all of these stages, oral and paraoral structures may be involved. The classic primary chancre begins at the site of inoculation and in homosexual men due to oral sex, the primary lesion may be found in the mouth where this painless lesion may remain unnoticed. The appearance of the primary lesion does not differ between HIV-positive and HIV-seronegative individuals. Chancres are mostly asymptomatic indurated ulcers with a brown crusted appearance that are usually seen on the lips, oral mucosa, tongue, palate, and posterior pharyngeal wall. Secondary syphilis is characterized by highly infectious mucosal ulcers with an appearance of white lesions surrounded by an erythematous base. Frank ulceration is most common in tertiary syphilis as a result of gummatous destruction. It is usually seen on the palate and tongue. The ulceration is often clinically indistinguishable from that due to tuberculosis, deep fungal infection or malignancy.

Dark field examination can be used to demonstrate Treponema Positive serological test, both Treponamal (TPHA, FTA) and non-treponemal tests (RPR) and histologic demonstration of *Treponema pallidum* are diagnostic. Patients should be referred to their physicians for evaluation and treatment. Treatment with Penicillin is treatment of choice, the dosage and duration of treatment depends on presence or absence of neurosyphilis.

9.4.3.5. Bacillary Epithelioid Angiomatosis (BEA)

This recently described lesion appears to be unique for HIV-infection and is often clinically indistinguishable from oral Kaposi's sarcoma (KS) since both may present as an erythematous, soft mass which may bleed upon gentle manipulation. Biopsy and histological examination are required to distinguish BEA from KS. The presumed etiological pathogen, *Rochalimae henselae*, can be identified using Warthin-Starry staining. Both KS and BEA are histologically characterized by atypical vascular channels, extravasated red blood cells and inflammatory cells. However, prominent spindle cells and mitotic figures occur only in KS. Erythromycin (500 mg four times daily for at least 10 days) is the treatment of choice for BEA. Clarithromycin and doxyciclin may also be used.

9.4.4. Neoplasm

9.4.4.1. Kaposi's Sarcoma (KS)

Kaposi's sarcoma (KS) is a low-grade vascular tumor associated with human herpes virus 8 (HHV-8). KS is an AIDS defining condition and the most common HIV associated neoplasm. The skin involvement is usual involved but extracutaneous spread of KS is common, particularly to the oral cavity, gastrointestinal tract and the respiratory tract. Sometimes only mucosal lesions are found while the skin is not affected. HHV-8 has been identified as the etiologic agent (Kaposi's sarcoma-associated herpes virus). The seroprevalence of HHV8 differs among the various populations in the world whereby the highest rates are found in Sub-Sahara Africa. KS can involve any oral site but most frequently involves the keratinized mucosa of the palate, gingiva, and dorsum of the tongue. The lesion may appear as a blue purple or red-purple macule, a nodule or mass that may ulcerate and cause local destruction (Figures 9.3 and 9.4). Progressing lesions can interfere with the normal functions of the oral cavity and become symptomatic secondary to trauma or infection.

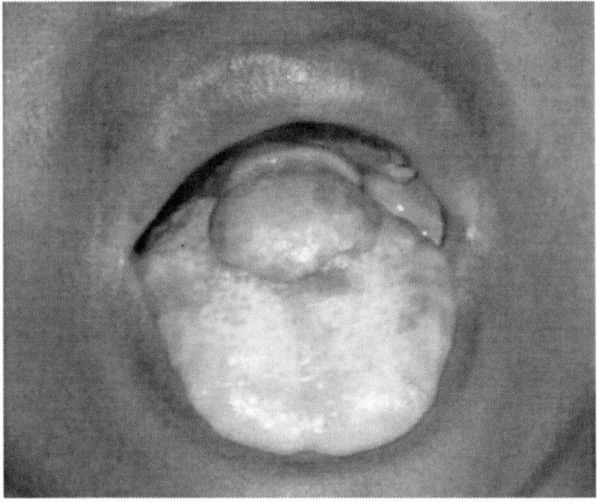

Figure 9.3. Kaposi's sarcoma tongue (a courtesy of O. Hamza).

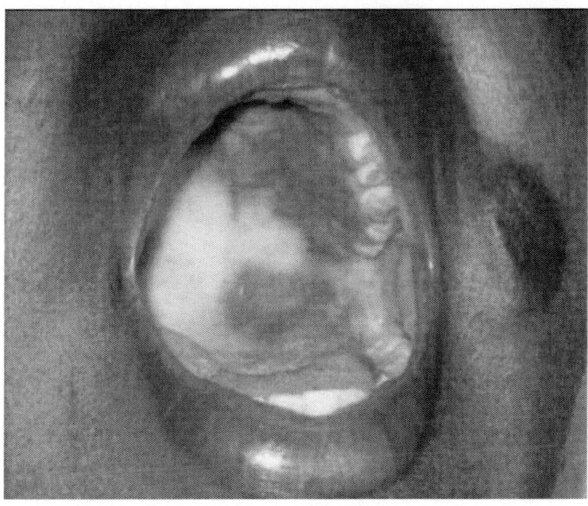

Figure 9.4. Kaposi's sarcoma palate and skin (a courtesy of O. Hamza).

The differential diagnosis includes ecchymosis, vascular lesions, and salivary gland tumors and the definitive diagnosis of KS requires therefore histological examination. There is no cure for KS, management is primarily palliative and directed towards alleviating pain and restoring normal function. Studies have shown reduction in incidence and prevalence of KS upon use of antiretroviral therapy (HAART). HAART is useful in management of HIV-related KS, as it reduces the HIV viral load and raises the CD4+ T-cell count, both of which contribute to the pathogenesis of KS. Treatment ranges from localized injections (intralessional) of chemotherapeutic agents such as vinblastine sulfate, to surgical removal. Small nodular lesions of the palate, not overlying neurovascular bundle, and lesions of the lips, tongue, or buccal mucosa/vestibule that interferes with speaking and eating may be surgically resected or debulked. Alternatively and for larger lesions that are not surgical candidates, intralesional injections of vinblastine sulfate or 3% sodium tetradecyl sulfate is recommended. Local therapy may be effective for limited disease, but systemic therapy is required for disseminated KS. Thus, referral to a medical specialist (for example, medical oncology, or radiation oncology) for evaluation and possible systemic chemotherapy or local radiotherapy may be warranted. Radiotherapy is can be used to control the size and number of lesions but stomatitis and glossitis are common side effects of radiation.

9.4.4.2. Non-Hodgkin's Lymphoma (NHL)

NHL is the second most common malignancy associated with HIV infection and is recognized as an AIDS-defining condition. NHL occurs in a younger age group of HIV-infected patients compared with NHL in non-HIV infected individuals. The risk to develop NHL is also increased in patients that are successfully treated with HAART and there is strong evidence for an etiological role of Epstein-Barr virus (EBV). Oral NHL presents with intra-oral soft tissue masses with or without ulceration and tissue necrosis whereby the palatal, gingival and alveolar mucosas are mostly involved (Figures 9.5 and 9.6). NHL may be indistinguishable from masses caused by KS or other diseases in HIV-infected patients and histological examination is therefore essential for the diagnosis. Treatment options include chemotherapy and radiotherapy for which the patient needs to be referred to a specialist.

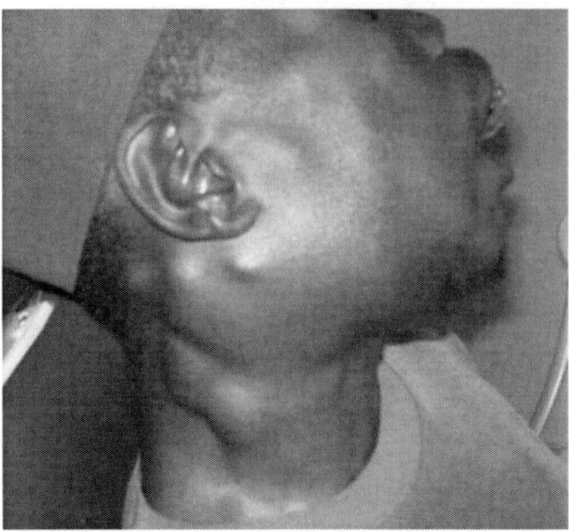

Figure 9.5. Non Hodgkin's lymphoma (a courtesy of O. Hamza).

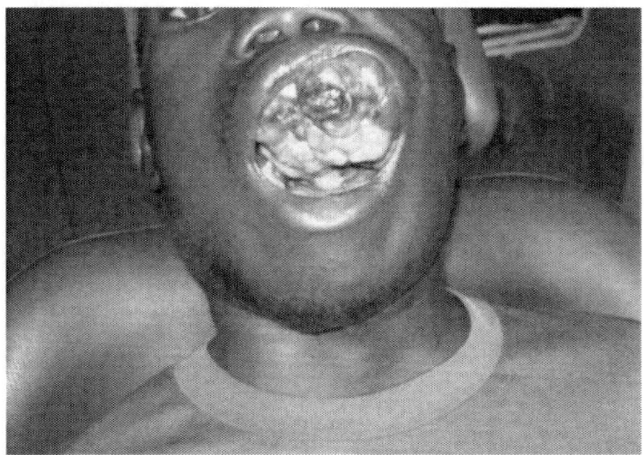

Figure 9.6. Non Hodgkin's lymphoma (a courtesy of O. Hamza).

9.4.5. Immune-Mediated Oral Lesions

HIV-infection is characterized by progressive cellular immunodeficiency making an individual more susceptible for certain infections. On the other hand, it has been suggested that some lesions appear as a result of an inflammatory response whereby the etiological agent may not be defined.

9.4.5. 1. Aphthous Ulcers (AU)

Recurrent aphthous ulcerations appear on non-keratinized, or non-fixed, tissues such as the labial or buccal mucosa, floor of the mouth, ventral surface of the tongue, posterior oropharynx, and maxillary and mandibular vestibule. There are three forms, Herpertiform, Minor and Major.

9.4.5. 2. Major Apthous Ulceration

Major apthous ulceration is the most common observed immune-mediated HIV related oral disorder. The large solitary or multiple, chronic, deep, painful ulcerations of major aphthae appear identical to those in non-infected patients, but they often last much longer and are less responsive to therapy. The lesions are characterized by a halo of inflammation and a yellow-gray pseudomembranous covering. Large aphthae are associated with advanced HIV infection (typically with CD4+ counts of less than 50 cells/mm^3). They are very painful, especially during consumption of salty, spicy, or acidic foods and beverages, or hard or rough foods. Due to its associated pain, it limits the patients' dietary intake. Diagnosis is mainly clinically, however, biopsy for histological examination may be indicated if the lesion mimics malignant disease.

Treatment requires topical corticosteroids such as clobetesol (0.05% ointment applied for 45 seconds 3 times daily) or dexamethasone oral rinse (0.5 mg/5 ml dexamethasone elixir 3 times daily, rinse for 1 minute and expectorate). Systemic corticosteroids therapy is required when multiple ulcers are present or response to topical treatment is incomplete Systemic prednisolone may however also lead to complications such as oral candidiasis and/or reactivation of tuberculosis. Alternative therapy such as dapsone 50-100 mg daily for 4 weeks can also be considered.

9.4.6. HIV-Related Salivary Gland Disease

HIV infection is affecting the salivary gland HIV-related salivary gland disease (HIV-SGD) describes xerostomia and benign (unilateral or bilateral) salivary gland enlargement in HIV-infected patients. The prevalence of HIV-SGD is reported to be higher in pediatric HIV-infected patients than adult patients.

9.4.6.1. Salivary Gland Enlargement

The parotid gland is mostly affected while the submandibular gland is rarely affected. Enlargement typically involves the tail of the parotid gland and is usually bilaterally (figure 9.7). Patients with salivary gland enlargement may present with or without xerostomia. The swelling arises as a consequence of a variety of etiologies, including reactive/inflammatory conditions, infections and neoplasms. While the appearance may raise suspicion of malignancy (salivary gland carcinoma or lymphoma), aspiration of a yellow mucinous secretion supports a non-malignant cause. Malignancy is suspected when lesion progressively increases in size and ulcerates and in these cases biopsy is necessary to make a proper diagnosis. Of particular concern are lymphoma and Kaposi's sarcoma, both of which have been reported in the salivary glands of HIV-infected individuals. Benign parotid hypertrophy is especially seen in children and may be a manifestation of diffuse infiltrative CD8+ lymphocytosis syndrome (DILS). Histology reveals hyperplastic lymph nodes, lymphocytic infiltrates and cystic cavities. Parotid enlargement may also occur after initiation HAART as part of an immune reconstitution inflammatory syndrome.

The treatment of the benign parotid hypertrophy remains non-specific and primarily symptomatic. Occasionally swelling can be managed by repeated aspiration, and rarely radical removal of the gland is necessary.

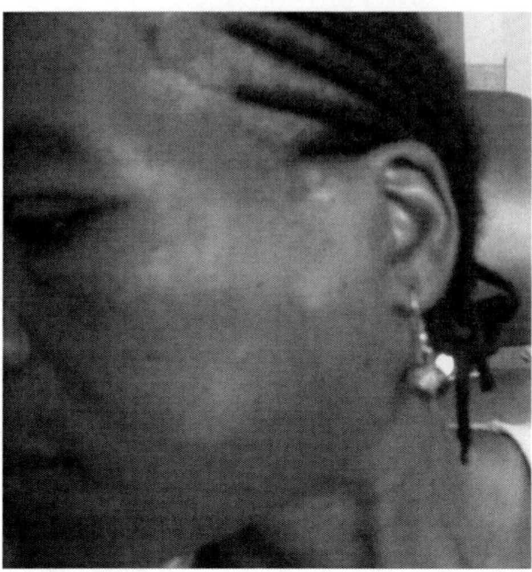

Figure 9.7. Parotid gland enlargement (a courtesy of O. Hamza).

9.4.6.2. Xerostomia

Reduced salivary flow, leading to xerostomia or dry mouth, is a common finding in HIV infected patients. Dryness present a significant risk factor for caries, periodontal diseases, oral candidiasis, mucosal injury, impaired ability to chew, dysphagia and reduced food intake.

Xerostomia can occur as result of side effects of medications, or because of significant major salivary gland disease. Several antiretroviral agents have been associated with impaired salivary flow, including didanosine, zidovudine and different protease inhibitors (PIs). The mechanism by which antiretroviral therapy causes xerostomia is not completely understood, but it has been speculated that PIs have an antisecretory effect upon acinar cells and/or induce parotid lipomatosis that alter salivary gland structure and function. Many other non-antiretroviral agents, such as antidepressants and antihypertensive may however also cause xerostomia as well as (previous) radiation therapy that included salivary glands in the field. Human immunodeficiency virus (HIV) infection is often accompanied by autoimmune phenomena such as Sjögren-like syndrome (SLS), characterized by subjective symptoms of xerostomia and xerophthalmia that may be accompanied clinically by unilateral or bilateral parotid gland enlargement. HAART may have reduced the occurrence of this syndrome.

The clinical diagnosis is made on the basis of little or no saliva pooling in the floor of mouth at rest and appearance of dry oral mucosa during clinical examination.

Symptomatic relief from oral dryness can be achieved by continuously sipping water or administration of saliva substitutes. Stimulation of saliva flow can sometimes be accomplished by chewing sugarless gum or sucking on sugarless candies. Cholinergic agonists such as bethanechol and pilocarpine can also be used. Discontinuation of xerostomia-inducing medications should also be tried after consultation with patient's physician. To prevent caries and periodontal diseases, fluoride rinse and oral hygiene instructions could be advised. The use of topical fluorides such as fluoridated toothpaste, fluoride rinses in HIV infected patients with xerostomia is critical to control dental caries.

9.4.7. Other Lesions

9.4.7.1. Melanotic Hyperpigmentation (HIV Oral Melanosis)

Melanotic hyperpigmentation of oral mucosa have been reported in 2-5% of HIV-infected patients. They appear as well defined brown-black macules. The buccal mucosa is the most frequently affected site, but the gingiva, palate, and tongue may also be involved. The etiology remains undetermined, but may be due to medications taken such as zidovudine, or as a direct result of the virus. Addison's disease is a rare cause of oral hyperpigmentation whereby infiltration of the adrenal glands by mycobacteria or fungi may underlie this process. Like all diffuse melanoses, HIV-associated pigmentation is microscopically characterized by basilar melanin pigment, with incontinence into the underlying submucosa. No treatment is needed.

References

Ampel NM (1996). Emerging disease issue and fungal pathogens associated with HIV infection. *Emerging Infect Dis.* 2: 109-116.

Brawner DL, Cutler JE (1989). Oral *Candida albicans* isolates from nonhospitalized normal carriers, immunocompetent hospitalized patients, and immunocompromised patients with or withoutacquired immunodeficiency syndrome. *J. Clin. Microbiol.* 27:1335-1341.

Campo J, Del Romero J, Castilla J, Garcia S, Rodriguez C, Bascones A (2002). Oral candidiasis as a clinical marker related to viral load, CD4 lymphocyte count and CD4 lymphocyte percentage in HIV-infected patients. *J. Oral Pathol. Med.* 31:5-10.

Cartledge JD, Middle J, Gazzard BG (1999). Non-albicans oral candidosis in HIV-positive patients. *J. Antimicrob. Chemother.* 43: 419-422.

CDC (1999). Guidelines for national human immunodeficiency virus case surveillance, including monitoring for human immunodeficiency virus infection and acquired immunodeficiency syndrome. *MMWR Morb. Mortal Wkly Rep.* 48(RR-13): 1-27, 29-31.

Cruz GD, Lamster IB, Begg, MD, Phelan JA, Gorman JM, and El-Sadr W. (1996). The accurate diagnosis of oral lesions in human immunodeficiency virus infection. *Journal of the American Medical Association*, 112, 68-73.

Coulter ID, Heslin KC, Marcus M, Hays RD, Freed J, Der-Martirosia C, et al., (2002). Associations of self-reported oral health with physical and mental health in a nationally representative sample of IIIV persons receiving medical care. *Quality of Life Research.* 11:57-60.

EC-Clearinghouse on Oral Problems Related to HIV Infection and WHO Collaborating Centre on Oral Manifestations of the Immunodeficiency Virus (1993). Classification and diagnostic criteria for oral lesions in HIV infection. *J. Oral Pathol. Med.* 22: 289-91.

Fichtenbaum CJ, Koletar S, Yiannoutsos C *et al.* (2000). Refractory mucosal candidiasis in advanced human immunodefficiency virus infection. *Clin Infect Dis.* 30: 749-56.

Greenspan D, and Greenspan JS. (1997). Oral manifestations of HIV disease. *AIDS Clinical Care*, 9(4), 29-33.

Greenspan D, Canchola AJ, MacPhail LA, Cheikh B, and Greenspan JS. (2001). Effects of highly active antiretroviral therapy on frequency of oral warts. *Lancet*, 357(9266), 1411-1412.

Hamza OJM, Matee MIN, Simon ENM, et al., (2006). Oral manifestations of HIV infection in children and adults receiving highly active anti-retroviral therapy [HAART] in Dar es Salaam, Tanzania. *BMC Oral Health.* 6,12.

Hamza OJM, Matee MI, Brüggemann RJ, Moshi MJ, Simon ENM, et al., (2008). Single-dose fluconazole versus standard 2-week therapy for oropharyngeal candidiasis in HIV-infected patients: A randomized, double-blind, double-dummy trial. *Clinical Infectious Diseases* 47: 1270-1276.

Hicks MJ, Flaitz CM, Cohen PR (1997). Perioral and cutaneous umbilicated papular lesions in acquired immunodeficiency. *Oral Surg., Oral Med., Oral Path., Oral Radiol. and Endod.* 83: 189-191.

Hodgson TA, Naidoo S, Chidzonga M, Ramos Gomez F, Shiboski C (2006). Identification of oral health care needs in children and adults, management of oral diseases. *Advances in Dental Research.* 19: 106-117.

King MD, Reznik DA, O'Daniels CM, Larsen NM, Osterholt D, Blumberg HM (2002). Human papillomavirus-associated oral warts among human immunodeficiency virus-seropositive patients in the era of highly active antiretroviral therapy: An emerging infection. *Clin Infect Dis*, 34: 641-648.

Matee MI, Scheutz F, Moshy J (2000). Occurrence of oral lesions in relation to clinical and immunological status among HIV-infected adult Tanzanians. *Oral Dis.* 6:106-111.

Manfredi R, Mazzoni A, Cavicchi O, Santini D, Chiodo F (1994). Invasive mycotic and actinomycotic orophayngeal and craniofacial infection in two patients with AIDS. *Mycoses.* 37:209-215.

Ministry of Health, the United Republic of Tanzania, NACP (2005). National Guidelines for Clinical Management of HIV/AIDS. 2:66-75.

Patton LL, McKaig R, Strauss R, Rogers D, and Eron JJ. (2000). Changing prevalence of oral. manifestations of human immunodeficiency virus in the era of protease inhibitor therapy. *Oral Surgery, Oral Medicine, Oral Pathology, Oral Radiology, and Endodontics*, 89(3), 299-304.

Ramirez-Amador V, Esquivel-pedraza L, Sierra-Madero J, Anaya-Saavedra G, Gonzalez-Ramirez I, Ponce-de-Leon S: The changing clinical spectrum of Human Immunodeficiency Virus [HIV]-related oral lesions in 1,000 consecutive patients: A 12-year study in a referral Center in Mexico. *Medicine- [Baltimore]* 2003, 82: 39-50.

Ramos-Gomez FJ, Flaitz C, Capatano P et al., (1999). Classification, diagnostic criteria, and treatment recomendations for orofacial manifestations in HIV-infected paediatric patients. *J. Clin. Pediatr. Dent.*; 18: 121-126.

Reznik DA. (1999). Recognition and management of the most common oral manifestations of HIV infection. Available: http://www.hivdent.org.

Samaranayake LP, Fidel PL, Naglik JR, Sweet SP *et al.* (2000). Fungal infections associated with HIV infection. *Oral Dis.* 8: 151-160.

Schiodt M, Bakilana PB, Hiza JF, Shao JF, Bygbjerg I, Mbaga I, Vestergaard BF, Nielsen CM, Lauritzen E, Lerche B, Kuijlen K (1990). Oral candidiasis and Hairy leukoplakia correlate with HIV infection in Tanzania. *Oral Surg. Oral. Med Oral Pathol.* 69:591-596.

Schmidt-Westhausen AM, Priepke F, Bergmann FJ, Reichart PA. Decline in the rate of oral opportunistic infections following introduction of highly active antiretroviral therapy. *J. Oral Pathol. Med.* 2000, 31:336–341.

Shetty K, Leigh J: The Changing Face of Oral Lesions in HIV/AIDS Patients Undergoing Highly Active Antiretroviral Treatment. *AIDS Patient Care STDS* 2000, 14: 627-635.

Singh A, Bairy I, Shivananda PG (2003). Spectrum of opportunistic infections in AIDS cases. *Indian J. Med. Sci.* 57: 16-21.

Tappuni AR, Fleming GJ (2001). The effect of antiretroviral therapy on the prevalence of oral manifestations in HIV-infected patients. A UK study. *Oral Surg. Oral Med. Oral Pathol. Oral Radiol. Endod.* 92: 623-628.

UNAIDS (2008): Report on the global AIDS epidemic.

WHO Acquired immunodeficiency syndrome (AIDS) (1990). Interim proposal for a WHO staging system for HIV infection and disease. *Wkly. Epidemiol. Rec.* 65: 221-228.

In: Oral Health Care for Socially Disadvantaged Communities   ISBN: 978-1-62948-287-3
Editors: F.K. Kahabuka, E.N. Kikwilu and I. Anderson © 2013 Nova Science Publishers, Inc.

Chapter X

Feasible Preventive Methods for Controlling Oral Diseases and Conditions in Socially Disadvantaged Comunities

Evelyn Wagaiyu[1] and Emil Kikwilu[2]
[1] College of Dental Sciences, Nairobi University
[2] School of Dentistry, Muhimbili University of Health and Allied Sciences

10.1. Introduction

The world today has witnessed many preventive methods or interventions for combating oral diseases that have been tested and proved useful in different settings. There is also ample evidence that point to the fact that for interventions to be successful, they must be attuned to suit the conditions or circumstances that prevail in a community in which they are being implemented. The aim of this chapter is to review the preventive interventions in oral health so as to sort out these that can suit the circumstances prevailing in socially disadvantaged communities.

It stresses the importance of common risk approach in the design and implementation of interventions in socially disadvantaged communities as a means of obtaining quick acceptance of the intervention by the community, as well as maximizing the merger resources in these communities which are usually hard hit by poverty. It is expected that this chapter will assist a reader to appreciate the importance of common risk approach in designing interventions, as well as assist him/her in identifying suitable interventions for use in socially disadvantaged communities to quicken the global goal of improving quality of life among all citizens of the globe.

10.2. Overview of the Burden of Oral Diseases

The most common oral diseases and conditions in the world include dental caries, periodontal diseases, oral cancers, dental trauma and developmental irregularities. The following few examples that were summarized by WHO in year 2007 show the magnitude of some of these diseases and conditions:

- 60-90% of school children worldwide had dental cavities.
- Severe periodontal (gum) disease, which may result in tooth loss, was found in 5-20% of middle-aged adults; the rate varies across geographical regions.
- Incidence of oral cancer ranged from one to 10 cases per 100 000 population in most countries.
- Birth defects such as cleft lip and palate occurred in around one per 500-700 of all births; the birth prevalence rate varies substantially across ethnic groups and geographical areas (http://www.who.int/mediacentre/factsheets/fs318/en/).

Recent literature indicate that in the majority of countries the greatest burden of oral diseases and conditions is among socially disadvantaged communities (Reisine et al 2001, Amaral et al 2005, Conway 2008, Clarke et al 2009, Mtaya et al 2009, Mashoto et 2010, Sabbah et al 2010, Mamai-Homata et al 2010). There is also indisputable evidence that the occurrence and severity of oral diseases and conditions are greatly influenced by the lifestyles of an individual person and the community in which he/she lives (Turnbull 1995, Locker D. 2000, Johnson et al 2004, Reichart et al 2008, Hujoel et al 2009, Ruxton et al 2010). Therefore a large proportion of the population could live to their old age without being afflicted by these diseases and conditions if they adopted lifestyles conducive to oral health as from their childhood. Sociologic and behavioural interventional approaches to prevention of oral diseases and conditions are required to attain this assertion.

10.3. Overview of Preventive
Methods in Oral Health

Scientists and public oral health specialists have, for decades, worked tirelessly to design and test methods for preventing oral diseases and conditions. These can be broadly classified into three levels: Primary, secondary and tertiary preventive methods.

10.3.1. Primary prevention includes all interventions aimed at preventing disease from occurring. These interventions aim at reducing or eliminating the etiologic, risk and predisposing factors, and promote factors that favour good oral health (Hu et al 1998, Chestnutt et al 1998, Petersen et al1999, Lopez et al 1999, Isokangas et al 2000, Kowash et al 2000). To achieve this aim, these interventions may target at individuals as in chair-side health education; community as in the mass media educational programmes, specific groups as in oral health education to school children (Petersen et al 2004) and mothers attending the reproductive and child health; environment as in promoting sugar free snack sales at school premises (Kwan et al 2005), and policies as in advocating reduction of taxes on toothpaste.

The key themes that feature in Ottawa Charter as pillar of health promotion fall under this level of prevention (WHO 1986).

10.3.1.1. In prevention of dental caries, interventions that fall under primary prevention include: reduction of consumption of in between meals sugary snacks; encouraging tooth brushing with fluoridated tooth paste at least twice a day – morning and evening before retiring to bed with minimal rinsing after brushing (Chestnutt et al 1998, Marinho et al 2003, Twetman et al 2003, Zero DT 2006); creating sugar free school environment by discouraging sales of sugary snacks, and offering alternative sugar free snack sales at school premises and provision of routine school meals (Belot et al 2011, Stevens et al 2011); instituting water fluoridation projects; reducing taxation for tooth brushes and fluoridated toothpaste in view of raising their routine use among populations (Goldmn et al 2008); educating communities on causes of tooth decay and available means for preventing dental caries to enable them make informed decisions about their oral health; and advocacy aimed at increased use of fluoridated tooth paste and tooth brushes.

10.3.1.2. In prevention of periodontal diseases, interventions that fall under primary prevention include: reinforcing daily and effective tooth brushing; advocating diets rich in vegetables and fruits; instituting measures to prevent diabetes; anti-smoking and anti-HIV/AIDS campaigns and discouraging excessive alcohol consumption (Petersen et al 2005).

10.3.1.3. In prevention of oral cancer, interventions such as anti-tobacco and anti-HIV/AIDS campaigns; discouraging excessive alcohol consumption; discouraging diets rich in fat; encouraging high intake of foods containing vitamin A or its precursor β-carotene; encouraging diets rich in fiber and vitamin C; and prevention of iron deficiency constitute primary prevention (WHO, 2005).

10.3.1.4. In prevention of Dentofacial irregularities (Malocclusions) the following interventions constitute primary prevention: provision of balanced diets to pregnant mothers and children to ensure optimal formation and maturation of the dentition; discouraging smoking and alcohol consumption among child bearing women to reduce risks for genetic aberrations to developing fetus; discouraging habits that may lead to distorted arrangement of teeth like thumb and finger sucking; avoiding early loss of primary teeth by preventing dental caries in primary dentition to allow natural exfoliation time to prevent loss of space for their successors.

10.3.1.5. Dental trauma is always accidental, and the majority of dental traumas seem to be non-preventable. Majority of dental trauma occur to the upper anterior teeth due to accidents leading to collisions, falls during normal play by children, and falls during causal home activities like moping smooth and slippery floors. Protruding anterior teeth due to thumb sucking or genetic variations is a predisposing factor. Information to communities about first-aid treatment to a trauma victim and immediate professional care appears to be essential.

10.3.2. Secondary prevention includes interventions that are targeted at stopping the progression of the disease that has already established itself. In dentistry secondary prevention mainly requires professional intervention. In dental caries prevention, interventions that fall under secondary prevention include: professional prophylaxis (professional tooth cleaning and application of fluoride varnishes to arrest rampant caries in children); fissure sealant application to pits and fissures with initial carious lesions. In prevention of periodontal diseases, interventions like scaling and root planning to patients with periodontal pockets constitute secondary prevention. In prevention of oral cancer, dental trauma and Dentofacial irregularities, secondary prevention does not exist in practice.

10.3.3. Tertiary prevention includes interventions that are targeted at reducing the disabilities caused by disease process. In dental caries prevention, interventions that fall under tertiary prevention include removal of carious tooth tissues and replacing it with appropriate filling material; root canal treatment and extraction of carious lesions. In prevention of periodontal diseases, interventions that fall under tertiary prevention include periodontal surgery and implants. In prevention of oral cancer, interventions that fall under tertiary prevention are mainly surgical interventions and radiotherapy. In the prevention of dental trauma, interventions that fall under tertiary prevention include prophylactic and treatment measures to trauma cases.

10.4. Merits and Demerits of Preventive Methods in View of Social Disadvantage

Socially disadvantaged communities are generally hard hit by resource limitations compared to socially advantaged communities. Families and individuals strive to earn a daily meal, and can hardly avail or save money for health care. Unemployment is rampart, and those employed, are usually deployed in risky tasks and manual labor with low wages. They are usually less educated, less able to assimilate health information, therefore more likely to indulge in health risky behaviors (Sounders et al 2006). Dentist is not well known by the majority of the people, therefore beliefs and misinformation about dentistry dominate (Kikwilu et al 2009). Majority of the people are not health insured, and seek care only when in intolerable pain. The general health is usually poor, with high prevalence of communicable and non-communicable diseases. The meager resource set for health care is usually used to treat people suffering from communicable life threatening diseases, therefore oral health care receive little budgetary attention. The oral health personnel as well as the oral health care facilities are usually sparsely distributed in these communities, thus not easily accessible by majority of people (Kikwilu et al 2008).

In view of the above description of the socially disadvantaged communities, the choice of any oral health intervention for such communities must take into consideration the resource limitations prevailing in socially disadvantaged communities and the associated factors that may hinder the adoption of oral health interventions. Given the menu of the available preventive interventions summarized under the Overview of preventive methods in section two above, interventions that fall under primary prevention seem to be of the first choice for these communities. To maximize the benefits of the selected interventions in view of limited resources, one needs to identify interventions that can address two or more oral health problems at once, or those interventions that address oral and general health problems simultaneously as advocated in the common risk approach (Sheiham A. 1992, Cinar et al 2009, Watt 2005, Cane et al 2004, Petersen PE 2004a, Petersen PE 2004b, dela Cruiz et al 2004, Petersen et al 2005).

The interventions falling under secondary and tertiary prevention in dentistry require trained oral health personnel as well as high investments in terms of resources. Expecting interventions under secondary and tertiary prevention to be fully implemented in socially disadvantaged communities in near future is being a bit overambitious. Therefore only interventions under secondary and tertiary prevention that target at pain relief should be undertaken as a matter of moral obligation to reduce suffering among socially disadvantaged communities. For example, governments could be urged to provide much cheaper restorative care by ensuring that the few dental practitioners available in socially disadvantaged communities are empowered with knowledge and skills on Atraumatic Restorative Treatment (ART) technique which use only hand instruments to clean the dental caries cavity by removing carious tooth tissues and subsequently restoring the cleaned cavity with an adhesive glass ionomer cement (Frencken et al 1996). Since ART do not require electricity and piped water supply, restorative care can easily be undertaken in dental clinics even if these clinics do not have dental equipment, instruments and utilities required by conventional restorative care. In addition to ART, dental clinics could also be supplied with tooth extraction forceps to allow dental practitioners undertake pain relieving by extracting teeth are hopelessly decayed and cannot be restored by ART.

Due to sparsely distributed dental clinics and dental personnel, outreach programs should be emphasized to enable few dental practitioners reach people in far distances to fulfill their moral obligation of relieving suffering from toothache. These dental practitioners could be facilitated by providing them with the cheapest means of transport to enable them carry along with them the dental extraction instruments and ART hand instruments. In this way, practitioners could take the essential dental services close to people in remote areas. Through ART, dental practitioners undertaking outreach programs would be able to save majority of socially disadvantage people from suffering due to pain arising from open dental carious cavities. These dental practitioners would also be able to relieve suffering arising from painful teeth that are hopelessly decayed to the extent that they cannot be saved through ART restoration by extracting them.

10.5. Suitable Combinations of Interventions That Can Be Applicable in Socially Disadvantaged Communities

All means should be taken to ensure that the intervention program proposed for socially disadvantaged community is cost effective and affordable by the community in question. As much as possible multi-sector approaches must be considered in first place over mono-sector approaches. The concept of common risk approach must be fully utilized to maximize resources There is accumulated evidence that improved oral hygiene practices prevent periodontal disease (van Palenstein et al 1991, Sheen et al 2001, Deery et al 2004), dental caries (Chestnutt et al 1998, van Loveren et al 2001) and adverse outcomes of pregnancy (Iida et al 2009, Heimonen et al 2009, Chan et al 2010, Han et al 2010). Tobacco control reduces the risk of periodontal disease (Iida et al 2009, Malhotra et al 2010), oral (Ljung et la 2011, de Souza et al 2011, Biazevic et al 2011, Jaber et al 2011, Scully C. 2010) and lung cancer (Cataldo et al 2010, Waller et al 2010, Kiyohara et al 2010, Klingerman et al 2011), heart (Pipe ct al 2010, Prassad et al 2009) and lung diseases (Washko et al 2011), adverse outcomes of pregnancy (Suter et al 2010, England et al 2010). Balanced diet has been shown to be important in proper development of dentition, reduced risks of systemic diseases and adverse outcomes of pregnancy (de Onis et al 1998, Theobald HE 2007, Yacoob et al 2009). Since the occurrence of oral diseases have common risk factors with several systemic diseases, oral and general health workers should team up to control multiple ill health using single interventional programs.

10.5.1. Common Preventive Interventional Programs against Frequent and Excessive Sugar Consumption for Control of Dental Caries and Chronic Systemic Diseases

Frequent sugar consumption has been associated with development and progression of dental caries in human population because sugar consumption provides substrate for microorganisms present in the oral cavity that is required for their metabolism. Lactic and acetic acids are the main by products of metabolism by these microorganisms that use sugar. These acids when produced are released in the oral environment. It is the presence of these acids in the vicinity of the tooth that cause mineral loss to the tooth surface. When the mineral loss happens for many times, the tooth surface becomes weak and subsequently breaks easily under mechanical pressure to form a defect known as dental caries or cavity. Frequent sugar consumption also provides excess energy to many individuals that is transformed and deposited as fat in various parts of the body leading to obesity. Obesity has been shown to have adverse consequences to general health. Obesity has strong association with development of type 2 diabetes, some cancers, and heart and liver diseases.

Both these diseases impose a burden to the wellbeing of populations including reduced productivity and financial costs for attending to persons who fall sick due to these diseases. Authorities taking care of socially disadvantaged communities should adopt interventions that will pool resources from both general and oral health budgets to spearhead the campaigns aimed at advocating judicious use of sugar to reduce both dental caries and obesity. Measures such as advocating for sugar free environment in schools, availing sugar free alternative snacks in public places, and promoting non-sugar sweeteners may save to reduce incidence of dental caries and obesity. Messages that inform communities on the detrimental effect of sugar consumption in a holistic way are likely to win attention of many people than messages implicating sugar and dental caries only.

10.5.2. Promoting Oral Hygiene Practices as Part of General Hygiene and Glooming for Control of Periodontal Disease, Dental Caries and Infectious Diseases Related to Poor Body Hygiene

In many societies, people clean their teeth not because they know the importance of oral hygiene in the control of periodontal disease and dental caries, rather they clean their teeth because they want to keep themselves clean, with nor bad breath from mouth as they interact with their members of the society. Information capitalizing cleanliness to improve social acceptability is likely to attract many of the people, rather than asking them to do so in order to prevent periodontal disease and dental caries.

Toothpaste manufacturers and distributors are of great importance in increasing the use of toothpaste among populations. They are well training in marketing strategies, and if assisted with key messages related to health they can be the best agents for improving oral and general hygiene, while at the same time improving the use of fluoridated toothpaste. This will in turn improve the prevention of periodontal disease and dental caries among the targeted communities.

Collaboration between distributors of toothpaste, national bureau of standards and dental professionals to ensure that the toothpaste distributed has therapeutic dose of fluoride will achieve the prevention of dental caries through toothpaste use. This can be reinforced by giving an approval seal to the toothpaste that meet the recommended free fluoride content in toothpaste.

Advocating use of toothpaste alone may not be a sufficient drive for majority of people who are socially disadvantaged to regularly use toothpaste at a rate that it can lead to dental caries prevention. This is because of the low purchasing power of majority of socially disadvantaged families and individuals. In view of this fact, dental professional associations should negotiate with the government to reduce taxes for toothpaste and tooth brushes to enable more people to purchase toothpaste. These efforts should be ascribed to toothpaste brands that meet the specified free fluoride content, and therefore certified by seal of approval.

This will increase the affordability, accessibility and acceptability of the toothpaste by majority of the population. In this way more and more socially disadvantaged individuals, families and communities can use the fluoridated toothpaste, with the ultimate goal of preventing dental caries and periodontal disease in these communities.

10.5.3. Interventions against Use of Different Forms of Tobacco and Excessive Alcohol Consumption to Prevent Periodontal Disease, Oral and Lung Cancer, Heart and Liver Diseases

There is ample evidence in literature on the association between tobacco use and oral and lung cancer, periodontal and heart diseases. There is also ample evidence in literature on the association between excessive alcohol consumption and liver and periodontal diseases, and oral cancer.

Campaigns against smoking and excessive use of alcohol should be undertaken jointly by both dental and medical profession and other social groups to ensure that advertisements that foster tobacco and alcohol use are kept to minimum if not abolished. Other efforts could be imposition of high taxes on tobacco and alcohol products to discourage indiscriminate use of these products among socially disadvantaged communities.

These campaigns when successful will reduce the prevalence and severity of periodontal disease, oral and other cancers, and morbidity and mortality among the socially disadvantaged communities.

All stakeholders should be made aware that instituting such campaigns that benefit the control of multiple diseases and conditions are more rewarding than single targeted campaigns especially in socially disadvantaged communities with limited resources.

10.5.4. Interventions to Raise the Nutritional Status of Individuals and Families in Socially Disadvantaged Communities for Controlling Dental Caries, Periodontal and Systemic Diseases, Oral and Other Cancers

Joint campaigns aimed at attaining balanced diets among families and individuals are a key to combating many oral and systemic diseases in communities. Balanced diets ensure optimal development and maturation of the body as a whole, and teeth and periodontium in particular. Well formed and matured dentition is more resistant to dental caries attack than dentition with hypoplastic teeth. Poorly nourished children have been shown to be more affected by Ulcerative Gingivitis including noma compared to well-nourished children. Deformed teeth may present various forms of malocclusion such as peg lateral, and hypodontia. Iron deficiency has adverse effects to general health. In addition, it is a risk factor for oral cancer. Balanced diet also provides essential nutrients for repair and renewal of body tissues including the periodontal tissues. In addition, it ensures sufficient supply of compounds essential for the maintenance of immune system for improved resistance of the body to infections as well as tumor proliferation. Vitamin A and its precursor β-carotene, for example, are important in prevention of oral cancer initiation and progression.

Oral health information to communities about oral health is an obligation of all oral health professionals. Correct oral health messages can easily reach populations who has habits for regular dental check-ups. In socially disadvantaged communities such habit is not developed, and as pointed above, the oral health professionals are usually sparsely distributed, making it difficult for these professionals to reach majority of the people. The feasible way to reach majority of the people in such communities is for the professionals to formulate simple accurate messages and let it be distributed to communities by using non-dental personnel. Mass media may be the easiest means to disseminate such important information in areas where mass media is reached by people in a given community. Both the two methods are cheaper than tasking the sparsely distributed dental professionals to send these messages to communities.

10.5.5. Interventions against Social Disadvantage as a Means to Control Oral and Systemic Diseases and Conditions

Numerous studies have shown strong relationships between social disadvantage and health of individual and families as detailed in Chapter 1. Socially disadvantaged individuals and families have been shown to exhibit more disease than their counterparts belonging to socially advantaged groups (Chapter 1). There is also ample evidence that social disadvantage affect negatively the utilization of health services including preventive services (Chapter 1). The best preventive interventional program for oral diseases in socially disadvantaged communities is reduction of factors precipitating social disadvantage. Studies on social disadvantage point to appropriation of means of production and poverty as the key factors in creating social class and thus social disadvantage. Governments and those interested in improving oral health need to play a key role in ensuring that socially disadvantaged communities are empowered to earn their living to enable them acquire the essentials or necessities of life. The global efforts to reduce poverty, illiteracy, and gender imbalance as stipulated in the Millennium Development Goals (UN 2000) clearly ascribe to this assertion.

References

Amaral MA, Nakama L, Conrado CA, Matsuo T. (2005) Dental caries in male young adults: prevalence, severity and associated factors. *Braz Oral. Res.*;19:249-255.

Baelum V, van Palenstein Helderman W, Hugoson A, Yee R, Fejerskov O. (2007) A global perspective on changes in the burden of caries and periodontitis: implications for dentistry. *J. Oral. Rehabil.*; 34:872-906; discussion 940.

Belot M, James J. (2011) Healthy school meals and educational outcomes. *J. Health Econ.* doi:10.1016/jhealtheco.2011.02.003.

Biazevic MG, Toporcov TN, Antunes JL, Rotundo LD, Brasileiro RS, Carvalho MB, Filho JF, Kowalski LP. (2011) Cumulative coffee consumption and reduced risk of oral and oropharyngeal cancer. *Nutr. Cancer*; 63:350-356.

Cane RJ, Butler DR. (2004) Developing primary health clinical teams for public oral health services in Tasmania. *Aust. Dent. J.;* 49:162-170.

Cataldo JK, Dubey S, Prochaska JJ. (2010) Smoking cessation: an integral part of lung cancer treatment. *Oncology*; 78:289-301.

Chan HC, Wu CT, Welch KB, Loesche WJ. (2010) Periodontal disease activity measured by the benzoyl-DL-arginine-naphthylamide test is associated with preterm births. *J. Periodontol.*; 81:982-991.

Chestnutt I.G., Schäfer F., Jacobson A.P.M., Stephen K.W. (1998) The influence of tooth brushing frequency and post-brushing rinsing on caries experience in a caries clinical trial. *Community Dent. Oral. Epidemiol.*; 26:406-411.

Cinar AB, Murtomaa H. (2009) A holistic food labelling strategy for preventing obesity and dental caries. *Obes. Rev.*; 10:357-361.

Clarke DD, Ward P, Truman W, Bartle C. (2009) A poor way to die: social deprivation and traffic fatalities. Behavioural research in road safety. Queen's printer and controller of Her Majesty's Stationery Office, London, UK.

Conway DI, Petticrew M, Marlborough H, Berthiller J, Hashibe M, Macpherson LM. (2008) Socioeconomic inequalities and oral cancer risk: a systematic review and meta-analysis of case-control studies. *Int. J. Cancer*; 15; 122:2811-2819.

de Onis M, Villar J, Gülmezoglu M. (1998) Nutritional interventions to prevent intrauterine growth retardation: evidence from randomized controlled trials. *Eur. J. Clin. Nutr.*;52 Suppl 1:S83-93.

de Souza DL, Bernal Pérez MM, Curado MP. (2011) Predicted incidence of oral cavity, oropharyngeal, laryngeal, and hypopharyngeal cancer in Spain and implications for cancer control. *Cancer Epidemiol.* doi:10.1016/j.canep.2011.02.012.

Deery C, Heanue M, Deacon S, Robinson PG, Walmsley AD, Worthington H, Shaw W, Glenny AM. (2004) The effectiveness of manual versus powered toothbrushes for dental health: a systematic review. *J. Dent.*; 32:197-211.

dela Cruz GG, Rozier RG, Slade G. (2004) Dental screening and referral of young children by pediatric primary care providers. *Pediatrics*; 114: 642-652.

England LJ, Kim SY, Tomar SL, Ray CS, Gupta PC, Eissenberg T, Cnattingius S, Bernert JT, Tita AT, Winn DM, Djordjevic MV, Lambe M, Stamilio D, Chipato T, Tolosa JE. (2010) Non-cigarette tobacco use among women and adverse pregnancy outcomes. *Acta. Obstet. Gynecol. Scand.*; 89:454-464.

Frencken J.E., Pilot T., Songpaisan Y., Phantumvanit P. (1996) Atraumatic Restorative Treatment (ART): rationale, technique, and development. *J. Public Health Dent.;* 56:135-140.

Han YW, Fardini Y, Chen C, Iacampo KG, Peraino VA, Shamonki JM, Redline RW. (2010) Term stillbirth caused by oral Fusobacterium nucleatum. *Obstet. Gynecol.*; 115:442-445.

Heimonen A, Janket SJ, Kaaja R, Ackerson LK, Muthukrishnan P, Meurman JH. (2009) Oral inflammatory burden and preterm birth. *J. Periodontol.*; 80:884-891.

Hu D, wan H, Li S. (1998) The caries inhibiting effect of a fluoride drop program: a 3-yearstudy on Chinese kindergarten children. *Chinese J. Dent. Res.* 3; 17-20.

Hujoel P. (2009) Dietary carbohydrates and dental-systemic diseases. *J. Dent. Res.* Jun; 88:490-502.

Iida H, Kumar JV, Kopycka-Kedzierawski DT, Billings RJ. (2009) Effect of tobacco smoke on the oral health of U.S. women of childbearing age. *J. Public Health Dent.*; 69:231-241.

Isokangas P, Soderling E, Pienihakkinen K, Alanen P. (2000) Occurrence of dental decay in children after maternal consumption of xylitol chewing gum, a follow-up from 0 to 5 years of age. *J. Dent. Res.* 79; 1885-1889.

Jaber L, Shaban S, Hariri D, Smith S. (2011) Perceptions of healthcare practitioners in Saudi Arabia regarding their training in oral cancer prevention, and early detection. *Int. J. Health Care Qual. Assur.*; 24:8-18.

Johnson GK, Hill M. (2004) Cigarette smoking and the periodontal patient. *J. Periodontol.;* 75:196-209.

Kikwilu E.N. , Frencken J.E., Mulder J., Masalu J.R. (2009) Barriers to restorative care as perceived by dental patients attending government hospitals in Tanzania. *Community Dent. Oral. Epidemiol.;* 37:35-44.

Kikwilu EN, Masalu JR, Kahabuka FK, Senkoro AR. (2008) Prevalence of oral pain and barriers to use of emergency oral care facilities among adult Tanzanians. *BMC Oral Health*; 8: 28. Published online 2008 September 29. doi: 10.1186/1472-6831-8-28

Kiyohara C, Ohno Y. (2010) Sex differences in lung cancer susceptibility: a review. Gend Med; 7:381-401.

Kligerman S, White C. (2011) Epidemiology of lung cancer in women: risk factors, survival, and screening. *AJR Am. J. Roentgenol.*; 196:287-295.

Kowash MB, Pinfield A, Smith J, Curzon MEJ. (2000) Effectiveness on oral health of a long-term health education programme for mothers with young children. *Br. Dent. J.;* 188:201-205.

Kwan SY, Petersen PE, Pine CM, Borutta A. (2005) Health-promoting schools: an opportunity for oral health promotion *Bull World Health Organ*; 83:677-685.

Ljung R, Martin L, Lagergren J. (2011) Oral disease and risk of oesophageal and gastric cancer in a nationwide nested case-control study in Sweden. *Eur. J. Cancer.* doi:10.1016/jhealtheco.2011.02.003.

Locker D. (2000) Deprivation and oral health: a review. *Community Dent. Oral. Epidemiol.*; 28:161-169.

Lopez L., Berkowitz R., Zlotnik H., Moss M., Weinstein P. (1999) Topical antimicrobial therapy in the prevention of early childhood caries. *Paediatric Dentistry*; 21:9-11.

Malhotra R, Kapoor A, Grover V, Kaushal S. (2010) Nicotine and periodontal tissues. *J. Indian Soc. Periodontol.*; 14:72-79.

Mamai-Homata E, Polychronopoulou A, Topitsoglou V, Oulis C, Athanassouli T. (2010) Periodontal diseases in Greek adults between 1985 and 2005--risk indicators. *Int. Dent. J.*; 60:293-299.

Marinho V.C., Higgins J.P., Sheiham A., Logan S. (2003) Fluoride toothpaste for preventing dental caries in children and adolescents. *Cochrane Database Syst. Rev.;* (1):CD00278.

Mashoto KO, Åstrøm AN, Skeie MS, Masalu JR. (2010) Socio-demographic disparity in oral health among the poor: a cross sectional study of early adolescents in Kilwa district, Tanzania. *BMC Oral Health*; 10:7 (http://www.biomedcentral.com/1472-6831/10/7).

Mtaya M, Brudvik P, Astrøm AN. (2009) Prevalence of malocclusion and its relationship with socio-demographic factors, dental caries, and oral hygiene in 12- to 14-year-old Tanzanian schoolchildren. *Eur. J. Orthod.* 2009 Oct;31(5):467-76.

Petersen P.E., Torres A.M. (1999) Preventive oral health care and health promotion provided for children and adolescents by the Municipal Dental Health Service in Denmark. *Int. J. Paed Dentistry*; 9:81-91.

Petersen P.E., Ogawa H. (2005) Strengthening the prevention of periodontal disease: the WHO approach. *J. Periodontol.*; 76:2187-2193.

Petersen PE, Peng B, Tai B, Bian Z, Fan M. (2004) Effect of a school-based oral health education programme in Wuhan City, Peoples Republic of China. Int. Dent. J.; 54:33-41.

Petersen PE, Yamamoto T. (2005) Improving the oral health of older people: the approach of the WHO Global Oral Health Programme. *Community Dent. Oral. Epidemiol.*; 33(2):81-92.

Petersen P.E. (2004) Challenges to improvement of oral health in the 21st century--the approach of the WHO Global Oral Health Programme. *Int. Dent. J.;*54(6 Suppl 1):329-343.

Petersen PE. (2003) The World Oral Health Report 2003: continuous improvement of oral health in the 21st century--the approach of the WHO Global Oral Health Programme. *Community Dent. Oral. Epidemiol.;*31 Suppl 1:3-23.

Pipe AL, Papadakis S, Reid RD. (2010) The role of smoking cessation in the prevention of coronary artery disease. *Curr. Atheroscler Rep.*; 12:145-150.

Prasad DS, Kabir Z, Dash AK, Das BC. (2009) Smoking and cardiovascular health: a review of the epidemiology, pathogenesis, prevention and control of tobacco. *Indian J. Med. Sci.*; 63:520-533.

Reichart PA, Nguyen XH. (2008) Betel quid chewing, oral cancer and other oral mucosal diseases in Vietnam: a review. *J. Oral. Pathol. Med.*; 37:511-514.

Reisine ST, Psoter W. (2001) Socioeconomic status and selected behavioral determinants as risk factors for dental caries. *J. Dent. Educ.*; 65:1009-1016.

Ruxton CH, Gardner EJ, McNulty HM. (2010) Is sugar consumption detrimental to health? A review of the evidence 1995-2006. *Crit. Rev. Food Sci. Nutr.*; 50:1-19.

Sabbah W, Sheiham A, Bernabé E. (2010) Income inequality and periodontal diseases in rich countries: an ecological cross-sectional study. *Int. Dent. J.*; 60:370-374.

Saunder P, Sutherland K, Davidson P, Hampshire A, King S, Taylor J. (2006) Experiencing poverty: the voice of low-income Australian. Towards new indicators of disadvantage project. Stage I: Focus group outcomes. *Social Policy Research Centre.* Sydney.

Scully C. (2011) Oral cancer aetiopathogenesis; past, present and future aspects. Med Oral Patol Oral Cir Bucal. Mar 28. http://www.medcinaoral.com/medoral/free01/aop/17238.pdf.

Semakula HM, Haq SM. (2010) Potential health effects of tobacco smoking in Uganda and how to overcome them through an appropraite communication strategy. *East Afr. J. Public Health*; 7:131-139.

Sheen S, Pontefract H, Moran J. (2001) The benefits of toothpaste--real or imagined? The effectiveness of toothpaste in the control of plaque, gingivitis, periodontitis, calculus and oral malodour. *Dent Update*; 28:144-147.

Sheiham A. (1992) The role of the dental team in promoting dental health and general health through oral health. *Int. Dent. J.*; 42:223-228.

Stevens L, Nelson M. (2011) The contribution of school meals and packed lunch to food consumption and nutrient intakes in UK primary school children from a low income population. *J. Hum. Nutr. Diet*; 21. doi: 10.1111/j.1365-277X.2010.01148.x.

Suter M, Abramovici A, Aagaard-Tillery K. (2010) Genetic and epigenetic influences associated with intrauterine growth restriction due to in utero tobacco exposure. *Pediatr Endocrinol Rev*; 8:94-102.

Theobald HE. (2007) Eating for pregnancy and breast-feeding. *J. Fam. Health Care*; 17:45-49.

Turnbull B. (1995) Smoking and periodontal disease. A review. *J. N. Z. Soc. Periodontol.*; 79:10-15.

Twetman S., Axelsson S., Dahlgren H., Holm AK., Källestål C., Lagerlöf F., Lingström P., Mejàre I., Nordenram G., Norlund A., Petersson L.G., Söder B. (2003) Caries-preventive effect of fluoride toothpaste: a systematic review. *Acta Odontol. Scand.*; 61:347-355.

UNNP (2000) Millennium Development Goals. http://www.undp.org/mdg/basics.shtml accessed on 29th April 2011.

Waller LL, Weaver KE, Petty WJ, Miller AA. (2010) Effects of continued tobacco use during treatment of lung cancer. *Expert Rev. Anticancer Ther.*; 10:1569-1575.

Washko GR, Hunninghake GM, Fernandez IE, Nishino M, Okajima Y, Yamashiro T, Ross JC, Estépar RS, Lynch DA, Brehm JM, Andriole KP, Diaz AA, Khorasani R, D'Aco K, Sciurba FC, Silverman EK, Hatabu H, Rosas IO; COPDGene Investigators. (2011) Lung volumes and emphysema in smokers with interstitial lung abnormalities. *Engl. J. Med.*; 364:897-906.

Watt RG. (2005) Strategies and approaches in oral disease prevention and health promotion. *Bull World Health Organ*; 83:711-718.

WHO. (2005) Strengthening the prevention of oral cancer: the WHO perspective, Guest editorial; 33: 397-399.

World Health Organization, 1986. The Ottawa Charter for Health Promotion. Geneva: WHO. http://www.who.int/hpr/hpr/documents/ottawa.html Accessed on 29th April 2011.

World Health Organization. (2007) Oral health fact sheet No 318. Common oral diseases and conditions. http://www.who.int/mediacentre/factsheets/fs318/en/. Accessed on 15th March 2011.

Yakoob M.Y., Menezes E.V., Soomro T., Haws R.A., Darmstadt G.L., Bhutta Z.A. (2009) Reducing stillbirths: behavioural and nutritional interventions before and during pregnancy. BMC Pregnancy Childbirth; 9 (Suppl 1):S3 doi:10.1186/1471-2393-9-S1-S3. http://www.biomedcentral.com/1471-2393/9/S1/S3.

Zero D.T. (2006) Dentrifices, mouthwashes, and remineralization/caries arrestment strategies. *BMC Oral Health*; 6:S9 dio:101186/1472-6-SI-S9.

D

E

F

G

H

I

N

Q

R

S

uninsured, 12
United Kingdom (UK), 5, 11, 13, 14, 29, 49, 68, 69, 72, 86, 126, 128, 148, 186, 228, 267, 277, 280
United Nations (UN), 2, 17, 221, 229, 231, 244, 277
United States, 12, 78, 85, 87, 124, 125, 128, 229, 254
upper respiratory tract, 188
urban, 8, 10, 11, 12, 14, 20, 28, 29, 30, 34, 79, 85, 129, 130, 131, 134, 161, 182, 201, 221, 225, 234, 235
urban areas, 10, 12, 134, 182, 221, 234
urban population, 10, 85
urban residents, 11
urbanization, 29
urinary tract, 186
urinary tract infection, 186
uvula, 188, 189

V

vacancies, 221
vaccine, 246
variations, 86, 164, 271
varieties, 43, 82, 89, 146
vasculature, 119
vegetables, 271
vehicles, 43, 44, 45, 53
velvet, 252
Vietnam, 28, 279
violence, 2, 10, 26, 134, 189, 221
viral infection, 25, 114
virus infection, 155, 156, 247, 249, 265
viruses, 148, 151, 153, 250
viscosity, 48, 49, 50, 51, 52, 53, 56, 59, 60, 62, 66, 67, 71, 74
vision, 136, 258
vitamin A, 154, 271
vitamin C, 88, 122, 271
vitamin D, 122
vomiting, 102, 183, 253

W

wages, 272
Wales, 86, 129
war, 86, 131
warts, 156, 246, 257, 266
Washington, 35, 77

water, 2, 7, 33, 42, 43, 45, 49, 53, 54, 55, 73, 76, 77, 87, 103, 106, 122, 135, 177, 182, 192, 193, 194, 195, 196, 201, 203, 204, 238, 254, 264, 271, 273
wealth, 2
wear, 7, 60, 102, 111, 234, 242, 244
weight gain, 39
weight loss, 90, 246
welfare, 12, 169
West Africa, 85
Western Australia, 126
wires, 110
witchcraft, 233
wood, 102
wool, 50, 64, 65
workers, 2, 31, 33, 220, 221, 222, 226, 249, 274
workforce, 33, 222, 224, 242
working conditions, 221
workplace, 221
World Bank, 27, 34
World Health Organization (WHO), 19, 20, 21, 23, 25, 26, 32, 33, 34, 35, 36, 44, 70, 71, 73, 74, 77, 78, 81, 87, 100, 129, 132, 153, 156, 159, 161, 175, 182, 203, 221, 222, 229, 238, 242, 243, 244, 246, 247, 248, 249, 265, 267, 270, 271, 279, 280
worldwide, 19, 21, 22, 23, 25, 32, 38, 49, 53, 153, 170, 186, 207, 216, 222, 245, 270
worms, 183
wound healing, 119, 121, 122, 149

X

xerophthalmia, 264
xerostomia, 246, 263, 264
x-rays, 148

Y

yeast, 251
yield, 70, 143, 192
young adults, 13, 15, 46, 80, 90, 152, 225, 235, 277
young people, 90

Z

Zimbabwe, 28, 74, 159, 245
zygoma, 136
zygomatic arch, 136
zygomycosis, 248